Cardiothoracic Care for Children and Young People

A Multidisciplinary Approach

Edited by

Kerry Cook
RGN, ITEC Dip, RN (child), BA (Hons), MSc (ANP), PGCHE, L/PE
Course Tutor, Postgraduate Certificate in Paediatric Cardiothoracic Care
Senior Lecturer, Children and Young People's Nursing
Faculty of Health and Life Sciences
Coventry University
Coventry

Professor Helen Langton
RGN, RSCN, RCNT, RNT, BA(Hons), MSc
Dean
Faculty of Education, Health and Sciences
University of Derby
Derby

(W)WILEY-BLACKWELL

A John Wiley & Sons, Ltd., Publication

This edition first published 2009
© 2009 John Wiley & Sons

Wiley-Blackwell is an imprint of John Wiley & Sons, formed by the merger of Wiley's global Scientific, Technical and Medical business with Blackwell Publishing.

Registered office
John Wiley & Sons Ltd, The Atrium, Southern Gate, Chichester, West Sussex, PO19 8SQ, United Kingdom

Editorial office
John Wiley & Sons Ltd, The Atrium, Southern Gate, Chichester, West Sussex, PO19 8SQ, United Kingdom

For details of our global editorial offices, for customer services and for information about how to apply for permission to reuse the copyright material in this book please see our website at www.wiley.com/wiley-blackwell.

The right of the author to be identified as the author of this work has been asserted in accordance with the Copyright, Designs and Patents Act 1988.

Wiley also publishes its books in a variety of electronic formats. Some content that appears in print may not be available in electronic books.

Designations used by companies to distinguish their products are often claimed as trademarks. All brand names and product names used in this book are trade names, service marks, trademarks or registered trademarks of their respective owners. The publisher is not associated with any product or vendor mentioned in this book. This publication is designed to provide accurate and authoritative information in regard to the subject matter covered. It is sold on the understanding that the publisher is not engaged in rendering professional services. If professional advice or other expert assistance is required, the services of a competent professional should be sought.

Library of Congress Cataloging-in-Publication Data
Cardiothoracic care for children and young people : a multidisciplinary approach / edited by Kerry Cook, Helen Langton.
    p. ; cm.
  Includes bibliographical references and index.
  ISBN 978-0-470-51841-0
  1. Congenital heart disease in children.   2. Congenital heart disease in children–Nursing.
I. Cook, Kerry, 1970-   II. Langton, Helen.
  [DNLM: 1. Cardiovascular Diseases–nursing.   2. Adolescent.   3. Child.   4. Infant.
5. Nursing Care–methods.   6. Thoracic Diseases–nursing.   WY 152.5 C26741 2009]
  RJ426.C64.C37 2009
  618.92′12–dc22

                                                                    2009005625

A catalogue record for this book is available from the British Library.

Set in 9.5/11.5pt Palatino by SNP Best-set Typesetter Ltd., Hong Kong
Printed in Singapore by Markono Print Media Pte Ltd

1 2009

Contents

Contributors

Imran Ali Btec, Cert Ed, BA (Hons), Masters E-commerce
Learning Technologist
Faculty of Health and Life Sciences
Coventry University
Coventry

Paula Banda SRN
Northern co-ordinator
GUCH Patients Association
Saracen's House
Ipswich

Christine Bearne MA, PGCert (Education) PG(Dip) Medical Ethics and Law
Senior Lecturer – Paramedics
Faculty of Health and Life Sciences
Coventry University
Coventry

Collette Clay RGN, RM Dip, BSc (Hons), MA
Senior Lecturer, Midwifery Team
Faculty of Health and Life Sciences
Coventry University
Coventry

Kerry Cook, RGN, ITEC Dip, RN (child), BA (Hons), MSc (ANP), PGCHE, L/PE
Course Tutor, Postgraduate Certificate in Paediatric Cardiothoracic Care
Senior Lecturer, Children and Young People's Nursing Team
Faculty of Health and Life Sciences
Coventry University
Coventry

Richard Crook ACP, LCCP
Senior Clinical Perfusionist, Perfusion Department
Great Ormond Street Hospital for Children NHS Trust
London

Michael Cumper
Chairman GUCHPA
Saracen's House
Ipswich

Rami Dhillon BMedSci (Hons), BM BS, FRCP, FRCPCH
Consultant Paediatric Cardiologist, Cardiac Unit
Birmingham Children's Hospital
Birmingham

Catherine Dunne Dip PT, MSc
Clinical Specialist, Physiotherapy Department
Great Ormond Street Hospital for Children NHS Trust
London

Caroline Green Dip Nursing, BSc (Hons), MSc, PGCE
Senior Lecturer, Childrens and Young Peoples Nursing Team
Faculty of Health and Life Sciences
Coventry University
Coventry

Rebecca Hill RGN, BA (Hons), RN (child), MSc (Clinical Nursing), ENB 415
Advanced Nurse Practitioner Critical Care, Paediatric Intensive Care Unit
Royal Liverpool Childrens Hospital Alder Hey NHS Trust
Liverpool

Suzie Hutchinson RGN, RSCN
Chief Executive, Little Hearts Matter
Edgbaston
Birmingham

Tim Jones MD FRCS (CTh)
Consultant Congenital Cardiac Surgeon, Cardiac Unit
Birmingham Children's Hospital
Birmingham

Fiona Kennedy BSc, RGN, RSCN, Cert Ed, ENB 160, 998
Grown Up Congenital Heart (GUCH) Nurse Specialist
The Heart Hospital
London

Helen Langton RGN, RSCN, RCNT, RNT, BA(Hons), MSc
Professor/Dean of Faculty of Education, Health and Sciences
University of Derby
Derby

Melanie Linzell BA (Hons), RN (child)
Sister, Ocean Ward
Southampton General Hospital
Southampton

Karen Miles
Community Children's Nurse, Hospital at Home Team,
Rugby

Jimmy Montgomerie FRCA
Consultant Anaesthetist, Anaesthetic Department
Birmingham Children's Hospital
Birmingham

Lorraine Priestley-Barnham RN (child), BSc
Clinical Nurse Specialist Paediatric Cardiothoracic Transplant
Great Ormond Street Hospital for Children NHS Trust
London

Anne Maree Robinson
Clinical Nurse Specialist
Inherited Cardiovascular Diseases Service
Great Ormond Street Hospital for Children NHS Trust
London

Gurleen Sharland MD FRCP
Consultant in Fetal Cardiology, Fetal Cardiology Unit
Evelina Children's Hospital
St Thomas' Hospital
London

Jean Simons BA (Hons), MSc, CQSW
Support and Education Manager
Foundation for the Study of Infant Deaths (FSID)
London

Doulas Wall
Consultant Cardiac Surgeon
The Prince Charles Hospital
Chermside
Australia

Julie Wootton BA (Hons)
Chair of Trustees, Children's Heart Federation and Max Appeal
Stourbridge
West Midlands

Jo Wray BSc, PhD, DHP (NC)
Health Psychologist, Cardiac Unit
Great Ormond Street Hospital for Children NHS Trust
London

1 An overview of new ways of working for the 21st century

Kerry Cook, Helen Langton, Imran Ali

This chapter sets the scene in relation to the remainder of this exciting new textbook. Whilst the care of children and young people with cardiac conditions is the context, it would not be right to dive in to looking at anatomy, physiology, treatment and care without identifying the current context within which health or social care practitioners find themselves working as part of this specialist area. Therefore, this chapter looks at both practice and educational context in order to develop the reader's awareness in this arena and therefore enable the reader to make sense of the rest of the book.

This chapter looks at the concepts and realities of patient journeys, e-based learning, interprofessional learning (IPL) and collaborative practice, and concludes by examining the controversial organisation of paediatric cardiac services within the UK and the role of the advanced practitioner in contemporary settings. All these areas are of current relevance to practitioners, and care is performed within this context.

Patient journeys

Over recent years, the term 'patient journey' has become a frequently used description of the experience of the patient (child, young person and their family), their 'journey', through the healthcare system, but the term may not necessarily mean the same thing to our patients. Perhaps we should consider why and how we use and develop 'patient journeys' and whether they are really based on the real lived experience of the patient or are just our description of a 'case' or our interpretation as healthcare professionals (HCPs) of what we think the patient experiences. Our patients, the service users, may for example view their whole life as the 'journey' and the episodes of contact with the healthcare system as alternative routes, diversions or hurdles within the much bigger picture. It is therefore imperative that we involve the 'patients' and of course their families in the development of what we know as 'patient journeys', to ensure that we consider reflexively the broader picture of their lives and the impact that contact with HCPs and the healthcare setting has (see Chapter 7). Throughout this book, we aim to utilise patient journeys – some written purely by HCPs, some written by patients and their families, and some written jointly – to illustrate the relationship of theory to practice and to illuminate the experiences of the service users as a learning opportunity.

Patient journeys may be written and utilised in a variety of ways, such as to allow us as HCPs to focus on the patient's experience of the chronic journey to enable changes to be made to long-term management; as an IPL tool for HCPs engaged in continual professional development (CPD); within publications of the 'one-off' medical or surgical situation; and by involving the patient in modelling their movements through a healthcare setting so that improvements can be made in specific parts of the process, care or treatment, or as an opportunity to explore and learn from the narrative of a clinical encounter.

Narrative could be viewed as a form of story-telling – outlining parts, the 'enacted narratives', of the wider patient journey, i.e. 'the wider narratives of people's lives' (Greenhalgh & Hurwitz, 1999, p. 48). In the narrative about our lives, we expect there to be a starting point, a series of incidents, encounters and occurrences, and a closing point or end. The way in which these narratives (our life stories) are interpreted then depends upon the listener(s), the person telling the story and the feelings of each of those individuals. The story-teller can modify the information given depending upon the interests or needs of the listener, and so the narrative provides a framework through which the character's story can be lived, from which clues can be elucidated, meaning can be discerned and problems and diagnoses can be considered holistically (Greenhalgh & Hurwitz, 1999).

Narratives could also be used to generate a picture of the patient's journey through a specific healthcare episode, system or process. Process mapping of the whole or part of a patient's journey will enable an exploration of what currently happens and any areas of inadequacy, duplication or unnecessary steps within the journey, whilst encouraging an understanding of the role of each HCP involved (NHS Institute for Innovation and Improvement, 2008). For example, the handover process from theatre to cardiac intensive care had been recognised as being a critical time for children who had just had cardiac surgery; the staff were aware that they 'needed to improve and speed up' the process (Darby, 2008). Staff at one large paediatric cardiac unit decided to review the current handover process and called on the Formula One team to assist them in their evaluation. The input of the Formula One pit technicians resulted in a major restructuring of their patient handover from theatre to the ICU (Darby, 2008).

For children, young people and adults with congenital heart disease, the patient journey may have begun at a variety of points and may have even begun for the parents before their baby was born. For some families, the 20-week prenatal scan may have been the beginning of a new but simultaneous journey. At a time when parents are expecting to visualise a healthy baby, a rollercoaster of emotions emerges for them as they discover that their unborn baby has a heart defect. For other parents and infants, the journey will have begun postnatally, either immediately after birth, in the first few weeks or occasionally later in the child's life. We cannot predict the starting point of any journey as there as so many variables; therefore, as practitioners, we need to remember that every story is different and additionally every child and family will cope with the experience in different ways.

Likewise, the end point of each child's journey will vary. Some children, particularly those who have corrective surgery, may have very little contact with healthcare once their initial treatment is complete; for many, however, their palliative journey will continue until their life ends. Many children and young people are now living into adulthood, due to the improvements in medical and surgical techniques, where their healthcare episodes continue following transition to the grown-up congenital heart services. Chapter 6 focuses on this transition process and the preparation that is required in order to support young people during this critical part of their overall journey or narrative.

Throughout this book, real episodes of patient journeys have been utilised to illustrate the effect of the contact with healthcare services and professionals. It is hoped that this will create a link between the theory and practice and will bring the book alive, demonstrating the importance of creating effective partnerships with children, young people and their families and listening to their stories to ensure that care is tailored to the needs of our client population. Chapter 7 has been written by professionals from support groups some of whom are parents of children and young people with congenital heart disease; it paints a picture of the journey from an alternative perspective. It is essential that practitioners have a clear understanding of the real journeys that are experienced on a daily basis as this will assist in the continual development of a service that is truly patient centred.

E-based learning

Universities are increasingly facing escalating competition in a global market, especially with the rapid developments in technology. E-learning in its various forms is seen to have the potential to provide learners with anywhere and anytime learning. The Higher Education Funding Council produced an e-learning strategy for the sector in 2005. Although it refrained from providing a specific definition of e-learning, suffice to say that it stipulates the government's definition as 'any learning using information communication technology' (ICT).

Although this broad definition promotes exploration and diversity, a more specific definition may be useful to provide an institutional context. Seale (2008) clarifies that in order to understand the correlation between learning and technology, it is important to identify the context. There also appears to be a lack of emphasis on other support services that may utilise technologies that enable learning. For example, learner support services such as libraries are increasingly making reading material available online, linking to library catalogues and other online resources such as online journals. This is becoming increasingly integrated in to institutional virtual learning environments (VLEs). This has presented opportunities for students to reduce their time spent searching for publications and has therefore provided more time to read and understand reading material.

New ways of learning

E-learning provides new ways of learning and innovative pedagogies through the use of ICT. This has included utilising web-conferencing to deliver live lectures. This has been a simulating method of learning for learners and lecturers because of the high level of interactivity. Learners and lecturers interact through the use of webcams and microphones. In addition to this, learners are able to take control of the teaching space and demonstrate their understanding. For example, during a lecture given by a perfusionist for a purely online CPD course, the focus of the teaching was in part on the heart–lung machine. Learners were given control of the learning environment and were then able to point out various parts of the machinery and engage the lecturer in discussion, which provided an opportunity to interact and met the learners' needs.

Usability and accessibility

The majority of learners enrolling on online and blended learning courses are expected to learn how to use and navigate the interface of the given VLE. Nielsen (2003) clarifies that 'Usability is a quality attribute that assesses how easy user interfaces are to use'. According to the IMS special interest group, 'accessibility' is defined 'as the ability of the learning environment to adjust to the needs of all learners' (IMS Global Learning Consortium, 2002). The VLEs currently available support to a certain degree this type of flexibility. For example, WebCT Vista allows users to adopt various high-colour contrast schemes, collapsible menus and keyboard shortcuts. Cooper et al explain that the accessibility and usability of an e-learning system are crucial for the success of teaching and learning online, and that they directly affect 'pedagogical effectiveness' (Cooper et al, 2008, p. 233).

Universities have created web pages and made them available via their chosen VLE. One higher education institution has created interactive web pages around 'Patient Journeys'. These web pages present the core part of the course content and have been designed with an authoring tool that produces accessible content. However, as Cooper et al point out, accessibility works on different levels. Although the standards stipulated by W3C's Web Content Accessibility Guidelines can be met from a technical perspective, for example checks can be made to identify whether alternative texts have been associated with images, this does not reflect how 'pedagogically meaningful' that text may be (Cooper et al, 2008, p. 234). Therefore accessibility in its broadest sense can refer to technical, pedagogical and learning design issues. These are all interlinked and impact each other within any given e-learning environment.

Flexibility

One of the key virtues of delivering the course through e-learning is the flexibility that it affords to both lectures and learners. Learners are able to access the course materials at any time during the day or night and engage by writing, reading, watching and listening. Although all study materials can be made available in their entirety, online courses can be delivered at a particular pace. For example, certain study materials can be released only when certain tasks have been completed, or every week. Although it can be argued that this restricts flexibility, evidence suggests that pacing students helps them to complete courses (Coldeway, 1986). Furthermore, pacing students is critical in preventing early dropouts (Gibson & Graff, 1992).

Cost-effectiveness

The higher education sector has been quick to adopt technology and invest in supporting e-learning. However, this has come at a cost, e.g. the appointments of learning technologists across the UK higher education sector to facilitate the development of courses that have an online presence. There is a question mark over the tangible benefits for learners, lecturers and institutions. A Joint Information Systems Committee (JISC) report in 2008 highlighted key benefits after working with 16 universities and eight subject areas to discover the tangible benefits (JISC, 2008). The report identified the following areas:

■ Cost savings/resource efficiency
■ Recruitment and retention

- Skills employment
- Student achievement
- Inclusion
- Widening participation and socially equality
- Other benefits.

In terms of cost savings/resource efficiency, online courses can provide savings in the area of online assessment where multiple choice questions can be presented and marked by the computer. This system of delivery and marking can be invaluable when managing large numbers of students.

Guest lecturers can be invited to deliver lectures. This can prove cost-effective because invited speakers deliver their presentations from their work or home and therefore eliminate the travelling time and associated costs that would be incurred were they to travel to the host institution to deliver the lecture.

Changes in service and organisational effectiveness

E-learning introduces challenges and opportunities to organisations that deliver education. By its very nature, it presents change to both people and business processes. The strength of e-learning lies above all in its ability to provide anytime, anywhere learning. In order to deliver this type of learning, various aspects of the learning organisation will be required to consider the impact of e-learning (Morris, 2005). The information technology infrastructure is required to provide the continuous stable and accessible network necessary to support staff in acquiring the skills needed to teach and facilitate effectively online.

Interprofessional learning and collaborative practice

The modernisation agenda for health, social care and education amongst other disciplines emphasises the need for professionals to adopt more flexible ways of working to make the best use of their skills (Department of Health [DH], 2000; NHS, 2007). Closer collaboration between health, social care, education and some science professionals is seen as essential in the delivery of more effective service provision. The NHS Workforce Strategy Document (DH, 2000) stated the need for 'genuinely multi-professional' education and training to promote effective teamwork and partnership, and collaboration between professions, in order to provide a seamless service for the user or patient. The Centre for the Advancement of Interprofessional Education (CAIPE, 2000) concluded that:

> The emerging evidence suggests that inter-professional education can, in favourable circumstances and in different ways, contribute to improving collaboration in practice.

Higher education institutes have been charged by the DH, strategic health authorities and workforce development directorates with promoting interprofessional leaning in preregistration health and social care courses.

Opportunities to develop collaborative ways of working amongst pre- and postgraduate students within higher education are not new. Many universities offering undergraduate and postgraduate curricula identify ways in which students on a variety of health and social care courses can learn together, and many utilise the CAIPE definition (2000) to underpin this:

2 or more students from different disciplines or professions learning with, from and about each other to improve quality in their field of practice.

In order to achieve this, staff are therefore encouraged to teach across disciplines in order to facilitate interdisciplinary understanding and engender mutual respect and an awareness of the unique and separate contribution that each profession makes in the delivery of health and social care. Many universities also are well placed to utilise an e-learning approach as already identified above.

The landscape of IPL continues to change and pose challenges for both learning and practice. This is evidenced in the recent publication from the Higher Education Academy detailing the progress made by the four pilot sites funded by the DH to trial interprofessional models in undergraduate education. The learning points generated from this work and work by other universities are summarised below.

Learning points from other higher education institutions

- IPL has more currency if based on service-users' experiences.
- The engagement of IPL activities is dependent on the development of IPL champions throughout all stakeholders (academic, practice and student).
- IPL outcomes should be based on capability rather than merely competence.
- The use of invented/virtual scenarios for student learning allows for flexibility but must be supplemented with real-life scenarios. This learning is different from the practice element in most programmes. The emphasis here is on collaborative working rather than meeting profession-specific competencies.
- IPL student groupings must reflect practice rather than every programme learning the same content at the same time.
- The facilitation of IPL student groups is different from that of teaching uniprofessional groups, and therefore staff development must be in place to enable this to happen successfully.
- A variety of mediums and environments can be utilised for IPL. Examples include virtual electronic approaches that rely on interprofessional interaction via an electronic discussion board, practice-based workshops and classroom events.
- Pedagogically, the approach to IPL has to be student-centred and defined by a student's field of practice.
- The Higher Education Academy subject centres have been instrumental in supporting the production of literature on interprofessional education (IPE) and evaluation of IPL. In particular, the Health Sciences and Practice (HSAP), Social Policy and Social Work (SWAP) and Medicine, Dentistry and Veterinary Medicine (MEDEV) subject centres have supported IPE as a strand in national conferences, festivals of learning and regional meetings. The three centres recently jointly funded the IPE Special Interest Group meeting on Interprofessional Competences. Occasional Papers on IPE can be found on the HSAP website for free download. The government-funded Centres for Excellence in Teaching and Learning project also includes a number of IPE projects. A summary of health and social care projects has been produced by the HSAP.

In developing new curricula, higher education institutions also have to take into account the widespread desire from user groups and government to provide more responsive health and social care services (see, for example, Beresford & Trevillion, 1995; Barnes et al, 2000; Braye, 2000; Newman, 2001; Glendenning et al, 2005) that are 'personalised' to the particular needs of individual users and patients. This aim was enunciated by the DH in the preface to the NHS Plan in 2000:

> The NHS will shape its services around the needs and preferences of individual patients, their families and their carers: The NHS of the 21st century must be responsive to the needs of different groups and individuals within society

and again in the NHS Improvement Plan (2004, Executive Summary, Para. 4):

> The next stage in the NHS's journey is to ensure that a drive for responsive, convenient and personalised services takes root across the whole of the NHS and for all patients. For hospital services, this means that there will be a lot more choice for patients about how, when and where they are treated and much better information to support that. For the millions of people who have illnesses that they will live with for the rest of their lives, such as diabetes, heart disease, or asthma, it will mean much closer personal attention and support in the community and at home.

More recently, the Darzi Report (DH, 2008, p. 23) has said that:

> making services more personal: designing and delivering services that fit with people's lives will help to reduce inequalities in health and social care outcomes.

It also identified the following key areas:

■ A fair NHS
■ A personalised NHS
■ An effective NHS
■ A safe NHS
■ A locally accountable NHS.

Such policy discourse, along with recent legislation including the NHS and Social Care Act 2001, has promoted the inclusion of users and patients, along with citizens more generally, in the shaping of health and social care provision. In a similar vein, higher education providers of health and social care programmes have increasingly included users' perspectives in the design and delivery of their courses.

Both the Quality Assurance Agency (QAA) for Higher Education and the Statutory bodies – the Health Professions Council (HPC) and the Nursing and Midwifery Council (NMC) – have confirmed their support for the inclusion of service users' perspectives in the development and delivery of higher education programmes. The QAA has articulated this in various documents and statements, including:

■ the Prototype Document for Approval and Ongoing Quality Monitoring and Enhancement (OQME) (2004)

▦ subject benchmark statements, not least those for dietetics, midwifery, nursing, occupational therapy and physiotherapy (all QAA, 2001).

The statutory bodies have similarly expressed their support for the development of professionals who place the needs and interests of users and patients at the centre of service provision; see, for example, Standards of Proficiency for dietetics (HPC, 2003a), midwifery (NMC, 2004a), nursing (NMC, 2004b), occupational therapy (HPC, 2003b) and physiotherapy (HPC, 2003c).

The above discourse identifies that there is increasing emphasis not only on learning to work together, but also on ensuring that this happens in practice and that the service user is seen as an integral collaborative member in the planning, delivery and evaluation of care for the future. Furthermore, these fundamental features reflect the key recommendations of the Kennedy Report (DH, 2001), the public inquiry that explored the tragic failures of surgery in Bristol and led to the Paediatric and Congenital Cardiac Services (PCCS) Review, which commenced in 2001 and will now be explored further.

Changes in health care

Cardiac surgery has seen instrumental advances over the last 70 years and 'in the developed world, it represents one of the flagships of successful high tech surgery' (Pawade, 2005, p. 15). However, the exposure of tragedies in Bristol that were blamed on a necessary learning curve for surgeons and the hope that improvements would be subsequently evident had a major impact on the whole specialty and healthcare in general across the UK and beyond. Following this exposure and the Kennedy Inquiry (DH, 2001), the government established the Paediatric and Congenital Cardiac Services (PCCS) Review Group in an attempt to assess service provision and make recommendations for the safe organisation and delivery of the paediatric and congenital cardiac service in the future. The review group considered a number of specific recommendations from the Kennedy Report, particularly recommendation 192:

> National standards should be developed as a matter of priority, for all aspects of the care and treatment of children with congenital heart disease (CHD). The standards should address diagnosis, surgical and other treatments, and continuing care. They should include standards for primary and social care, as well as for hospital care. The standards should also address the needs of those with CHD who grow into adulthood. (DH, 2001, p. 460)

In order to develop these standards, the PCCS Review Group considered the core principles of the NHS Plan (www.dh.gov/Publications) and the philosophy developed by the Children's Taskforce (www.dh.gov/Publications), as well as numerous other reports and studies that were relevant.

Two generic care pathways (Figures 1.1 and 1.2) were devised to assist in the exploration of current practices and service provision. The first outlines the process from identification of a congenital abnormality to diagnosis, and the latter the process from diagnosis to outcome. These were used to identify areas where standards might be necessary and to ensure that these standards contained all of the required aspects (DH, 2002).

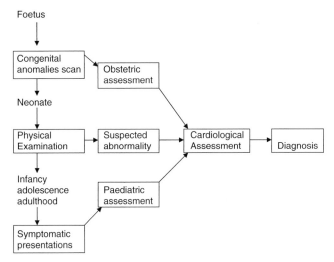

Figure 1.1   Care pathway 1: Identification to diagnosis (from DH, 2002)

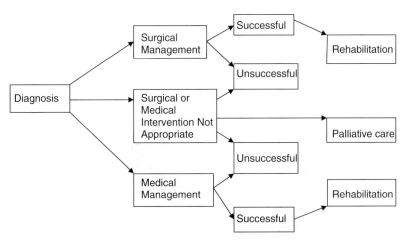

Figure 1.2   Care pathway 2: Diagnosis to outcome of intervention (from DH, 2002)

The standards focused on the following key areas, which have been summarised; full details of these can be found in the PCCS Review document (also known as the Munro Report; DH, 2002).

The context of care

■ The environment should be within a paediatric setting.
■ Use of audit is necessary – the Central Cardiac Audit Database.
■ The report suggested the development of a review group similar to the Safety and Efficacy Register for New Interventional Procedures – to have responsibility for approving a new surgical, medical or interventional procedure, rather than restricting the rarer procedures to two units.

Information and consent

- More information is required at diagnosis.
- It is vital for parents to receive written information.
- Good evidence-based information with treatment is appropriate.
- The relevant consent documents issued by the DH should be used. These are available from the DH website (www.dh.gov.uk/consent) and are:
  - *The Good Practice in Consent Implementation Guide*, which contains a model consent policy and four consent forms together with an accompanying information leaflet.
  - The *Reference Guide to Consent for Examination or Treatment*, which provides a comprehensive summary of the current law on consent and includes requirements of regulatory bodies such as the General Medical Council where these are more stringent.
  - The *12 Key Points on Consent: The Law in England*, which has been distributed widely to health professionals working in England. This one-page document summarises those aspects of the law on consent that arise on a daily basis.
  - Specific guidance, incorporating both the law and good practice advice, that is available for health professionals working with children, people with learning disabilities and older people.
- Clear information is required by parents when a coroner's post mortem is necessary. The Code of Conduct for communication can be found at www.dh.gov.uk/tissue

The patient's journey

- Early antenatal identification allows choice and the opportunity to make plans for management.
- Referral to a paediatric cardiologist should occur without delay.
- There are recommendations for minimum numbers of staff: cardiologists, surgeons and cardiac liaison nurses.
- Practitioners should refer to *Paediatric Intensive Care: A Framework for the Future* (DH, 1997), which makes recommendations for the staffing of paediatric intensive care units.
- There has been an impact of the European Working Time Directive – this allows an imaginative use of services and innovative new roles (as discussed in the next section of this chapter).
- There is limited evidence to support the implementation of the framework or to help determine what the minimum level of procedures should be in each centre despite the recommendations of the Kennedy Report.
- The threshold for cardiac surgery in children should be set at 300 cases per centre per year based on one American study of paediatric congenital cardiac surgery which concluded that the mortality risk was lower at an institution performing more than 300 cases annually (Jenkins et al, 1995). It also showed that hospitals that were carrying out fewer than 100 paediatric cardiac procedures annually had significantly higher mortality rates than hospitals with volumes of 100 or more (Hannan et al, 1998). The evidence to support the relationship between volume and outcome is continuing to grow (Gauvreau, 2007), with further American studies

demonstrating similar results in more recent years (Sollano et al, 1999; Chang & Klitzner, 2002; Bazzani & Marcin, 2007).

■ Ensuring a minimum of four operating sessions per week will prevent occasional practice for surgeons.
■ It is unsafe for any surgeon to be performing fewer than 40 open heart procedures a year on neonates and infants.
■ There is no minimum number for surgical procedures carried out with the grown-up congenital heart disease population.
■ There need to be minimum standards for the training and experience of anaesthetists working in the specialty.
■ Interventional cardiologists should undertake a minimum of 40 procedures per year, with the lead interventional cardiologist undertaking a minimum of 80 procedures per year.

Joined-up care

■ Care should be linked in with local services and ensure that staff in these areas are capable of caring for these children and providing parents with the relevant support.
■ Some paediatric cardiac units should have an immediate-access service.
■ Good communication between cardiac centre and community teams is essential.
■ The role of cardiac liaison nurses is critical in maintaining the interface between teams.
■ A key worker should be identified for each child/family.
■ Outreach clinics should deliver the same quality of care.

Growing up

■ Parents' support is needed to enable teachers to have an understanding of the child's condition; cardiac liaison school visits should be encouraged.
■ An improvement in transition services is required.
■ A close partnership is required between adult and paediatric centres.
■ Appropriate environments are needed for the care of young people.

Support to parents and families

■ Parents' facilities need to be improved.
■ Appropriate bereavement support, which includes the needs of siblings, is required.
■ There must be an opportunity for the parents to talk to the professionals involved when their child dies unexpectedly.

Congenital Cardiac Services Workshop June 2006

In 2006 a workshop was organised by the DH in response to concerns about the pressures on paediatric cardiac surgical centres. The aim was to reflect upon the aesthetics of an optimum centre, the logistics of moving to an optimum service and the identification of steps required in order to achieve this. It was concluded that there should be large centres of excellence with a minimum of five surgeons and eight cardiologists. In the interim period of transition, it was suggested that there should be joint alliances between centres. The workshop report was subsequently delivered to NHS specialised services commissioners to facilitate decision-making regarding the optimal configuration of congenital cardiac services in England. The report was also used in DH briefings for government ministers.

The suggested move to larger centres of excellence has been controversial amongst the varied professional groups, with varying beliefs about the appropriateness and feasibility of these plans. At the time of writing this chapter, the British Congenital Cardiac Association is reviewing the results of a poll of members regarding the reconfiguration process that has recently taken place. The nature of service delivery in this country is likely to remain dynamic despite the plans of the DH, and therefore the future will surely be one of major change and innovation despite the geographical location of the centres involved. All of the issues discussed in the previous sections will have a considerable impact upon staffing these units in the future; the new and advancing roles that practitioners are increasingly working towards will be further investigated in the next section.

Advancing roles

The changes outlined within this chapter have without doubt led to the cultivation of an environment in which nurses and allied health professionals have been able to develop and advance their roles. Essentially, this has been under the guise of attempts and initiatives to improve the health and wellbeing of children, young people and their families – in other words, the streamlining of aspects of service delivery – but also without doubt it relates to the personal reward and increased job satisfaction of those practitioners involved (Jane, 2008).

The changed political climate culminated in the DH document *Making a Difference* (DH 1999), which made explicit the contribution that nurses and professionals allied to medicine make to the patient journey, embracing this with the advent of consultant roles. Changes in nursing education, historically quick at an in-house level to embrace the concept of expanded roles, have demonstrated an ad hoc approach to how to consistently develop and advance the role of non-medical professionals to take on responsibility for aspects of patient management that have previously been the remit of doctors. Despite this, advanced practice roles have become integral not only to defined parts of the patient journey, but increasingly also along the whole trajectory.

However, in establishing roles of greater autonomy and patient responsibility, has the gap between the bedside nurse and the 'maxi nurse' widened (Royal College of Nursing, 2005)? Autonomy within nursing practice lies in directing and managing patient care, but it seems this is no longer the remit of the bedside nurse, as concerns over professional liability are increasingly overriding the willingness to make clinical decisions regarding the management of children in his or her care. The role of the ward manager, who directed and supervised care for all patients on the ward, has been replaced with individual nurses taking an allocation of patients (often not prioritised by dependency or workload), resulting in nurses feeling isolated, frustrated and exposed, and furthermore lacking a clinical role model on which to focus the development of their own practice. Advanced practice roles are increasingly being looked upon to meet these shortcomings. However, the majority of nurses will choose to view these roles as 'medicalised', so will not see them as doing so. Consequently, there is a tendency for these roles to be dismissed as 'not nursing', with the knowledge that we have, as a profession, struggled to provide a robust definition of what exactly nursing is, providing a source of cognitive dissonance.

Changes to junior doctors' working hours (NHS Management Executive, 1991), and more recently the changes being implemented as part of the European Working Time Directive, have, and will continue to have, a major impact on service delivery. These workforce issues have directly resulted in the timing and opportunity to invest in advanced practice roles as a means of making important contributions to achieving the goal of providing quality, cost-effective seamless care (Cox, 2000). However, there is a real risk that such roles will be pioneered in areas without the vital commitment to the practitioners' academic preparation (generally accepted to be a Master's level programme), on-the-job training and clinical supervision.

The essence of the role lies within expert clinical practice. Jasper (1994) defines the attribute of the expert as the possession of a specialised body of knowledge or skill, seen as a combination of the analytical ability of the practitioner and the nature of the individual's clinical experience (Woods, 2000), in addition to extensive experience in a field of practice, acknowledgment by others and highly developed levels of pattern recognition.

These ideas can be equated to the 'knowing that' and the 'knowing how' (Carper, 1978). It combines propositional knowledge, which deals with theories, facts and concepts that are known, with the practical and experiential knowledge that has previously been referred to as 'tacit' knowledge (Polyani, 1966). Calkin (1984) identified that advanced practitioners use deliberative reasoning processes to draw on their substantial theoretical knowledge base, which in turn informs their clinical practice – this concept of reflective practice is not new to nursing. The amalgam between experience and academic qualification assists in the development of expertise in nursing practice (Woods, 2000).

From the literature, however, there appears to be a failure to clarify sufficiently, and communicate to all relevant parties, the boundaries and objectives of advanced roles (Lloyd Jones, 2005). This can impede role transition, contributing to feelings of stress and role ambiguity for advanced practitioners (Glen & Waddington, 1998). As specialist and advanced roles generally involve contact with a range of HCPs, effective interprofessional relationships are important (Lloyd Jones, 2005) and are seen as facilitating or impeding role transition, with conflict in particular impairing the ability to set realistic work targets, thus creating job dissatisfaction (Glen & Waddington, 1998). Advanced practitioners who are not in line management can only influence change through collaborative relationships with key stakeholders such as senior managers (Flanagan, 1998), who in turn may themselves view advanced practice roles as a 'panacea' to the immediate needs of their respective institutions (Woods, 2000).

There will always be an aura of uncertainty when one tries to define advanced practice. To some extent this uncertainty will come from an inability to understand the role, especially if you are not in a position to perform it. Perhaps more fundamentally, it reflects the difficulty in managing these roles – clinical supervision has to be from medical colleagues, with knowledge, skills and attitudes on a par as autonomous practice and decision-making is more at a medical level. As a nurse, within traditional nursing hierarchies, managers must be of nursing origin. This, in its essence, poses a conflict of interest. Resistance to role development has generally been from within the nursing profession, rather than from outside it (Flanagan, 1998; Glen & Waddington, 1998; Ball, 1999; Tye & Ross, 2000).

Therefore, understanding the phenomenon of advanced practice can be problematic – colleagues may think they know what the role consists of, and will certainly have definite ideas about what the role should be, but in reality there is a spectrum of generalist and specialist practice to most advanced roles, especially those involved with the delivery of paediatric cardiac surgical services, which will make them as individual as the children being treated. The essence of most advanced roles is the skill set and experiences practitioners bring along with them and, importantly, the service in which the role will need to be established.

However, the advantage of these roles within paediatric cardiac surgery is clear to foresee. Experienced senior clinical nurses transitioning into advanced roles can reduce the peaks and troughs in the quality of care delivered to children with rotational trainee medical posts, as well as address some of the shortfalls in service provision. Within the clinical team, advanced practitioners can support and orientate both medical and nursing staff new to the clinical area, thereby maintaining high standards of care. Involvement at the time of preadmission, perhaps taking the first stage of consent, introduces to the child and parents a nurse clinician who will be constantly involved in the management decisions made throughout the child's entire hospital admission. This nurse clinician, along with the specialist cardiac liaison nurse role, can provide emotional and psychological support during the entire patient journey.

Conclusion

So what lies ahead? Interestingly, the debate around advanced practice within nursing looks likely to culminate once again in bi-level nursing registration, with the expectation that advanced practice will soon be registrable with the NMC. This will no doubt lead to a requirement for increased professional indemnity, as role transition requires the nurse to change the nature of decision-making in terms of outcome for patients; therefore, decision autonomy is increased. For experienced and knowledgeable practitioners, reluctant to undergo transition into management as a means of career progression, it provides a new, challenging and ultimately rewarding clinical career pathway – the ability to conduct comprehensive clinical assessments and prescribe management, remain in a position to research and evaluate care, and act as consultant and educator within their chosen field. These are exciting possibilities for a non-medical professional, but ones that needs careful planning and preparation for, not least in terms of the individual, but also for the organisation, which will ultimately benefit from these highly knowledgeable, highly trained advanced practitioners.

References

Ball, C. (1999). Revealing higher levels of nursing practice. *Intensive and Critical Care Nursing, 15*, 65–76.

Barnes, D., Carpenter, J. & Dickinson, C. (2000). Interprofessional education for community mental health: attitudes to community care and professional stereotypes. *Social Work Education, 19*, 565–583.

Bazzani, L.G. & Marcin, J.P. (2007). Case volume and mortality in pediatric cardiac surgery patients in California, 1998–2003. *Circulation, 115*, 2652–2659.

Beresford, P. & Treveillion, S. (1995). *Developing skills for community care: A collaborative approach.* Aldershot: Arena.

Braye, S. (2000). Participation and involvement in social care: an overview. In Kemshall, H. & Littlechild, R., eds. *User involvement and participation in social care: Research informing practice.* London: Jessica Kingsley.

Calkin, J. (1984). A model for advanced nursing practice. *Journal of Nursing Administration, 14,* 24–30.

Carper, B. (1978). Fundamental patterns of knowing in nursing. *Advances in Nursing Sciences, 1,* 13–23.

Centre for the Advancement of Interprofessional Education (2000). Information available at: http://www.caipe.org.uk

Coldeway, D. (1986). Learner characteristics and success. *Distance Education in Canada,* pp. 81–87.

Chang, R.K. & Klitzner, T.S. (2002). Can regionalization decrease the number of deaths for children who undergo cardiac surgery? A theoretical analysis. *Pediatrics, 109,* 173–181.

Cooper, M., Colwell, C. & Anne, J. (2008). Embedding accessibility and usability: considerations for e-learning research and development projects. *ALT-J, 15,* 231–245. Available from: http://www.informaworld.com/smpp/title~content=t713605628~db=all~tab=issueslist~branches=15-v15

Cox, C. (2000). Nurse consultant: the advanced nurse practitioner? *Nursing Times, 96,* 48.

Darby, G. (2008). *How can Formula 1 be useful for healthcare?* NESTA. Available from: http://www.nesta.org.uk/how-can-formula-1-be-useful-for-healthcare/ [Accessed 12 March 2009].

Department of Health (1997). *Paediatric intensive care: A framework for the future. Report from the National Coordinating Group on Paediatric Intensive Care to the Chief Executive of the NHS Executive.* London: DH.

Department of Health (1999). *Making a difference: Strengthening the nursing, midwifery and health visiting contribution to health and healthcare.* Leeds: DH.

Department of Health (2000). *The NHS plan: A plan for investment, a plan for reform.*

Department of Health (2001). *The report of the public inquiry into children's heart surgery at the Bristol Royal Infirmary: learning from Bristol* [The Kennedy Report]. London: DH.

Department of Health (2002). *Report of the Paediatric and Congenital Cardiac Services Review Group* [The Munro Report]. London: DH.

Department of Health (2004). *NHS improvement plan. Putting people at the heart of public services.* London: DH.

Department of Health (2008). *Our NHS, our future: NHS next stage review.* London: DH.

Flanagan, M. (1998). Factors influencing tissue viability nurse specialists in the UK: 2. *British Journal of Nursing, 7,* 690–692.

Gauvreau, K. (2007). Reevaulation of the volume-outcome relationship for pediatric cardiac surgery. *Circulation, 115,* 2599–2601.

Gibson, C. & Graff, A. (1992). Impact of adults' preferred learning styles and perception of barriers on completion of external Baccalaureate Degree Programs. *Journal of Distance Education, 7,* 39–51.

Glen, S. & Waddington, K. (1998). Role transition from staff nurse to clinical nurse specialist: a case study. *Journal of Clinical Nursing, 7,* 283–290.

Glendinning, C., Hudson, B. & Means, R. (2005). Exploring the troubled relationship between health and social care. *Public Money and Management, 25,* 245–251.

Greenhalgh, T. & Hurwitz, B. (1999). Narrative based medicine. Why study narrative? *British Medical Journal, 318,* 48–50.

Hannan, E.L., Racz, M., Kavey, R.E., Quaegbeur, J.M. & Williams, R. (1998). Pediatric cardiac surgery: the effect of hospital and surgeon volume on in-hospital mortality. *Pediatrics, 101,* 963–969.

Health Professions Council (2003a). *Standards of proficiency for undergraduate dietetics education.* London: HPC.

Health Professions Council (2003b). *Standards of proficiency for undergraduate occupational therapy education*. London: HPC.

Health Professions Council (2003c). *Standards of proficiency for undergraduate physiotherapy education*. London: HPC.

Higher Education Funding Council (2005). *Strategy for e learning*. March 2005/12.

IMS Global Learning Consortium. (2002). *Guidelines for developing accessible learning applications*. Available from: http://www.imsglobal.org/accessibility/accv1p0/imsacc_guidev1p0.html [Accessed 12 March 2009].

Jane, K.S. (2008). Developing e-learning experiences and practices: the importance of context. *ALT-J, 16*, pp. 1–3. Available from: http://www.informaworld.com/smpp/title~content=t713605628~db=all~tab=issueslist~branches=16-v16

Jasper, M. (1994). Expert: a discussion of the implications of the concept as used in nursing. *Journal Advanced Nursing, 20*, 769–776.

Jenkins, K.J., Newburger, J.W., Lock, J.E., Davis, R.B., Coffman, G.A. & Iezzoni, L.I. (1995). In-hospital mortality for surgical repair of congenital heart defects: preliminary observations of variation by hospital caseload. *Pediatrics, 95*, 323–330.

Joint Information Systems Committee (2008). *Tangible benefits of e-learning. Does investment yield interest?* Bristol: JISC.

Lloyd Jones, M. (2005). Role development and effective practice in specialist and advanced practice roles in acute hospital settings: systematic review and meta-synthesis. *Journal of Advanced Nursing, 49*, 191–209.

Morris, D. (2005). E-learning strategy at Coventry University to 2010.

Newman, K. (2001). Loss, grief and bereavement in interprofessional education, an example of process: anecdotes and accounts. *Nurse Education in Practice, 5*, 281–288.

NHS (2007). *Putting people first: A shared vision and commitment to the transformation of adult social care*. London: DH.

NHS Institute for Innovation and Improvement (2008). *ILG 1.2 process mapping, analysis and redesign*. Available from: http://www.institute.nhs.uk/index.php?option=com_joomcart&Itemid=194&main_page=document_product_info&products_id=295 [Accessed 12 March 2009]

NHS Management Executive (1991). *Junior doctors: The new deal*. London: NHSME.

Nielsen, J. (2003). Usability 101: Introduction to usability. Available from: http://www.useit.com/alertbox/20030825.html [Accessed 12 March 2009]

Nursing and Midwifery Council (2004a). *Standards of proficiency for midwifery*. London: NMC.

Nursing and Midwifery Council (2004b). *Standards of proficiency for pre-registration nursing*. London: NMC.

Pawade, A.K. (2005). Accountability and quality assurance in paediatric cardiac surgery, *Annals of Cardiac Anaesthesia, 8*, 15–20.

Polyani, M. (1966). *The tacit dimension*. London: Routledge & Kegan Paul.

Royal College of Nursing (2005). *Maxi nurses – nurses working in advanced and extended roles promoting and developing patient centred health care*. London: RCN.

Seale, J.K. (2008). Developing e-learning experiences and practices: the importance of context. *ALT-J, 16*, 1–3.

Sollano, J.A., Gelijns, A.C., Moskowitz, A.J., Heitjan, D.F., Cullinane, S., Saha, T. et al (1999). Volume-outcome relationships in cardiovascular operations: New York State, 1990–1995. *Journal of Thoracic and Cardiovascular Surgery, 117*, 419–428.

Tye, C.C. & Ross, F.M. (2000). Blurring boundaries: professional perspectives of the emergency nurse practitioner role in a major accident and emergency department. *Journal of Advanced Nursing, 31*, 1089–1096.

Woods, L.P. (2000). *The enigma of advanced nursing practice*. Wiltshire: Quay Books.

2 Presentation and diagnosis

Rami Dhillon, Gurleen Sharland, Anne-Maree Robinson, Collette Clay, Christine Bearne

Fetal diagnosis of congenital heart disease

Antenatal diagnosis of congenital heart disease (CHD) has become well established over the last 25 years, although there remain large variations in prenatal detection rates (Allan et al, 1994; Bull, 1999). There are several reasons for performing cardiac scans in the fetus, the main being to detect major forms of cardiac abnormality as early as possible. A recent study has shown that a significant number of infants (25%) with potentially life-threatening malformations of the heart were undiagnosed at the time of discharge from hospital (Wren et al, 2008). An antenatal diagnosis could help to reduce the morbidity and mortality in some of these cases by making an earlier diagnosis. Detection in early pregnancy also allows parental choice and time for parents to be prepared for the likely course of events after delivery. Additionally, examining the fetal heart during pregnancy can be of great benefit, if normality can be confirmed, in providing reassurance to parents at high risk of having a child with CHD, in particular where a previous child has been lost because of CHD. An example of the options available for parents with a fetal diagnosis of transposition of the great arteries (TGA) can be seen in Boxes 2.1–2.5.

A high degree of diagnostic accuracy is now expected in the diagnosis of fetal CHD, and most of the major malformations of the heart, as well as some minor forms, are detectable during fetal life (Allan et al, 2000). However, fetal series are still skewed towards the severe end of the spectrum of cardiac abnormality, particularly those that will result in single-ventricle palliation rather than a corrective procedure. This is a reflection of the way in which patients are currently selected for fetal echocardiography, with the vast majority of fetal cardiac abnormalities being initially detected by obstetric screening. As a result of this, abnormalities associated with an abnormal four-chamber view are still much more common in fetal series.

In the early years of fetal echocardiography, there were significant proportions of referrals because of extracardiac malformations in the baby or associated non-immune fetal hydrops. As a result, there was a high incidence of associated anomalies, particularly chromosomal anomalies (Sharland & Allan, 1992). In more recent years, however, the rate of chromosomal anomalies seen with prenatal CHD has fallen. This is partly related to improved obstetric screening of the low-risk population, so that more isolated cardiac abnormalities are detected, and is partly attributable to the introduction of the nuchal translucency measurement in the first trimester (Hyett et al, 1999, Pandya et al, 1995). This latter method has led to the detection of trisomies earlier in pregnancy, and although a significant number of these may be associated with heart disease, many may no longer be referred for detailed evaluation of the fetal heart.

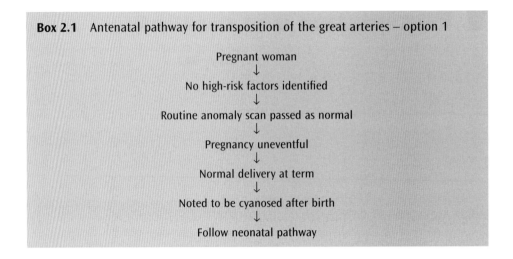

Box 2.1   Antenatal pathway for transposition of the great arteries – option 1

Pregnant woman
↓
No high-risk factors identified
↓
Routine anomaly scan passed as normal
↓
Pregnancy uneventful
↓
Normal delivery at term
↓
Noted to be cyanosed after birth
↓
Follow neonatal pathway

Prenatal screening for congenital heart disease

High-risk groups
High-risk pregnancies, as listed below, are usually referred for specialised fetal cardiology assessment.

Maternal factors identified at booking
A *family history of CHD* is significant. If one previous child has had CHD, the risk of recurrence in any subsequent pregnancy is in the region of 2–3%, but is higher for some lesions than others. Where there have been two affected children, the risk increases to about 10%, and this rises to 50% if three children have previously been affected. If one of the parents has CHD, there is an increased risk in the baby of between 2% and 5% (Gill et al, 2003).

Maternal diabetes is associated with a risk of cardiac malformation of about 2–3% (Meyers-Wittkopf et al, 1996). Good diabetic control in early pregnancy is thought to diminish this risk.

Exposure to *teratogens* such as lithium, phenytoin or steroids in early pregnancy is reported to be associated with about a 2% risk of heart malformation.

Fetal high-risk factors
The detection of an *extracardiac fetal anomaly on ultrasound* should lead to a complete examination of the fetal heart as many types of abnormality, for example exomphalos or diaphragmatic hernia, may be associated with CHD (Copel et al, 1986). Abnormalities in more than one system in the fetus should arouse the suspicion of a chromosome defect.

Some *fetal arrhythmias*, particularly complete heart block, are associated with structural heart disease (Machado et al, 1988). Evaluation of a fetal arrhythmia must therefore include examination of the cardiac structure.

Non-immune fetal hydrops can be due to CHD or a fetal arrhythmia (Skoll et al, 1991).

The detection of *increased nuchal translucency* in the first trimester is associated with a high risk of CHD, even when the fetal karyotype is normal (Hyett et al, 1999).

Box 2.2 Antenatal pathway for transposition of the great arteries (TGA) – option 2

Pregnant woman
↓
No high-risk factors identified
↓
Concern about fetal heart at time of anomaly scan at 20 weeks
↓
Referred for specialist fetal cardiac assessment at 21 weeks
↓
Diagnosis of TGA made in specialist centre
↓
Parents counselled regarding problem and management options. Treatment options and current results from surgery discussed. Parents given option to talk with other parents who have had a child with TGA, and also with a cardiac surgeon, if they wish
↓
Parents decide whether or not to continue with pregnancy
↓
If continuing, arrange follow-up appointments including an appointment in a fetal medicine unit. Arrange follow-up fetal cardiology scans
↓
Discuss site of delivery with parents and referring obstetrician
↓
For diagnosis of TGA, recommend delivery at or near paediatric cardiac centre
↓
Prepare parents for what will happen after delivery
↓
Aim for delivery at or near term
↓
After birth transfer to neonatal/paediatric intensive care unit
↓
Follow neonatal pathway from point of diagnosis of TGA by paediatric cardiologist

If parents elect to stop pregnancy:

– request post mortem
– arrange post-termination counselling

Low-risk groups

Although high-risk groups form the largest numbers of cases referred for fetal cardiology assessment, the majority of cases of CHD will occur in a low-risk population. These can only be detected if the low-risk population is screened. The concept of prenatal screening for CHD was introduced in the UK in 1986 (Allan et al, 1986) following the results of a French study (Fermont et al, 1986). Obstetric sonographers were initially taught to incorporate and examine the four-chamber view of the fetal heart at the time of the routine obstetric anomaly scan. Although this is an effective method of detecting some of the severe forms of cardiac malformation before birth (Sharland et al, 1992; Tegnander et al, 1995), there is no doubt that including examination of the arterial connections of the heart will greatly improve the detection rates

Box 2.3 Antenatal pathway for transposition of the great arteries (TGA) – option 3

Pregnant woman
↓
Family history of congenital heart disease
↓
Referred for specialist fetal cardiac assessment at 21 weeks
↓
Diagnosis of TGA made in specialist centre
↓
Parents counselled regarding problem and management options. Treatment options and current results from surgery discussed. Parents given option to talk with other parents who have had a child with TGA, and also with a cardiac surgeon, if they wish
↓
Parents decide whether or not to continue with pregnancy
↓
If continuing, arrange follow-up appointments including an appointment in a fetal medicine unit. Arrange follow-up fetal cardiology scans
↓
Discuss site of delivery with parents and referring obstetrician
↓
For diagnosis of TGA, recommend delivery at or near paediatric cardiac centre
↓
Prepare parents for what will happen after delivery
↓
Aim for delivery at or near term
↓
After birth transfer to neonatal/intensive care unit
↓
Follow neonatal pathway from point of diagnosis of TGA by paediatric cardiologist

If parents elect to stop pregnancy:

– request post mortem
– arrange post-termination counseling

(Wigton et al, 1993; Kirk et al, 1994). Although views of arterial connections have additionally been incorporated into the obstetric scan by some centres, this is not the case in all.

The normal fetal heart

A systematic approach to the examination of the fetal heart will enable the easy confirmation of normality and in cases with congenital heart malformations will ensure an accurate diagnosis (Allan et al, 2000). As with postnatal cardiac assessment, this is best achieved by checking the connections of the heart. Additional cardiac anomalies, such as defects in the interventricular septum, can be excluded once the major connections have been checked.

Box 2.4 Antenatal pathway for transposition of the great arteries (TGA) – option 4

Pregnant woman
↓
No high-risk factors at booking
↓
Found to have increased nuchal on first-trimester screening
↓
Referred for specialist fetal cardiac assessment at 13–14 weeks
↓
Diagnosis of TGA made in specialist centre
↓
Parents counselled regarding problem and management options. Treatment options and current results from surgery discussed. Parents given option to talk with other parents who have had a child with TGA, and also with a cardiac surgeon, if they wish
↓
Parents decide whether or not to continue with pregnancy
↓
If continuing, arrange follow-up appointments including an appointment in a fetal medicine unit. Arrange follow-up fetal cardiology scans
↓
Discuss site of delivery with parents and referring obstetrician
↓
For diagnosis of TGA, recommend delivery at or near paediatric cardiac centre
↓
Prepare parents for what will happen after delivery
↓
Aim for delivery at or near term
↓
After birth transfer to neonatal/paediatric intensive care unit
↓
Follow neonatal pathway from point of diagnosis of TGA by paediatric cardiologist

If parents elect to stop pregnancy:

– request post mortem
– arrange post-termination counselling

In the fetus, it easiest to first check the abdominal situs and ensure that the heart and stomach are both on the left. One can then examine the four-chamber view and proceed to obtain a view of the great vessels.

The four-chamber view

This view is achieved in a transverse section of the fetal thorax just above the diaphragm. Examination of this view will demonstrate the pulmonary veins and atria, the atrioventricular (AV) connections and the two ventricles. The interventricular septum can also be examined in this view, as can the AV septum. An example of a normal four-chamber view is shown in Figure 2.1. The pulmonary venous drainage to the left atrium can be confirmed with colour Doppler ultrasonography.

Box 2.5 Antenatal pathway for transposition of the great arteries (TGA) – option 5 (rare in TGA but can happen)

Pregnant woman
↓
No high-risk factors at booking
↓
Found to have an extracardiac abnormality at time of anomaly scan
↓
Referred for specialist fetal cardiac assessment at 20–22 weeks
↓
Diagnosis of TGA made in specialist centre
↓
Parents counselled regarding problem and management options. Treatment options and current results from surgery discussed. Parents given option to talk with other parents who have had a child with TGA, and also with a cardiac surgeon, if they wish
↓
Parents decide whether or not to continue with pregnancy
↓
If continuing, arrange follow-up appointments including an appointment in a fetal medicine unit. Consider amniocentesis. Arrange follow-up fetal cardiology scans
↓
Discuss site of delivery with parents and referring obstetrician
↓
For diagnosis of TGA, recommend delivery at or near paediatric cardiac centre
↓
Prepare parents for what will happen after delivery
↓
Aim for delivery at or near term
↓
After birth transfer to neonatal/paediatric intensive care unit
↓
Follow neonatal pathway from point of diagnosis of TGA by paediatric cardiologist

If parents elect to stop pregnancy

– request post mortem
– arrange post-termination counselling

Arterial connections
The aorta and pulmonary artery can be imaged in both transverse and longitudinal projections. A view of the aorta arising from the left ventricle is shown in Figure 2.2. Figure 2.3 illustrates a transverse view showing a normal pulmonary artery, the transverse view being commonly used in fetal life. In this view, the aorta and superior vena cava can also be seen. A view comparable to the short axis view used in postnatal life showing the right heart structures can also be obtained in the fetus, but this view is less routinely used in fetal life. There are two arches to consider in fetal cardiac assessment, the aortic arch and the ductal arch. An example of a normal aortic arch is shown in Figure 2.4.

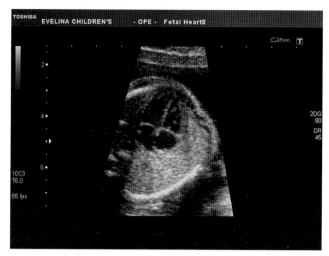

Figure 2.1 A normal four-chamber view

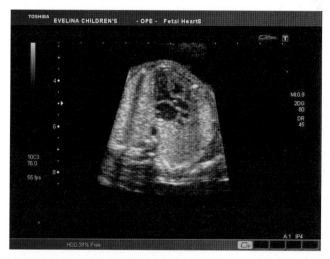

Figure 2.2 A view of the aorta arising from the left ventricle

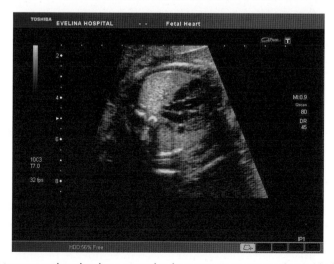

Figure 2.3 A transverse view showing a normal pulmonary artery, commonly used in fetal life

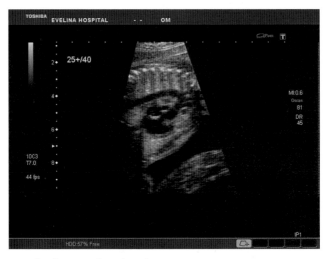

Figure 2.4 An example of a normal aortic arch

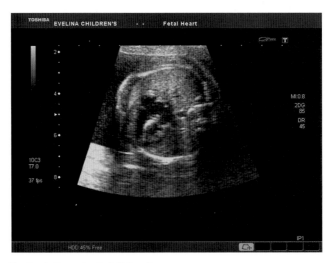

Figure 2.5 Aortic atresia/hypoplastic left heart

What can and cannot be detected prenatally?

The major forms of CHD, as well as some of the minor forms, can be detected in the fetus in experienced centres (Allan et al, 1994, 2000; Sharland, 2001). The most common lesions in fetal series are those associated with an abnormal four-chamber view, the two most common lesions being hypoplastic left heart syndrome (Figure 2.5) and AV septal defect (AVSD). Figures 2.6–2.8 show further examples of other major abnormalities associated with an abnormal four-chamber view. An example of a double-inlet left ventricle is shown in Figure 2.6. Figure 2.7 shows an example of Ebstein's anomaly of the tricuspid valve. The four-chamber view of an example of pulmonary atresia with an intact ventricular septum is seen in Figure 2.8. In contrast, Figures 2.9

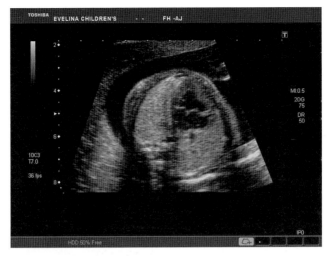

Figure 2.6 A double-inlet left ventricle

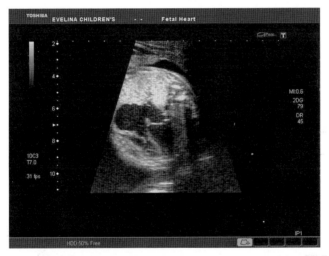

Figure 2.7 Ebstein's anomaly of the tricuspid valve

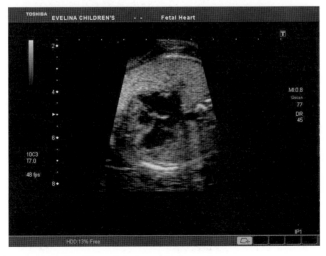

Figure 2.8 Pulmonary atresia with an intact ventricular septum

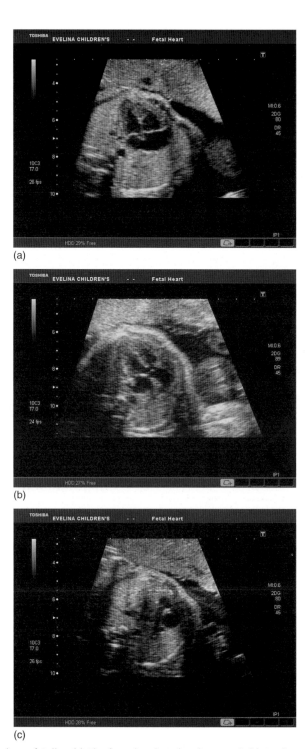

Figure 2.9 Tetralogy of Fallot. (a) The four-chamber view is normal. (b) Aortic override. (c) A small pulmonary artery from the right ventricle

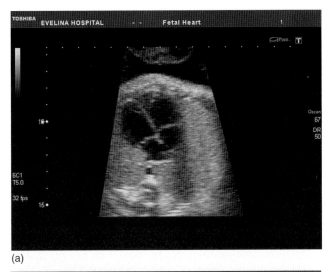

(a)

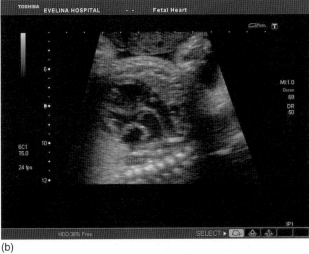

(b)

Figure 2.10 Simple transposition of the great arteries. (a) A normal four-chamber view occurs in transposition. (b) Parallel great arteries are seen

and 2.10 show examples of great artery abnormalities associated with a normal four-chamber view. An example of tetralogy of Fallot is shown in Figure 2.9, and an example of simple transposition in Figure 2.10.

There are, however, some lesions that cannot be predicted from fetal life. These include a secundum type of atrial septal defect and a persistent ductus arteriosus, since all fetuses should have a patent foramen ovale and a patent duct. In addition, some types of ventricular septal defect (VSD) may also be difficult to detect, because of either their size or their position. The milder forms of obstructive lesions of the aorta and pulmonary artery can develop later, and there may be no signs of obstruction during fetal life. It is important to make the parents aware of the types of lesion that are not detectable at the time of fetal cardiac assessment.

Management and outcome following prenatal diagnosis of congenital heart disease

Information to parents
Following the diagnosis of a cardiac malformation, the parents should be provided with detailed information about the problem and its implications. This includes an accurate description of the anomaly, along with information about the type of treatment available for the condition, the need for surgical or catheter intervention, the number of procedures likely to be required, the mortality and morbidity associated with these, and the overall long-term outlook for the child. The parents need to understand all these facts before they can make any decisions about how to proceed.

Support following diagnosis
It is normal for parents to be extremely distressed at the time of disclosure of an abnormality, and further information is likely to be required after the initial explanations. A single consultation with the parents often does not resolve parental anxiety or may not provide them with adequate understanding of the problem. The majority of parents require continuing support and are likely to need more than one consultation in order to absorb and understand the implications of the ultrasound findings. Information leaflets and contact with other parents who have had a child affected with a similar problem are invaluable. In order to help deal with the needs of the parents, many units have a nurse counsellor or specialist nurse practitioner as part of the team, who can be present during any consultations with the parents and can provide continuing support for them throughout pregnancy and in some instances after delivery.

Options and further management
A major decision that has to be made by the parents, if the diagnosis is made early enough, is whether they wish to continue with the pregnancy or whether they wish to interrupt it. Termination of pregnancy is an option available before 24 weeks of gestation, but the parents should have accurate and adequate information before making their final choice. Should a termination take place, it is important to try and obtain permission for autopsy wherever possible, in order to confirm the diagnosis and to look for any associated malformations. This information is important when counselling parents for recurrence risks in future pregnancies.

In continuing pregnancies, appropriate arrangements should be made to restudy the fetal heart in later pregnancy. Some types of lesion may progress to a more severe form as pregnancy advances (Sharland et al, 1991; Hornberger et al, 1995a, 1995b; Simpson & Sharland, 1997), and some will be at risk of developing non-immune fetal hydrops (Knilans, 1995). In some lesions, such as TGA and hypoplastic left heart syndrome, evaluation of the atrial septum, looking for signs of restriction, is important in later pregnancy, as this will influence the immediate postnatal outcome (Bonnet et al, 1999; Glatz et al, 2007). The parents can meet with the paediatricians, paediatric cardiologists and paediatric cardiac surgeons likely to be looking after their baby after birth. In some types of cardiac diagnosis, it may be beneficial to transfer antenatal care to allow delivery in a unit with paediatric cardiology facilities available on site or nearby. The advantage of having a prenatal diagnosis is that it allows immediate cardiac assessment of the neonate and avoids late diagnosis after an infant has become cyanotic or acidotic.

Outcome

Although the overall outlook for CHD diagnosed prenatally has been poor, there has been a significant improvement in the numbers of babies surviving. The outcome for prenatally diagnosed CHD is influenced by several factors. A different spectrum of disease is still detected in prenatal compared with postnatal life, with those lesions that can be easily picked up during obstetric screening being dominant. There is also a higher incidence of associated abnormalities. In addition, a significant number of affected pregnancies may result in a spontaneous intrauterine loss.

In the early days of fetal echocardiography, the termination rate after prenatal diagnosis of CHD was very high. However, there has been a significant fall in the number of parents electing to terminate the pregnancy in more recent years, with many units now finding that under 30% of parents choose this option.

Fetal arrhythmias

There are three main groups of rhythm disturbance encountered in the fetus. These are irregular heart rhythms, fast heart rhythms (tachycardias) and slow heart rhythms (bradycardias). Arrhythmias in fetal life can be evaluated by the use of various echocardiographic methods to examine the relationship of the atrial and ventricular contractions. This can be achieved by M-mode echocardiography or Doppler methods, which can be used either independently or in combination (Jaeggi et al, 1998; Fouron et al, 2003; Carvalho et al, 2007).

Irregular heart rhythms

An irregular heart rhythm is the most common form of fetal arrhythmia and usually causes a great deal of anxiety to midwives, obstetricians and the pregnant mother, even though this type of rhythm disturbance is usually benign. Irregularity of the fetal heart rhythm is most frequently due to multiple atrial premature contractions, but ventricular extrasystoles may rarely also occur. Multiple blocked beats can produce a slow ventricular rate that can sometimes be difficult to distinguish from complete heart block.

The natural history of ectopic beats is to resolve spontaneously, either prenatally or early in the postnatal period. However, in a small number, particularly in cases where there are frequent multiple ectopics or blocked ectopic beats, there is a risk of a fetal tachycardia developing (Simpson et al, 1996). Echocardiographic assessment should be performed in all cases to exclude structural heart defects. Providing this is normal, the parents can be reassured that this is generally a benign form of rhythm disturbance and not likely to cause any compromise. In the relevant cases, the risk of a tachycardia developing should be discussed.

Bradycardias

Variation in the fetal heart rate with brief periods of sinus bradycardia occurs in normal fetuses and is of no consequence. However, a sustained bradycardia should always be evaluated further. This may be due to a prolonged sinus bradycardia and be a sign of severe fetal distress. More rarely, congenital long QT syndrome can present with a fetal sinus bradycardia (Hofbeck et al, 1997). In cases of persistent fetal bradycardia of less than 80 beats per minute, the most likely diagnosis is of complete heart block, but this should be confirmed with M-mode or Doppler studies, which will show complete dissociation between atrial and ventricular contractions.

Complete heart block may occur in isolation or in association with structural heart disease. There is an association between isolated complete heart block and maternal connective tissue, and in particular with circulating maternal anti-Ro and anti-La antibodies (Groves et al, 1996). When heart block occurs with structural heart disease, the most commonly associated abnormality is left atrial isomerism.

Cases of complete heart block associated with structural heart disease generally have a poor outlook with very few long-term survivors (Jaeggi et al, 2005). The outlook for isolated complete heart block is better, but this does not always carry a good prognosis (Groves et al, 1996; Jaeggi et al, 2005). There are some adverse prognostic factors that can be identified in this group, which include the presence or development of fetal hydrops, a heart rate less than 50 beats per minute at presentation and a negative maternal anti-Ro antibody status.

The management of immune-mediated heart block remains controversial. Jaeggi et al (2004) report improved mortality and a reduced incidence of late complications for fetuses treated with dexamethasone with or without sympathomimetic agents compared with untreated fetuses. This group report an improvement in 1-year survival from 44% in an era where no treatment was given, to 80% in a later time period where a treatment protocol was initiated. Data from Rosenthal et al (2005), however, do not support the benefits of such a treatment protocol as this group report an increased 1-year survival from 77% to 93% during time periods identical to those in the study of Jaeggi et al, but with no change in the use of intrauterine therapy.

Tachycardias

A fetal tachycardia is defined as a heart rate above 180 beats per minute, but in most cases of a significant tachycardia the heart rate will be above 200 beats per minute. The tachycardia can be intermittent or sustained and may be a sinus tachycardia, a supraventricular tachycardia (SVT) or atrial flutter; much more rarely, there may be atrial fibrillation (AF), chaotic atrial tachycardia or a ventricular tachycardia (VT) (Simpson & Sharland, 1998).

The prenatal management of fetal tachycardia remains controversial, with no unified protocols regarding which cases should be treated, which drugs should be used and which is the optimal route of administration. The options when faced with a fetus with a tachycardia are as follows:

■ *Observation only* may be appropriate in a small group of fetuses when the pregnancy is near term, the episodes of tachycardia are short-lived and there is no evidence of intrauterine cardiac failure.
■ In general, the results of *premature delivery* have been disappointing (Maxwell et al, 1988), and this should only be considered if there is intrauterine cardiac failure and there has been no response to antiarrhythmic therapy.
■ *Prenatal drug therapy* can be employed. Antiarrhythmic drug therapy has been advocated prenatally to control the rhythm disturbance before delivery, and to prevent or treat cardiac failure. The decision to treat a tachycardia will depend on the gestational age of the fetus, signs of cardiac failure, the duration of the tachycardic episodes and parental wishes.

Various drugs have been used in the management of fetal tachycardia, including digoxin, adenosine, amiodarone, flecainide, procainamide, propranolol, propafenone, quinidine, sotolol and verapamil. Various routes of administration have also been used, which include transplacental therapy by giving maternal oral or intravenous doses of drugs, or direct fetal therapy via the umbilical vein, intramuscular, intraperitoneal or intra-amniotic routes. For fetuses with atrial flutter or re-entry SVT and no signs of fetal hydrops, maternal digoxin therapy has been used widely. However, digoxin therapy alone is not very effective in fetuses with hydrops due to poor placental transfer. In these cases, therapies widely used have included flecainide, sotalol and amiodarone.

Despite the various forms and route of therapy, the overall results in the larger series are similar (Hansmann et al, 1991; Van Engelen et al, 1994; Frohn-Mulder et al, 1995; Simpson & Sharland, 1998). The most important prognostic factor for an individual fetus is the presence or absence of fetal hydrops, with mortality being much higher if there is associated fetal hydrops. However, the outcome in this group is significantly improved if the rhythm is controlled prior to delivery.

Fetal intervention

Fetal cardiac intervention for structural heart disease was first reported by Maxwell et al (1991), who reported the results of a fetal aortic balloon valvuloplasty. Before this, in 1986, Carpenter et al (1986) had attempted to pace a fetus with complete heart block associated with non-immune fetal hydrops. However, although these early reports and others subsequently have shown that fetal cardiac intervention is possible, the benefits of such procedures are still under evaluation and the role for fetal intervention remains to be fully established.

To date, intervention for structural heart disease in the human fetus has been confined to severe obstructive lesions of the aortic or pulmonary valves, or cases of hypoplastic left heart syndrome with an intact or very restricted atrial septum (Kohl et al, 2000; Tulzer et al, 2002; Marshall et al, 2004, 2005). The rationale for intervention in severe obstructive lesions is to restrict secondary ventricular damage and to promote growth of the cardiac structures on the affected side of the heart.

Echocardiographic studies have shown that the evolution of some forms of cardiac lesions is a dynamic process during fetal life, and this is particularly true of the obstructive lesions. For example, critical aortic stenosis can develop into hypoplastic left heart syndrome, and severe pulmonary stenosis can develop into pulmonary atresia. In cases where there is an obstruction to the arterial valve, the corresponding ventricle is likely to show a reduced rate of growth as pregnancy advances. Intervention in fetal life has been proposed to alter the natural history and to try to promote growth of the cardiac structures, so that the surgical treatment after birth might be definitive rather than palliative. In cases of hypoplastic left heart syndrome with an intact or severely restricted atrial septum, the outlook is poor because of the damage caused to the pulmonary vasculature (Stasik et al, 2006). In cases of fetal diagnosis, an atrial septostomy has been advocated (Vida et al, 2007) to decompress the left atrium and reduce pulmonary congestion.

Overall, the results of fetal intervention have been disappointing, although better in some centres than others. This is partly explained by poor case selection and the fact that most centres, with a few exceptions, have reported an experience of only a small number of cases (Matsui & Gardiner, 2007). In 2006, guidelines for fetal intervention were produced by the National Institute for Health and Clinical Excellence in the UK (2006a), which recommended a multicentre approach to define criteria for patient selection and to evaluate the effectiveness of prenatal cardiac intervention. It is likely that improved patient selection and technical modifications in interventional methods will improve outcome in the future. Concentration of procedures in a few centres is also likely to improve the outcome and benefits of a fetal intervention.

Neonatal presentations

One of the health professionals best placed for detecting and screening newborn infants is the midwife. Over the ages, midwives have been the most common birth attendants in the world. A practising midwife is responsible for providing women and their babies with safe, effective care with optimal outcomes (Nursing and Midwifery Council, 2004). The European Union Second Midwifery Directive 80/155/ECC in article 4 states that the activities of a midwife should include the examination and care of the newborn infant and monitoring the progress of the baby during the postnatal period.

Before identifying what the midwife may detect during a cardiac assessment of the newborn, it is important to outline the context in which the midwife will be examining the newborn infant. The National Institute for Health and Clinical Excellence guidance on postnatal care (2006b) and the Child Health Promotion Programme (Department of Health, 2008) set the context for the newborn and infant examinations. The midwife is primarily responsible for the initial newborn examination that is performed shortly after delivery and for the daily examination of the baby that is carried out for the duration of the woman's postnatal care. The routine newborn examination is the continuation of child health screening that commenced during the antenatal period. These examinations have been carried out by healthcare professionals for many decades, traditionally the neonatology team, paediatric senior house officer and general practitioner (GP). The recent review and reconfiguration of service provision within the National Health Service has impacted upon the expansion of the roles of many healthcare professionals in this field (the NHS Plan; Department of Health, 2000). Midwives have been encouraged to acquire the relevant skills and competencies to undertake the routine physical examination of the newborn infant.

Aside from the midwife's detection of CHD in the newborn in hospital or at home, this may be picked up by the health visitor or the GP (including at the routine 6-week check). Newborns with CHD can also present in an emergency fashion (see 'Unscheduled care', below). Modes of presentation include symptomatic presentation with signs of cardiac failure – breathlessness, poor feeding, failure to thrive or cyanosis – or being asymptomatic on routine screening, with the detection of a heart murmur, accepting that most heart murmurs heard in infants are innocent.

Timing of the newborn examinations

The overarching aims of the initial newborn examination are to assess the baby's transition from intrauterine to extrauterine life and to provide physical examination to confirm normality in a term baby. Surveillance of the baby in a logical and systematic sequence from head to toe enables the midwife to detect any abnormality or any obvious visible unexpected features. The Apgar scoring system is used to assess the baby's condition at birth. This involves the assessment of five variables: respiratory effort, heart rate, colour, muscle tone and reflex irritability (Medforth et al, 2006). The midwife is responsible for understanding the physiological, pathological, sociological, ethical and cultural factors that underpin accurate assessment, examination,

Box 2.6   The beginning of Beth's patient journey

For the sixth time in the last 3 weeks of pregnancy, I arrived at the district hospital, hoping to have my baby. Each time so far I had been given injections to stop the labour and sent home again, but this time luckily the doctor said let's get on with it.

Five hours later we had a beautiful little girl called Beth. She weighed in at 5 lb 10 oz and seemed fine. We were sent back to our local hospital and on the fifth day there I decided it was time to go home. The midwife realised Beth hadn't had her health check so continued to do one. On listening to Beth's heart, she said she could hear a murmur but would get the on-call doctor to have a listen. He came straight away and said he could hear a murmur and thought she might, from what he could hear, need a balloon put in. I was very worried but I had a few friends whose babies had had heart murmurs and they grew out of them.

The doctor let us go home, and the next morning we received a call from the district hospital asking us to take Beth down there to be checked. When we arrived, the doctor decided she needed her pressures done. These showed that there was a big difference between her left and right side, the right being weaker. He then sent us for an ECG; we took the results back to him, and while he checked them he sent us for an X-ray. We had literally just got through the doors to X-ray when he came running down the corridor after us shouting that we had to go straight to the children's hospital as he was very concerned about her. I felt physically sick; what was happening? Our little girl's heart murmur was about to become something much bigger. It would have helped if he could have explained but he didn't have time to, so we didn't know what to think.

investigation and management of the newborn baby. Box 2.6 demonstrates the feelings of Beth's parents as they begin their healthcare journey with their newborn daughter following the healthcare check conducted by their midwife. The daily examination of the baby provides an opportunity for the midwife to provide information and address parental concerns about caring for their baby, whilst delivering health education about what to expect from their baby and transition to becoming a family.

The routine examination of the newborn continues the process of newborn screening in the postnatal period and involves a more detailed examination of the baby (Baston & Durward, 2001). The routine physical examinations of the neonate and 6–8-week infant are an integral part of the universal Child Health Promotion Programme (UK National Screening Committee, 2008). The UK National Screening Committee (2008) launched national guidance on the standards and competencies necessary to deliver a high standard of care to women and their babies. This examination is established as being good clinical practice for newborn health assessment, screening for abnormality and providing reassurance to parents that their baby is healthy and fully developed (Hall, 1999; Watts, 2003; UK National Screening Committee, 2008). The routine examination is for babies who are thought to be well, without significant problems and being cared for in the postnatal period (NHS Quality Improvement Scotland, 2008).

This routine examination is a comprehensive, physical clinical examination of the newborn baby usually performed within the first 72 hours of life (UK National Screening Committee, 2008). It should be conducted in a structured manner using observation, inspection, palpation and auscultation skills. The newborn examination will be performed either in a hospital or a home environment, depending on the woman's chosen place of birth and obstetric history.

Table 2.1 Differences between respiratory and cardiac cyanosis

	Respiratory cyanosis	Cardiac cyanosis
History	Prematurity, presence of meconium, risk of infection	Family history of congenital heart disease
Cardiovascular system examination	Normal	May have clear signs
Response to oxygen	Cyanosis likely to improve	Unlikely to improve
Chest X-ray	Obvious pathology	No respiratory pathology, abnormal heart shadow or lung vasculature
ECG	Usually normal	May be abnormal
Blood gases	Raised carbon dioxide	Normal or low carbon dioxide

Cardiovascular assessment

Any examination must be preceded by taking a history. The first consideration in the cardiovascular system is to review any problems arising from antenatal screening, family history or events in labour. The overarching aims of the newborn examination are to detect any abnormal cardiovascular features and to screen for specific target conditions such as CHD.

With an increased incidence of CHD in low-birthweight infant and an increased risk of patent ductus arteriosus (PDA) in premature infants, baseline observations including birth weight, gestational age and gender will be taken into consideration (Tappero & Honeyfield, 2003). The initial assessment will include general observation of the infant's appearance and behaviour. Consideration will be given to the infant's feeding pattern and ability to feed, whether this is breastfeeding or artificial feeding. Within the first few days of life, it is quite common for normal infants to sometimes become dusky or cyanosed around the mouth during feeds. Difficulty feeding, breathlessness, episodes of cyanosis and tachypnoea often occur in both respiratory and cardiac problems (Tappero & Honeyfield, 2003). It is therefore important to distinguish between the two systems. Table 2.1 illustrates features of respiratory and cardiac cyanosis.

Examination of the cardiovascular system should include the heart rate, heart rhythm, heart position, pulse volume, heart sounds and murmurs. Continuing with the cardiovascular assessment, the midwife (skilled in newborn infant physical examination) locates the apex beat and palpates the praecordium for thrills or heaves. With a paediatric stethoscope, the midwife auscultates the heart over the apex, left sternal edge, aortic and pulmonary areas. This allows the midwife to confirm normal heart sounds, detect any abnormal sounds and detect heart murmurs. The opportunity is taken to listen for breath sounds at the same time. Breath sounds should be assessed for pitch, intensity and duration. Care is taken during auscultation to listen for symmetry of breath sounds and air entry on both sides. Both the anterior and posterior chest walls should be auscultated for breath sounds.

An essential aspect in the cardiovascular assessment is the palpation of the femoral pulses. Weak or absent femoral pulses imply coarctation of the aorta. The pulse rate, rhythm, volume and character should be determined.

It is expected that immediate referral is made to the neonatology team where an abnormality is suspected so that an accurate diagnosis may be made and prompt treatment or referral can be planned (Box 2.7). The UK National Screening Committee

Box 2.7 Timmy's patient journey: neonatal presentation of an infant with tetralogy of Fallot

After a straightforward pregnancy and birth, Timmy presented with a 'blue' episode when he was 20 hours old. I was still at hospital as I was having problems breastfeeding him. He took a spell in my arms and went totally stiff. I rang the buzzer at the side of my bed (I don't know how I remained so calm) and the nurse arrived in seconds and whisked Timmy away. I walked in the direction that she had gone and saw my baby in an incubator looking a strange blue/dark pink colour. (I now know that this colour is referred to as 'dusky'.) Apart from his colour, he looked fine. The paediatrician said that he wanted to move Timmy to SCBU. At this point, I can remember feeling as if I was in a dream. My husband was at home with my daughter (then 20 months), and they were both due to be coming to the hospital in the next few hours.

SCBU was situated up some stairs. I went up the stairs and after waiting for some time was able to see my baby. I couldn't help but see the other babies in the unit. The paediatrician said that Timmy had a heart murmur and was being transferred to the children's hospital for an echo examination. The next few hours consisted of preparing Timmy for the journey. This is all a blur now. I remember my husband arriving amid all of this, as well as my sister and aunty. My aunty bought a huge balloon with congratulations written on it, and I remember thinking how out of place it looked.

The journey to the children's hospital is again a blur. Timmy travelled in the ambulance, and we were told to drive down separately. When we arrived, we went to the intensive care unit. We waited in the parents' waiting room for what seemed like ages until the cardiac consultant came to explain what he had found. He used a model of a heart to explain that Timmy had a tetralogy of Fallot. He also went on to explain that he also felt that Timmy showed signs of DiGeorge syndrome. This was way too much information. I can remember thinking 'right, let's deal with the heart problem first'. Little did I know that the heart defect was a result of the DiGeorge. The doctor said that Timmy would experience blue spells until he was about a year old, then he would need surgery.

We stayed at the ITU until the next day, when we were transferred to the baby ward. We stayed in hospital for a further 3 days and then went home. We had a follow-up appointment for 2 weeks' time. At the follow-up appointment, it was decided that Timmy needed surgery sooner rather that later, so was booked in to have a shunt inserted at 9 weeks. He had a full repair at 12 months and is now a healthy, very active little boy.

The aspects that I feel were negative were:

- not being able to travel in the ambulance with him;
- being overloaded with information;
- phrases like 'dysmorphic facial characteristics' being used and not explained;
- being given information whilst the consultants were doing their rounds so not having a lot of time.

The positives are that we have come through the experience and I have a very tough, caring lovely child who plays football, attends gymnastics, does tae kwon do, swims unaided and participates in athletic activities.

(2008) has developed competencies and standards for aspects of the newborn infant physical examination and pathways of referral including CHD. Healthcare professionals and parents need to understand that the initial, daily or routine examination cannot identify all abnormalities that present in the neonatal period as many may only present at a later date.

Neonatal arrhythmias

Tachyarrhythmias in utero can, if left untreated, lead to the development of hydrops fetalis and an increased risk of mortality and morbidity (Wren, 1998; Oudijk et al, 2000). Therefore, intrauterine management is often initiated with the maternal oral intake of antiarrhythmic agents, such as digoxin, flecainide and amiodarone (see the section above on fetal tachycardias). The presence of hydrops fetalis is reported to be associated with a higher mortality rate and may also dictate the choice of pharmacological agents or even dual therapy (Krapp et al, 2003). Naturally, fetal arrhythmias bear much similarity to neonatal arrhythmias and, of course, one can translate into the other after birth. First-line treatment is dictated by the mechanism underlying the arrhythmia, although the exact physiological mechanisms behind fetal arrhythmias are often not fully understood; neither are the long-term outcomes of children who present with arrhythmias at such an early age and require intrauterine management.

The precise identification of the mechanism underlying an arrhythmia is important since the pharmacological approach can be quite different. The most common arrhythmia in early childhood is SVT, accounting for approximately two-thirds of reported cases (Wakai et al, 2003). This is an abnormal heart rhythm that originates above the ventricles and can generate a heart rate greater than 220 beats per minute. The most common cause of an SVT is a re-entry circuit, often relying on an accessory pathway and the normal conduction system.

Atrial flutter is reported to be the second most common cause, affecting one-third of cases (Krapp et al, 2003). This is also an abnormal heart rhythm that originates in the atria and can cause a tachycardia. The other recognised fetal and neonatal arrhythmias include atrial ectopic tachycardia, bradycardia and atrioventricular (AV) block, and VT.

Unscheduled care

When ambulance crews respond to an incident that involves neonates, infants or children, this is in an out-of-hospital environment that is diverse and relatively uncontrolled. Therefore, the most basic of diagnostic tasks may be rendered more problematic by the simplest of issues, such as poor lighting (Jewkes, 2006).

The successful management of out-of-hospital paediatric cardiac emergencies requires an accurate assessment and diagnosis to establish an appropriate care plan. This may not always be clear cut, as the patient with congenital heart defects can present a non-specific clinical picture that contradicts the underlying severity of their illness (Lee & Mason, 2001). The causes of childhood illness can be wide ranging, and at times it is difficult to distinguish the exact diagnosis (Horrax, 2002). This is pertinent when considering the symptoms of cardiac disease in children; presentations vary with age, and the textbook manifestations of congestive heart failure and arrhythmias are often discreet or absent (Sharieff & Wylie, 2003). This is particularly relevant in the out-of-hospital setting, where symptoms of breathlessness can appear for many different reasons and cardiac signs may remain undetected. In contrast with adults, cardiac ischaemia is rare in children (Ochsenschlager et al, 2005).

Scene safety is of paramount importance, with the practitioner exerting a gentle command in order to manage the intrusion of loud televisions, errant siblings and unruly animals (Jewkes, 2006). It is against this potentially disquieting background that the paramedic must endeavour to establish the cause and initiate effective treatment without delaying conveyance to definitive care if required. Ambulance crews are frequently privy to a wealth of social, domestic and environmental information that eludes those practitioners who care for patients further along their journey through the healthcare system, and a comprehensive patient handover should make reference to this.

A primary survey is performed to establish the presence and adequacy of the airway, breathing and circulation, and the absence of exsanguinating haemorrhage. The purpose of the primary survey is to identify life-threatening problems that require immediate intervention in the field in order to effectively manage the patient. Whilst cardiac arrest in children is thankfully rare in the out of hospital setting, it is associated with high mortality rates (Pitetti et al, 2002) and a dismal prognosis for neurological morbidity (Schindler et al, 1996). Prompt recognition and initiation of appropriate therapy is essential in paediatric cardiac arrest for a favourable outcome.

History-taking and examination remain the foundation of assessment to help distinguish the cause of the problem, once vital functions have been assessed and the initial treatment of life-threatening conditions has been started. The secondary survey must be structured, logical and concise as it takes place in an arena where time is limited, and a focused approach is essential. Transfer to definitive care should not be delayed; consequently the secondary assessment may take place en route. On completion of this assessment, the practitioner should have a better understanding of the illness affecting the child and may have formulated a differential diagnosis. The history often provides the vital clues that help the practitioner identify the disease process and provide the appropriate emergency care (Advanced Paediatric Life Support Group, 2005). Children may present with acute exacerbations of pre-existing conditions such as asthma, bronchiolitis and epilepsy, all of which tend to centre the treatments to that particular condition, but the practitioner should be careful of disregarding new pathologies in such patients, and using a structured approach will prevent this (Advanced Paediatric Life Support Group, 2005).

So how can we establish the presence of cardiac problems in the very young? These can be categorised loosely into three groups: structural abnormalities, inflammatory reactions and arrhythmias (Ochsenschlager et al, 2005). Structural abnormalities include native and operated CHD and hypertrophic cardiomyopathy (HCM). Dilated cardiomyopathy or myocarditis in an infant or child, whilst uncommon, can be the cause in the patient who displays signs of shock and heart failure, and there may not be a history of CHD. These conditions can manifest in a variety of ways, will increase myocardial oxygen needs or decrease flow to the coronary arteries or both, and may result in cardiac ischaemia (Schindler et al, 1996; Archer & Burch, 1998; Pitetti et al, 2002; Advanced Paediatric Life Support Group, 2005; Ochsenschlager et al, 2005).

What do you look for? Cardiac pain is rare in childhood, although chest pain is a common symptom that is usually explained by musculoskeletal, gastrointestinal or anxiety problems. Children old enough to give a clear account may, during inflammatory or arrhythmic episodes, describe the characteristics of pericardial or cardiac pain. On the rare occasions that true angina presents in childhood, it is normally attributable to severe left ventricular outflow obstruction or congenital or acquired abnormalities of the coronary arteries (e.g. Kawasaki disease with giant coronary aneurysms; see Box 2.8 for a different presentation of Kawasaki disease). Rarely, angina from coronary artery disease may be present in infants who exhibit pallor, appear quiet (or inconsolable) and suffer sweating episodes. This may result from anomalous origin of the left coronary artery from the pulmonary artery, which is rare.

Box 2.8 Jamie's patient journey: the pre-hospital presentation of an infant with Kawasaki disease

A 6-month-old baby boy – Jamie – was referred by an emergency care practitioner (ECP) from the urgent care service (UCS) at the local hospital. His mother had phoned during the night stating that Jamie had been unwell for several days and was now screaming inconsolably. The ECP had given advice and reassurance and arranged further contact by the UCS that morning to reassess Jamie. His mother was contacted within an hour and reported that Jamie was more settled but was generally not well and was feeding less. A visit was arranged for later that morning.

On initial assessment, Jamie had been unwell for 6 days with a pyrexia, had red eyes and was generally miserable. Three days previously, he had been taken to see the GP, who had diagnosed a viral illness. Since then, Jamie had continued to have a high pyrexia despite paracetamol and was taking fewer feeds with only 2–3 oz each feed. His eyes had been red but not sticky. His feet had been swollen earlier in the week. There was no significant past medical history or birth history, and Jamie appeared to be developing normally. He had two siblings aged 4 years and 18 months.

On examination, Jamie was pale and quiet but responsive. A rash was evident on his trunk: pale pink spots that blanched. His temperature was 39.2 °C, his pulse 180 beats per minute, his respiratory rate 40 per minute, his oxygen saturations 100% and his throat only slightly red. Cervical lymphadenopathy was noted. Jamie's chest sounded clear, and his abdomen was soft, no obvious discomfort. Jamie did not look dehydrated despite his reduced fluid intake. His lips appeared very red (a few days earlier they had actually been cracked and bleeding), but there was no obvious 'strawberry tongue'.

Jamie's urine was tested using routine nitrite dipsticks and was found to be normal. Anti-pyretics were continued. He was taken to the hospital for review but was later sent home with the diagnosis of a probable viral infection, his mother being asked to obtain a repeat urine sample.

Three days later, Jamie's fingers had started to peel so he was taken back to hospital. He was still pyrexial and unwell, but it was a further 5 days before Jamie was given intravenous immunoglobulin with high-dose aspirin and a cardiac echo examination was performed. Unfortunately, Jamie had numerous large coronary artery aneurysms, and his parents were informed that the next few weeks would be a critical time for him. He was subsequently transferred to the children's hospital for specialist cardiological care.

A much more common symptom of acute cardiac problems in children is breathlessness, which in turn is related to cardiac failure. As mentioned, this symptom is rather non-specific and may of course be related to respiratory disease, rather than cardiac.

Hypercyanotic episodes can occur in patients with dynamic pulmonary outflow obstruction and VSD, typically in tetralogy of Fallot. They typically occur as the infant wakes or stops crying. At this point, instead of the colour returning to normal, the infant may remain unresponsive, cyanosed, drowsy and limp with rapid and deep respiration. Extreme cyanotic episodes should be treated as a time-critical emergency as this patient is in need of urgent vascular reassessment and treatment (Archer & Burch, 1998).

Infectious agents such as bacteria, fungi and viruses can cause pericarditis or myocarditis. This can present with pericardial pain that is aggravated by deep breathing, coughing, straining or leaning forward, and there may be associated symptoms such as fever, fatigue and shortness of breath. Arrhythmias, especially tachyarrhythmias such as SVT, can cause chest pain, palpitations or feelings of discomfort, even though children can usually endure rapid heart rates for a number of hours. In due course, they will exhibit symptoms such as weakness and dizziness and shows signs associated with congestive heart failure. It is important to recognise that tachyarrhythmias may be paroxysmal in nature; therefore, the practitioner may observe a normal rate, rhythm and electrocardiogram (ECG) as part of the patient's assessment.

Determining this type of problem in the field may be difficult if a diagnosis has not already been confirmed; however, observations for generic signs and symptoms are probably a more effective way of not missing vital clues. A conundrum exists when there are signs and symptoms compatible with both a respiratory and a cardiac problem. The reason for this is that respiratory symptoms may be a sign of associated cardiac abnormalities rather than directly attributable to respiratory pathology; consequently, breathlessness may be as a result of cardiac or respiratory causes. Hypoxia often results in tachycardia in the older infant and child, with severe or prolonged hypoxia leading to the preterminal bradycardic stage. In addition, vasoconstriction and skin pallor are evident; by the time this is visible, the child is close to respiratory arrest. Skin becomes mottled, cold and pale with a markedly slow capillary bed refill time, indicative of poor perfusion and impending circulatory failure (Archer & Burch, 1998; Advanced Paediatric Life Support Group, 2005).

Peripheral cyanosis is relatively common, predominantly in the newborn period, but can be apparent in all age groups. It may be normal if it occurs without central cyanosis and there is no obvious distress, ill health or discomfort. Peripheral cyanosis can also be found around the mouth of young babies, is often observed after feeding and may be identified as slight cyanosis or grey discoloration. Providing no related abnormal behaviour or distress is evident, the discoloration is no cause for concern and is often referred to as 'innocent perioral cyanosis'. Neonates may appear distressed, cry or grunt whilst undergoing the exertion of feeding. In the young patient, words like 'pain' and 'hurt' may be used to describe cardiac symptoms such as palpitations or dyspnoea, due to the limitations of children's vocabulary.

In the full-term newborn baby, breathing creates a rise in circulating oxygen that causes constriction of the ductus arteriosus tissue. The PDA is a normal structure that connects the systemic and pulmonary circulations in utero and permanently closes within 2–3 weeks of birth. However, in some infants, the ductus arteriosus remains patent and the left-to-right (aortic-to-pulmonary artery) shunting of blood may be significant when the PDA is large, resulting in cardiac failure (Schindler et al, 1996; Archer & Burch, 1998; Advanced Life Support Group, 1999). Conversely, the acute closure of the PDA in systemic or pulmonary duct-dependent circulations will result in haemodynamic collapse. Infants with severe life-threatening congenital heart lesions such as coarctation of the aorta, TGA, hypoplastic left heart syndrome and pulmonary atresia thus rely on the patency of the PDA for survival. Therefore, oxygen therapy will have little benefit in the treatment of duct-dependent CHD; administering oxygen may accelerate the closure of the duct.

In the UK, CHD affects approximately 8 in every 1000 live births. Out-of-hospital management of the infant or child is generically aimed at restoring haemodynamic stability through early attention to adequate oxygenation and ventilation, coupled with circulatory support where required. It is imperative in the critically ill child that these interventions do not compromise or delay transportation to definitive care, as the majority of cardiac arrests are secondary to hypoxia or, less commonly, circulatory failure rather than primary cardiac arrest (Schindler et al, 1996; Jewkes, 2001).

Late presentations

School health checks

In recent years, there has been a move away from routine childhood surveillance of all children at around school entry age, when they are 4–5 years old. Such surveillance is not statutory, and primary care trusts have some latitude in how such surveillance is delivered. In some areas, it is principally the higher-risk children (e.g. looked-after children) who are subjected to detailed preschool checks. When this takes place, it is called the School Entry Health Check and requires parental consent. It consists of three separate elements (see 'School checks' in the list of websites at the end of the chapter):

- *Growth.* A school nurse measures the height and weight of the child, and if either are found to be abnormally high or low, a referral is made to the GP or a community paediatrician for further investigation. The National Child Measurement Programme, again non-statutory, was launched in August 2008 (see the end of the chapter).
- *Hearing.* Most cases of hearing impairment are detected before school entry. The school nurse will assess the hearing at school entry using a sweep hearing test, to confirm that hearing is normal at different frequencies of sound. A referral to the GP for further investigation will be made if evidence of a hearing impairment is found.
- *Vision.* A trained orthoptist conducts the examination, which may take the form of a standard vision acuity test, with the child being asked to read lines of letters from a chart. A referral to the GP for further investigation will be made if evidence of visual impairment is found.

The Children's National Service Framework now includes a Child Health Promotion Programme to replace the current Child Health Surveillance Programme (see the end of the chapter) ensuring that immunisations are up to date, children have access to primary and dental care and general development is reviewed. Other physical assessment may include heart sounds and murmurs, and it is in this way that childhood cardiac disease may be detected. It is important to remember, however, that the vast majority of heart murmurs detected during the routine surveillance of school-age children, and even incidentally for that matter, will be innocent.

Cardiac arrhythmias and sudden death

Cardiac arrhythmias

A cardiac arrhythmia is defined as a disturbance of the normal electrical rhythm within the heart. This disturbance can be classified as too fast (tachycardia) or too slow (bradycardia) and can be a regular or irregular rhythm. Arrhythmias can originate from any part of the heart's conduction system, and the clinical manifestations are dependent on where the arrhythmia originates and the underlying heart condition.

Arrhythmias can occur in fetal life, within the neonatal period (see above) and beyond. Patients with CHD can experience arrhythmias in both the pre- and postoperative periods, as can those with primary heart muscle disorders (cardiomyopathies). Arrhythmias can also be of an inherited nature, these mostly presenting in the adolescent period. However, all arrhythmias can, if unrecognised and untreated, lead to cardiogenic shock and, in some cases, the sudden and unexpected death of a patient.

The symptoms experienced by the patient are very varied and, within the paediatric population, symptom reporting is very dependent on the child's age and cognitive understanding. Young children may appear pale, tired and sweaty during an episode of abnormal heart rhythm. Generally, the recognised symptoms range from palpitations, chest pain, dizziness and syncope to congestive heart failure and cardiogenic shock. The treatment options are very varied, from pharmacological management to medical devices, such as pacemakers and internal cardioverter-defibrillators and non-surgical procedures such as radiofrequency catheter ablation.

Arrhythmias in congenital heart disease

The improved survival rates and clinical outcomes post cardiac surgery have led to an increase in the number of CHD patients presenting with arrhythmias in adolescence and early adulthood. Arrhythmias are the most common cause of hospitalisation within this patient group. They can be a consequence of the native structural disease itself, or the substrate for the arrhythmia can be the surgical intervention undertaken to repair the defect. Due to this, the number of patients who require catheter ablation has increased over the last few years, both for re-entry tachycardias and for atrial arrhythmias such as atrial flutter and AF, although this latter arrhythmia is rare in children.

Ebstein's anomaly

Ebstein's malformation of the tricuspid valve is a relatively rare defect accounting for less than 1% of all CHD (Carpentier & Brizard, 2006). The tricuspid valve is displaced downwards into the right ventricle, thereby causing a reduction in effective right ventricular cavity size. In addition, the valve is often significantly regurgitant. The outcome in newborn infants who present with severe cyanosis is relatively poor. Adults and young teenagers who are diagnosed later into life often do not require surgical intervention.

Approximately 25% of patients with this defect also have Wolff–Parkinson–White (WPW) syndrome (Figure 2.11) due to the presence of an accessory pathway between the atria and ventricles called the bundle of Kent. This pathway can cause a re-entry SVT with very fast rates. In the neonatal period, this rhythm can drastically reduce cardiac output and result in the collapse of the newborn. Incessant arrhythmias require medical management, such as intravenous adenosine and possible cardioversion in the collapsed and shocked infant in whom medical management has failed to convert to sinus rhythm.

Older children can undergo an electrophysiology study and catheter ablation of the accessory pathway. However, this may prove difficult if the patient has undergone insertion of a prosthetic tricuspid valve as the placement of the new valve may obscure the pathway and prevent termination during radiofrequency catheter ablation.

Congenitally corrected transposition of the great arteries

Usually abbreviated as ccTGA, this is also a relatively rare cardiac defect, accounting for about 1% of CHD. This disorder is characterised by AV and ventricular–arterial discordance. Over time, this may result in late failure of the systemic right ventricle

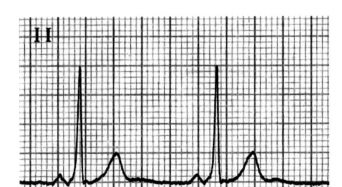

Figure 2.11 Wolff–Parkinson–White syndrome. Note the short PR interval and slurred upstroke of the R wave (delta wave)

Table 2.2 Known causes of arrhythmias in the postoperative period

Causes of tachyarrhythmias post cardiac surgery	Causes of conduction delay and bradyarrhythmias post cardiac surgery
Electrolyte disturbances	Inflammation around the sinoatrial node causing a junctional rhythm
Atriotomy may cause atrial flutter and atrial fibrillation	Right ventriculotomy causing conduction delay
Atrial dilatation before surgery may contribute to atrial tachycardias	Inflammation around AV node and AV bundles causing AV delay and/or block
Pyrexia and infection causing sinus tachycardia	Ischaemia post bypass
Pain after surgery may cause sinus tachycardia	Hypothermia post cardiopulmonary bypass

AV, atrioventricular.

if corrective surgery is delayed or a diagnosis is not made until later in adult life. As with Ebstein's anomaly, this defect is associated with accessory conduction pathways. Furthermore, there is a high incidence of heart block and patients may require a pacemaker insertion for rate control.

Arrhythmias post cardiac surgery

During the first 24 hours following cardiac surgery, there is a recognised and documented risk that the patient may develop heart rhythm and conduction disturbances. The reasons are multifactorial, but most are related to the effects of the surgical intervention rather than the inherent heart defect (Table 2.2). These disturbances can range from irregular extrasystoles, such as premature atrial and ventricular contractions (Figures 2.12 and 2.13 respectively) to more serious rhythm disturbances such as junctional ectopic tachycardia, atrial ectopic tachycardia, atrial flutter and AF. Sustained ventricular arrhythmias are very uncommon after cardiac surgery, with a reported incidence of less than 1% (Chung, 2000). However, they may be precipitated by ischaemia after cardiopulmonary bypass.

The congenital heart defects that mostly present with arrhythmias within the postoperative period are tetralogy of Fallot, repair of VSD and AVSD. The surgical repair

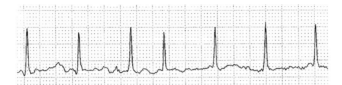

Figure 2.12 Premature atrial contractions. The atrial ectopic beats occur prematurely but have the same basic narrow QRS morphology as the normal beats

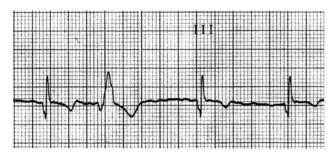

Figure 2.13 Premature ventricular contractions. The ventricular ectopic is premature and has a broad morphology, quite different from the normal complexes

of these cardiac lesions involves suturing the ventricular septum, which accommodates the AV conducting bundle. Junctional ectopic tachycardia is thought to be related in part to injury and oedema involving the bundle of His. It can be quite difficult to control and is associated with significant morbidity and mortality. Whilst surgical techniques have improved over the last 50 years, the physiology of these lesions predisposes the patient to develop arrhythmias and conduction disorders during the postoperative period.

Sudden cardiac death

Sudden cardiac death is described as the sudden and unexpected natural death of a cardiac cause in an individual with no previous symptoms or known underlying heart condition. The reported incidence in the USA is approximately 1 in 200,000–400,000 adult deaths and is mostly attributed to coronary artery disease. Sudden cardiac death amongst the paediatric population is an extremely rare occurrence. However, due to an increase in media interest and coverage in this subject, there has been a rise in the reported incidence of such events. In addition, there is a close link developing between sudden infant death syndrome and several of the known conditions related to sudden cardiac death in adults and children.

More research and development is needed in this area. There is also a national incentive to raise awareness amongst the pathology and coroner communities in order to provide further education and medical updates on the cardiac conditions that are so often responsible for the sudden cardiac death of both adults and children.

These cardiac conditions can be classified into two categories: structural and electrical. Over the last 50 years, there have been huge developments in understanding of the aetiology of the known conditions in each classification, and there is a growing awareness that many of these conditions are of an autosomal dominant inheritance. Continued research and development is needed to examine the physiological mechanisms that can lead to sudden cardiac death and the preventative measures and interventions required.

Electrical
Within this classification, the underlying heart disease is of an electrical nature and is often not diagnosed during a post mortem examination, as there is no evidence of structural heart disease in the individuals and an ECG can only be performed on a beating heart. In addition, the ECG of a child and young person alters slightly every year until after puberty, when the body is of adult size and the heart has taken its permanent position in the left side of the chest. During this period of growth, interpretation of the ECG changes in individuals with symptoms and is often difficult, and the diagnosis of electrical disturbances such as long QT syndrome often relies on such subtleties being assessed by an expert practitioner.

Long QT syndrome
This is a genetic condition, of which there are currently 12 known genetic types, each causing different ECG changes and phenotypical presentations. The reported incidence is approximately 1 in 5000 individuals. The electrical changes alter and ultimately lengthen the time taken between depolarisation and repolarisation of the heart (the QT interval). This increased QT interval can cause symptoms ranging from dizziness and syncope to sudden cardiac death caused by fatal ventricular arrhythmias such as ventricular fibrillation and VT. However, many individuals may not experience symptoms before their death.

The circumstances surrounding the death of an individual can assist with ascertaining a cause of death when there is no evidence of a structural cardiac abnormality. Long AQ type 1 (LQT1) is often exacerbated by exercise and the individual is at a higher risk of ventricular arrhythmias during strenuous exercise, in particular swimming. LQT2 should be suspected in individuals who experience ventricular arrhythmias or sudden death following auditory stimuli, such as loud noises or stress. Sudden cardiac death during sleep and rest suggests possible LQT3.

Brugada syndrome
This is also of autosomal dominant inheritance, affecting up to 14 per 1000 people, with high incidences reported in Asia. It was first described in 1992 by the Brugada family and, similarly to long QT syndrome, it causes electrical changes that can, if undiagnosed, lead to sudden cardiac death through ventricular arrhythmias. Sudden cardiac death from this condition often occurs when the heart is slow, especially during sleep. It is more commonly reported in individuals aged between 30 and 40 years; however, there are increasing number of case reports in which it has been diagnosed in a babies. It is currently being investigated for a link with sudden infant death syndrome.

Unlike long QT syndrome, the electrocardiographic subtleties of right bundle branch block and ST segment elevation in leads V1–V3 are often not evident, even amongst the adult population in symptomatic individuals. Occasionally, these changes may become evident during a period of fever in an individual, but it is extremely difficult to diagnose without further tests. It is now widely accepted that these ECG changes can be unmasked or further diagnosed using short-acting drug therapy, such as with flecainide and ajmaline. These two intravenous medications can be administered in an environment containing emergency equipment and an external defibrillator, and many specialist centres have established protocols for their administration in individuals suspected to have or carry a gene for Brugada syndrome. The interpretation of these tests and ECG changes within the paediatric population still remains difficult. Currently, children who have negative responses to these drugs will need a repeat test once they have completed their growth, as it is theoretically possible to have a false-negative result. Once again, further research is required to fully understand this condition.

Structural

Both adults and children may experience sudden cardiac death due to structural abnormalities, in particular 'cardiomyopathy'. This term refers to a disease of the heart muscle, and there have been great improvements over the last 20 years in classifying this condition further. There are currently four known and recognised types of cardiomyopathy, and the risk of sudden cardiac death varies with each type. As with electrical disturbances, it is standard practice to assess each individual known to have these conditions in terms of their risk of having fatal heart rhythms that may lead to sudden cardiac death. This process is called risk stratification and was first initiated in the early 1990s by William McKenna and colleagues. This process has been adopted by many centres worldwide and can save the lives of many individuals affected with these conditions. However, there are many individuals, both adult and paediatric, who are unaware that they have a heart condition, and a small but significant number of them will suffer premature death.

Hypertrophic cardiomyopathy

HCM was first described in various case studies in the 1950s by Donald Teare. This condition causes excessive thickening of the left side of the heart, more commonly in the septal region, although it can be seen in the apex and ventricular wall. It is known to be of autosomal dominant inheritance, and there are currently 11 genes known to cause this condition, with hundreds of documented mutations in these genes.

In addition to the thickening of the heart, this genetic condition causes the heart muscle cells at a microscopic level to disalign and become disorganised. It is this process which causes fibrosis or scar tissue to develop within the thickened areas of the heart and ultimately impacts upon the transmission of the heart's electrical impulses along the Purkinje fibres. Unfortunately, this disarray can only be diagnosed with a cardiac magnetic resonance imaging (MRI) scan and is not evident on a standard ECG. This fibrosis predisposes the individual to develop ventricular arrhythmias at some stage in their life, which obviously places them at risk of sudden cardiac death. With increasing knowledge of the genetic causes of this condition, it is becoming clear that there are certain genetic mutations that purely cause fibrosis whilst the heart remains of normal thickness. In particular, the gene for troponin T has been shown to cause higher incidences of sudden cardiac death with minimal hypertrophy evident.

Sudden cardiac death due to HCM can also be caused as the thickened muscle may cause left ventricular outflow tract obstruction. This blockage to forward blood flow can cause syncope and dizziness. However, more seriously, it can also cause ischemia of the heart if prolonged, leading to ventricular arrhythmias and, if untreated, sudden cardiac death.

The risk stratification process identifies individuals who are at high risk, and if deemed appropriate, an internal cardioverter-defibrillator may be implanted to treat such rhythm disturbances.

Dilated cardiomyopathy
Dilated cardiomyopathy is a disease that affects the function of the heart and causes it to become very enlarged and 'dilated'. Until recently, it was not felt to be genetically linked. However, it is now reported that approximately 30% of cases have a genetic cause. Individuals with this condition often develop heart failure and require many medications to preserve their heart function. Whilst they may experience chest pain, palpitations, shortness of breath and fatigue, the risk of sudden cardiac death is extremely low in this group of patients, although not zero per cent. As with hypertrophic cardiomyopathy, great progress has been made in examining the genetic causes of this condition. Approximately five of the same genes that can cause HCM have been found to cause dilated cardiomyopathy at different mutation points. There have also been a small number of reported cases in which a troponin T mutation has been discovered to cause dilated cardiomyopathy. Further research is required in this field of work to assist with risk stratification of these patients.

Restrictive cardiomyopathy
Restrictive cardiomyopathy affects the relaxation of the heart muscle and can lead to increased pulmonary pressures and heart failure. Sudden cardiac death connected to this condition is extremely rare, and individuals with this condition often require heart transplants.

Arrhythmogenic right ventricular cardiomyopathy
Arrhythmogenic right ventricular cardiomyopathy is the latest described cardiomyopathy. This disease is also autosomal dominant and causes severe ventricular arrhythmias through a process that replaces right ventricular muscle with fatty fibrous deposits. As with HCM, these deposits affect the electrical signals of the heart and patients can develop VT and fibrillation. Whilst the documented symptoms include palpitations, breathlessness and syncope, sudden cardiac death may be the first manifestation of the condition.

As with any genetically linked condition, family screening is of great importance to establish the risk factors and to prevent the unnecessary and unexpected death of both children and adults.

Cardiac investigations

Whilst history and examination are the mainstays of diagnosis, and experienced clinicians can in this way gain much information to guide the treatment of potential heart disease in children and young adults, specific cardiac investigations add a great deal to this process, particularly when it has been established that cardiac disease is present. Furthermore, recent years have seen a rapid development of newer, more specific modalities of cardiac assessment, particularly in the areas of cardiac imaging and electrophysiology. In this section, we shall expand on the standard diagnostic techniques and examine the more specialised ones, in illustration of what can currently be offered.

Electrocardiography

Although there are earlier examples of the recording of cardiac electrical activity from the surface of the human body, it was Willem Einthoven (1860–1927) who first formally employed basic electrocardiography in the form of a string galvanometer in 1901 (Einthoven, 1901). Further development of this technique was to earn him the Nobel Prize for Medicine in 1924 (Gottlieb, 1961).

Since then, use of the ECG has become commonplace, although its utility in paediatric practice perhaps remains underestimated. There are many reasons for this, including the greater challenge of obtaining good quality recordings in children, who may be more mobile and possibly less cooperative than their adult counterparts. Moreover, there is considerably less familiarity with the paediatric than the adult ECG. However, there are many publications currently available that highlight the differences between adult and paediatric ECG interpretation and, importantly, the ECG changes that take place with normal growth (Deal et al, 2004; Mehta & Dhillon, 2004; Park & Guntheroth, 2006), allowing practitioners from diverse medical and nursing disciplines access to the information this tool can provide. The investment in gaining familiarity with the rudiments of paediatric ECG interpretation is well worthwhile for any professional routinely involved in the medical care of children, given the ready availability of this investigation compared with other specialised cardiac investigations, for example echocardiography.

Basic principles of the ECG

The basic physical principle of ECG signal recording is that electrodes are used to measure the electrical activity of the heart from the surface of the body. Electrodes are positioned on the surface of the body in a variety of positions, most commonly in a 12-lead (or 13-lead if lead V4R is included) pattern. Whilst the leads relate to physical leads placed on the body, they also refer to unique perspectives or 'views' obtained of cardiac electrical activity in the coronal plane (leads I, II, III, AVR, AVL and AVF) and the transverse plane (leads V1–V6). In this way, the ECG records a net or 'average' vector in relation to the activation of heart muscle from the perspective of the 'viewing' positive electrode (lead). Depolarisation of heart muscle towards a positive electrode results in a positive deflection (above the isoelectric line), and conversely depolarisation away from a positive electrode produces a negative deflection. The greater the electric potential (voltage), the greater the deflection, and this can be used to determine abnormal, particularly increased, cardiac voltages. Thus, it is possible to define increased voltages relating to particular chambers of the heart as a result of chamber hypertrophy and/or dilatation. The normal range of cardiac voltages varies with age, and there are fortunately reference tables readily available for this purpose (Rijnbeek et al, 2001). Nevertheless, an appreciation of the changes that normally take place with growth is essential for paediatric ECG interpretation.

ECG changes with growth

In utero, the lungs of the fetus are filled with amniotic fluid, the vascular resistance within the pulmonary vessels is high and, by virtue of the placenta, the systemic vascular resistance is low. Whilst the pulmonary vascular resistance falls at birth and continues to fall in subsequent weeks, there is right ventricular dominance at birth, gradually changing to left ventricular dominance with increasing age. In the newborn period (up to 1 month of age), there are prominent right ventricular voltages with tall

R waves in lead V1 and typically a dominant S wave in V6, although this may not be seen in very preterm infants. After 3 years of age, there is an adult-type RS progression with the opposite pattern to that described in the newborn – a dominant S wave in V1 and a dominant R wave in V6. Between these two age ranges, the R wave is usually dominant in V1 and V6.

Praecordial ventricular voltages are relatively large, particularly in the mid-praecordial leads, in relation to the relatively thin chest walls of children, with better transmission of cardiac electrical voltages to the praecordial surface electrodes. The mean frontal QRS axis is more rightward (more positive) than in adults, generally greater than 90° at birth and becoming more leftward with increasing age. Children's hearts beat faster than adults, with correspondingly shorter durations (P waves and QRS complexes) and intervals (PR and QT).

Common patterns of abnormality

The ECG is best assessed in a systematic fashion and should always be assessed in the light of background clinical information, in particular why the investigation was carried out in the first place. There are subtly different methods suggested in the standard texts (Deal et al, 2004; Mehta & Dhillon, 2004; Park & Guntheroth, 2006) but also effective alternatives, and it is up to individual practitioners to find a method that is, for them, quick, thorough and therefore efficient. Traditionally, ECG interpretation begins with an assessment of rate, rhythm and QRS axis. Whilst this text is not intended to act as a comprehensive treatise on paediatric ECG interpretation, several ECG abnormalities occur commonly enough and provide a shortcut to identifying significant cardiac abnormalities in childhood as to be worthy of special mention:

■ *Superior QRS axis*: dominant S wave in lead AVF. This is abnormal in early childhood, although in adults up to −30° is permitted (a left superior axis), and this pattern may therefore also be seen in normal teenagers. A right superior axis (>180°) should be regarded as abnormal in any age group (even if occasionally found to be a normal variant after specialist evaluation). Superior QRS axes are associated with AVSDs, ventricular hypertrophy (directed towards the hypertrophied ventricle) and tricuspid atresia, and may be seen with right bundle branch block.

■ *Right ventricular hypertrophy*: upright T waves in lead V1 between 7 days and 10 years of age. This is usually accompanied by tall R waves in lead V1, deep S waves in V6 and right axis deviation. This pattern is associated with a multitude of cardiac malformations in children and, importantly, also the presence of longstanding or severe pulmonary hypertension.

■ *Increased left ventricular forces*: characterised by an inverse pattern to that described above, with deep S waves in lead V1, tall R waves in V6 and left axis deviation. Note that in paediatric practice this commonly describes left ventricular dilatation, rather than left ventricular hypertrophy. There may be abnormally deep Q waves in the left praecordial leads (V5 and V6). The range of normal voltages varies with age, and tables of normal values can be consulted in cases where there is doubt (Rijnbeek et al, 2001).

■ *Increased left or right atrial forces*: broad or tall P waves respectively, signifying left and right atrial enlargement respectively. Left atrial enlargement may be associated with congenital left-to-right shunts at an arterial or ventricular level (e.g. PDA or VSD) or more rarely cardiomyopathy or mitral stenosis. Right atrial enlargement is commonly seen in children with haemodynamically significant atrial septal defects and in those with significant longstanding pulmonary hypertension (e.g. associated with cor pulmonale).

■ *Appearance of Q waves*: in the right praecordial leads – V1 and V2. This is almost always abnormal and may be associated with severe right ventricular hypertrophy, ccTGA or double-discordance, or a functionally univentricular heart (true anatomically univentricular hearts being rare).

Arrhythmias and conduction abnormalities

Arrhythmias in children, as in adults, can be divided into fast and slow rhythm disturbances (tachyarrhythmias and bradyarrhythmias). These are described in relation to fetal rhythm disturbances above. There are a number of excellent textbooks specifically devoted to this topic (Walsh et al, 2001; Zeigler & Gillette, 2001). However, a number of specific entities are worthy of mention.

Narrow complex tachycardias are usually thought of as SVT (Figure 2.14), although narrow complex tachycardias may rarely represent a form of VT (Sarubbi et al, 2002). In childhood they are most commonly due to AV (including AV nodal) re-entry and an accessory AV pathway (Ko et al, 2004; Paul et al, 2000). When this is manifest on the surface ECG in sinus rhythm, typically with a short PR interval and a slurred upstroke of the R wave (a delta wave), it is described as WPW syndrome. Most individuals with an appearance of WPW on their surface ECGs will not experience SVT. Accessory AV pathways that are not evident from the surface ECG are described as 'concealed'.

There has been an increasing amount of interest in recent years in long QT syndrome that is associated with multifocal VT, typically torsades de pointes and, importantly, syncope and sudden death. Prolongation of the QT interval can be congenital or acquired (particularly in the presence of profound hypocalcaemia or hypomagnesaemia). It is abnormal if longer than 0.44 seconds (except in the first 6 months of life, when it may be normal up to 0.45 seconds). It is usually calculated using Bazett's formula (Bazett, 1920):

$$QTc = QT/\sqrt{(RR\ interval)}$$

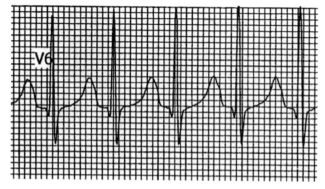

Figure 2.14 Supraventricular tachycardia. This example from an adolescent is quite subtle, with a rate of around 150/minute. Rates of over 180/minute are more typical, and in infants the rate is often over 220/minute. Note the lack of clearly definable P waves

where QTc = corrected QT interval, QT = measured QT interval and RR interval = interval between the R waves preceding the measured QT interval (Figure 2.15).

Brugada syndrome is another inherited cause of VT and sudden death, but is uncommon in the paediatric age range. Other inherited causes of VT include catecholamine-dependent VT and arrhythmogenic right ventricular cardiomyopathy (Figure 2.16).

Heart block, as in adults, has three degrees ranging from first-degree (PR prolongation) through second-degree (intermittent failure to conduct P waves to the ventricles) to third-degree or complete heart block, where there is complete AV dissociation (Figure 2.17). Symptomatic complete heart block usually requires the implantation of a permanent pacemaker. Second-degree heart block may occasionally require permanent pacing, and first-degree heart block does not usually require anything other than observation to ensure that the degree of block is not deteriorating (Gregoratos et al, 2002; Carlson et al, 2006).

Utility in assessing innocent murmurs

A final note about the utility of the ECG in assessing whether heart murmurs in children are significant or innocent. Whilst a conclusive study to determine the

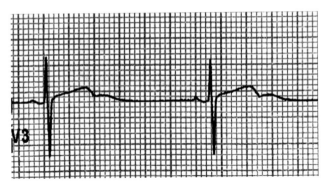

Figure 2.15   Long QT syndrome. See the main text for calculation of the corrected QT interval

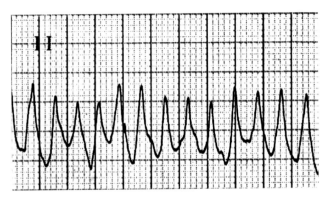

Figure 2.16   Ventricular tachycardia. This is characteristically a broad complex tachycardia, and in this example the rate is well over 300/minute

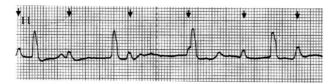

Figure 2.17 Complete heart block. Note the completely dissociated P waves

incidence of heart murmurs in childhood is lacking, the available evidence suggests that they are very common in early childhood (Amaral & Granzotti, 1999; Danford et al, 2002; Yi et al, 2002). It is likely (though unproven) that an innocent heart murmur will be audible at some point in at least 50% of children, although clearly this is very dependent on who is listening and how carefully. Given that structural heart disease is relatively uncommon (less than 1% of children), it can be seen that the vast majority of heart murmurs in childhood are innocent.

To an increasing extent, responsibility for deciding whether a heart murmur is innocent or significant is moving from primary and secondary care into tertiary care. Nevertheless, it is currently not feasible for paediatric cardiology services in the UK to see each and every child with a heart murmur, particularly if transient, and whilst it used to be recommended that these patients be investigated with an ECG and chest X-ray, the more useful of these is the ECG. Indeed, in the presence of history and examination findings consistent with an innocent heart murmur, and accepting that there are several different forms, a normal ECG is usually the only investigation required in order to make a confident diagnosis of an innocent murmur (Smythe et al, 1990). Pulse oximetry is non-invasive and a useful diagnostic adjunct, particularly in infants and babies. In most tertiary centres, echocardiography is reserved for those patients without history and signs consistent with innocence of the murmur, and for those with an abnormal ECG (Newburger et al, 1983; Geva et al, 1988).

Echocardiography

Echocardiography is the clinical application of ultrasound to observe the structure and function of the heart. Since 1953, when Inge Edler and Hellmuth Hertz first obtained time-varying echoes from within the heart using an industrial ultrasonic detector positioned on the skin overlying the heart, there have been rapid advances in this diagnostic modality (Lindstrom, 1991). Indeed, it is now the diagnostic mainstay for structural heart disease.

In its earliest clinical applications, it took the form of M-mode echocardiography, used to observe the timing of motion of cardiac structures in relation to a single pulsed ultrasound beam. Two-dimensional echocardiography was a logical development in the late 1950s and early 1960s, and has perhaps had the most impact in relation to the diagnosis of CHD, closely followed by the routine use of pulsed-wave Doppler (1970s) and colour Doppler (1980s) echocardiography. There have been steady advances in the development of better software and smaller ultrasound transducers. Trans-oesophageal echocardiography, initially suitable only for use in adults, has become a standard paediatric tool (Stumper et al, 1991). More recently, tissue Doppler and contrast echocardiography have emerged as important tools in the evaluation of regional myocardial function and blood flow (Kapusta et al, 2001). Three-dimensional echocardiography is currently undergoing a transition from being an attractive and interesting alternative method of viewing the heart to a being practical tool in its own right (Heusch et al, 2006).

Basic principles of echocardiography

Ultrasound, by definition waves of high-frequency sound, is created by the vibrations in a piezoelectric crystal. The beam of ultrasound thus produced is transmitted into the chest. When the waves pass an interface, such as between the heart wall and the adjoining blood in a cardiac chamber, or the surface of a heart valve, some of the sound is reflected. This is the echo after which echocardiography is named. The crystal also receives the echo, and the distance between the crystal and the surface that was the source of the echo is proportional to the time taken for the sound wave to bounce back to the crystal. In this way, multiple surfaces can be coded for distance and other more complex properties, allowing a detailed real-time picture of the heart in motion to be displayed (Roelandt et al, 1974).

Practical applications

As mentioned above, echocardiography has developed through M-mode to two-dimensional and now three-dimensional modes, each offering complementary and overlapping elements in imaging the structure and function of the heart. Two-dimensional echocardiography is currently the favoured mode in most centres but may be superseded by three-dimensional echocardiography at some point in the future, especially when computerised processing power enables clear real-time transthoracic images in children. The anatomical information thus obtained is greatly enhanced by physiological information from colour and spectral Doppler in the analysis of flow patterns in all of these modes. Tissue Doppler imaging, initially employed as a research tool, is now enjoying a role in the day-to-day assessment of myocardial function in clinical practice (Kapusta et al, 2001).

As illustrated earlier in this chapter, echocardiography is an ideal tool for assessment of the fetal heart. It is however, most widely used in the form of transthoracic echocardiography and, in certain circumstances, sedation of the patient may be required to obtain information of sufficient quality as to be clinically useful (Heistein et al, 2006; Yildirim et al, 2006; British Medical Association et al, 2007). Transoesophageal echocardiography has been in routine clinical use in children for around 20 years and usually requires general anaesthesia in the paediatric age range (Stumper et al, 1991). It is widely used on intensive care units, during conventional cardiac surgery and in interventional endovascular (transcatheter) procedures (Wolfe et al, 1993; Elzenga, 2000). It is particularly suited to viewing the posterior aspect of the heart, namely the atria, their venous connections and the AV valves. It has a higher sensitivity than transthoracic echocardiography in the detection of vegetations, particularly in older children.

Cardiac magnetic resonance imaging

In 1937, Isidor Rabi (Columbia University, New York City, USA) observed that atomic nuclei absorb or emit radio waves when exposed to a sufficiently strong magnetic field (Rabi, 1948). This phenomenon has become known as nuclear magnetic resonance. In 1973, Paul Lauterbur (State University of New York, Stony Brook, USA), produced the first nuclear magnetic resonance image (Brownell et al, 1982). Peter

Mansfield (University of Nottingham, UK), subsequently further developed this technology into a useful imaging technique, known as magnetic resonance imaging (MRI). He and Paul Lauterbur were jointly awarded the Nobel Prize for Medicine in 2003 for their work in this field.

Basic principles of magnetic resonance imaging

In MRI, the human body is exposed to a steady strong magnetic field and then pulsed radiofrequency waves to change the steady-state orientation of protons in the nuclei of hydrogen atoms in the body. When the radiofrequency signal is switched off, the protons in question eventually emit their absorbed radiofrequency energy, and this forms the MRI signal. That signal is then used to construct internal images of the body in a series of planes. MRI does not use ionizing radiation (X-rays).

Practical applications

Contrast enhancement is used to highlight the difference between adjacent but differing tissues, for example blood and the great vessels and the chambers through which it flows. This modality is therefore particularly suited to demonstrating vascular structures. The most commonly used cardiovascular MRI contrast agents are gadolinium-based, and as they do not contain iodine, they are less likely to cause an allergic reaction. Concerns have been raised, however, about the potential nephrotoxicity of these agents, although it is likely that this is only important in those patients with impaired renal function.

Real-time cardiac MRI is now available, although expensive and still relatively bulky. Whilst its use is currently mainly a research tool, in some centres it has been used for cardiac intervention, the patient being moved on rails between a standard cardiac catheterisation suite and an adjoining MRI suite (Horvath et al, 2007).

Practical limitations

In order to generate the images, the patient needs to lie still, within an enclosed space, with the magnet encircling. Some patients, both children and adults, experience claustrophobia. As a result of this, and the fact that a breath-hold is necessary for image acquisition, anaesthesia is usually required for studies in small children. On occasion, children as young as 6 years have been known to cooperate with the breath-hold.

Because of the very powerful magnetic fields involved, metal and electronic objects are not allowed in the examination room, and everyday objects such as credit cards can be irreversibly damaged. The use of MRI is contraindicated in patients with cardiac pacemakers or defibrillators, although it is safe with most other types of cardiac implant (e.g. artificial heart valves and septal occlusion devices).

Computed tomography

Computed tomography (CT) was invented by a British engineer, Godfrey Hounsfield, in 1972 (Ambrose & Hounsfield, 1973). His work earned him the Nobel Prize for Medicine in 1979. The basic principle involves taking X-ray images of a particular part of the body at multiple angles and then reconstructing an image of the area in question using powerful computing. The earliest CT scanners took hours to acquire imaging data and days to reconstruct this into a clinically useful image, and exposed the patient to a relatively high dose of radiation. Current CT scanners take seconds to acquire data and produce multiple images. Furthermore, they can now do this at relatively low radiation doses.

Practical applications

The heart and great vessels can be clearly imaged using CT, particularly with the latest multislice technology and the use of contrast agents to mark their internal dimensions. The relationship of these structures to the airways and lungs can be clearly demonstrated, and cardiac CT has a particular utility when airway compression is clinically important, for example with a vascular ring. The relationship to other thoracic structures may be important and can be demonstrated, for example, in thoracic neoplasia. Rapid advances in spatial and temporal resolution have permitted the development of three-dimensional CT (Ou et al, 2007). Although less commonly applicable in paediatric practice, these advances have made imaging of the coronary arteries by CT a practical alternative to coronary angiography. This technique may, by virtue of its non-invasive nature, have applications in paediatrics, particularly in older children.

Practical considerations

The relatively fast acquisition times compared with cardiac MRI provide a practical alternative to that modality. As a result, cardiac CT can usually be carried out without the need for general anaesthesia, although sedation may still be required. In similarity to cardiac MRI, CT is non-invasive. It is generally quicker than cardiac catheterisation and carries far less radiation exposure for the operator. As an advantage over cardiac catheterisation, cardiac CT allows assessment of not only the lumens of vessels and internal aspects of cardiac chambers, but also their walls.

Angiography and radiology

From Wilhelm Roentgen's discovery of X-rays in 1895 (Roentgen, 1959), they quickly came to be applied in clinical practice. He received the Nobel Prize in Physics in 1901 for his discovery. Fluoroscopy, the production of an X-ray image by projection onto a fluorescent screen, followed shortly afterwards and remains in use today, albeit with many refinements, such as image intensification and the ability to digitally record and play back dynamic images. This real-time imaging of internal structures, importantly the heart and great vessels, has permitted the development of cardiac catheterisation.

Plain chest X-radiographs are extremely useful in answering specific questions about a patient with known cardiac disease, and given the high incidence of the coexistence of cardiac and respiratory disease, they have a firm place in assessing the airways and lungs in 'cardiac patients'. However, they have been largely supplanted by ECG and echocardiography in the initial assessment of children with suspected cardiac disease.

Whilst cardiac catheterisation and angiography was originally a diagnostic modality, in most centres it now plays a mainly interventional role. Given the wealth of information that can now be obtained non-invasively, it is neither desirable nor justifiable to subject patients to the risks of an invasive procedure simply for diagnostic purposes, with some important exceptions. Notably, whilst the alternative methods give excellent information about the geometry of cardiovascular structures (including volume and therefore flow), it is not currently possible to measure pressure non-invasively. Therefore, we still rely upon this invasive technique in the assessment of vascular resistance, especially pulmonary vascular resistance, and in the assessment of the response to a potential intervention (e.g. the test occlusion of PDA or septation defect). Cardiac catheterisation may on occasion be the best way to obtain critical physiological information, for example (left-to-right) shunt size, and influence when deciding whether to close a native or residual lesion (e.g. residual VSD following surgical repair).

Practical applications

Broadly speaking, vascular access can be gained through any vessels, either venous or arterial, that are of sufficient calibre to permit the entry of a cardiac catheter or vascular sheath. For practical purposes, these are most commonly the femoral vessels, although the central neck veins (internal jugular and subclavian) are the second most common site in use. Access through the central veins and arteries allows access to the cardiac chambers and the main vessels to which they are connected. In this way, the pressure can be directly measured from the tip of the catheter positioned in these various sites, by use of an electronic pressure transducer connected to the cardiac catheter. Blood samples can be taken for oximetric readings, and angiographic contrast medium delivered to show dynamic images of the chambers of the heart and the great vessels.

Central venous access permits right heart catheterisation and arterial access left heart catheterisation in subjects with normally connected hearts. However, the most challenging patients in current cardiac practice in childhood are often those with abnormal cardiac connections, and the basis of 'right' or 'left' heart catheterisation does not necessarily apply. Indeed, in the functionally 'univentricular' heart, for practical purposes, there may not be a right or left heart as such. In these cases, note should be taken of which vessels have been entered to optimally provide access to the heart and great vessels. A great deal of diagnostic information is thus generated, although, as mentioned above, cardiac catheterisation nowadays has a chiefly interventional role. This is covered in the following chapter and will not be considered in detail in this section.

Practical limitations and considerations

Vascular injury is the most common significant complication following diagnostic cardiac catheterisation. Whilst the incidence of clinically important injury is relatively low (Vitiello et al, 1998; Ruud et al, 2002), it is more common in arterial than venous catheterisations, and the incidence of arterial problems rises as the age (and therefore weight) of the child falls, with correspondingly smaller arteries. The monitoring of pulses distal to the arterial puncture and the site of vascular entry is a mandatory aspect of aftercare, and whilst many centres will discharge older children with solely venous access on the day of the procedure, children who have experienced an arterial puncture will often be kept in hospital overnight.

Following the procedure, new medications may be required for a period of time. Where a device has been implanted, intravenous antibiotics are routinely administered, both at the time of the implant and typically for one or more doses during aftercare. Other drugs, for example antiplatelet agents such as aspirin, are usually administered for several months after the implantation of an intracardiac device, such as a septal occluder. Trials are currently being undertaken of the role of alternative antiplatelet agents in children, for example clopidogrel (Finkelstein et al, 2005; Li et al, 2008), and these agents may in due course come into routine use following intracardiac device implantation.

Postprocedural investigations are of more relevance to interventional than diagnostic procedures, but when, for example, a device has been implanted, its position and effects will need to be checked using echocardiography or plain radiography. The nature of the intervention will also determine the timing of follow-up after discharge from hospital and must be tailored to the individual patient and procedure.

Summary

In this chapter, we have reviewed the several different ways in which CHD can manifest in the young. It can first come to light antenatally, either as a result of detailed assessment in high-risk pregnancies or as a result of a population screening programme. Postnatally, a diagnosis of CHD may be established following routine newborn examination, and the now widespread use of pulse oximetry has the potential to be a particularly valuable tool in the cardiovascular assessment of the newborn. Babies can also present with symptoms and signs of major CHD in the form of cyanosis, cardiac failure or both. In later life, less acute CHD can present with failure to thrive or the detection of a heart murmur, although most heart murmurs are innocent.

We have also examined the various modalities available for diagnosing and assessing CHD. The development of diagnostic cardiology is proceeding rapidly, as evidenced by the emergence of non-invasive cardiology as a subspecialty in its own right. Diagnostic equipment is continuing to become more technologically refined and safe, with higher resolution. Many conditions that would previously have demanded invasive cardiac investigation can now be assessed non-invasively, and this trend is set to continue. As with many other areas of medicine, the discovery of genetic markers of disease is a developing field with the potential to guide the diagnosis of cardiac disease in selected cases.

References

Advanced Life Support Group (1999). *Pre-hospital paediatric life support*. London: BMJ Publishing Group.

Advanced Paediatric Life Support Group (2005). *The practical approach*. 4th edn. Oxford: Blackwell Publishing.

Allan, L.D., Crawford, D.C., Chita, S.K. & Tynan, M.J. (1986). Prenatal screening for congenital heart disease. *British Medical Journal*, 292, 1717–1719.

Allan, L.D., Sharland, G.K., Milburn, A., Lockhart, S.M., Groves, A.M.M., Anderson, R.H. et al (1994). Prospective diagnosis of 1,006 consecutive cases of congenital heart disease in the fetus. *Journal of the American College of Cardiology*, 23, 1452–1458.

Allan, L., Hornberger, L. & Sharland, G. (2000). *Textbook of fetal cardiology*. London: Medical Media.

Amaral, F. & Granzotti, J. A. (1999). Cardiologic evaluation of children with suspected heart disease: experience of a public outpatient clinic in Brazil. *Sao Paulo Medical Journal*, 117(3), 101–107.

Ambrose, J. & Hounsfield, G. (1973). Computerized transverse axial tomography. *British Journal of Radiology*, 46, 148–149.

Archer, N. & Burch, M. (1998). *Paediatric cardiology: An introduction*. London: Chapman & Hall/ Lippincott-Raven.

Baston, H. & Durward, H. (2001). *Examination of the newborn: A practical guide*. London: Routledge.

Bazett, H.C. (1920). An analysis of the time-relations of electrocardiograms. *Heart*, 7, 353–370.

Bonnet, D., Coltri, A., Butera, G., Fermont, L., Le Bidois, J., Jouvet, P. et al (1999). Fetal detection of transposition of the great arteries reduces morbidity and mortality in newborn infants. *Circulation*, *99*, 916–918.

British Medical Association, Royal Pharmaceutical Society of Great Britain, Royal College of Paediatrics and Child Health, & Neonatal and Paediatric Pharmacists Group (2007). *British National Formulary for Children*. London: Pharmaceutical Press.

Brownell, G.L., Budinger, T.F., Lauterbur, P.C. & McGeer, P.L. (1982). Positron tomography and nuclear magnetic resonance imaging. *Science*, *215*, 619–626.

Bull, C., on behalf of British Paediatric Cardiac Association (1999). Current and potential impact of fetal diagnosis on prevalence and spectrum of serious congenital heart disease at term in the UK. *Lancet*, *354*, 1242–1247.

Carlson, M.D., Wilkoff, B.L., Maisel, W.H., Carlson, M.D., Ellenbogen, K.A., Saxon, L.A. et al (2006). Recommendations from the Heart Rhythm Society Task Force on Device Performance Policies and Guidelines Endorsed by the American College of Cardiology Foundation (ACCF) and the American Heart Association (AHA) and the International Coalition of Pacing and Electrophysiology Organizations (COPE). *Heart Rhythm*, *3*, 1250–1273.

Carpenter, R.J., Strasburger, J.F., Garson, A., Smith, R.T., Deter, R.L. & Engelhardt, H.T. (1986). Fetal ventricular pacing for hydrops secondary to complete atrioventricular block. *Journal of the American College of Cardiology*, *8*, 1434–1436.

Carpentier, A. & Brizard, C. (2006). Malformations of the tricuspid valve and Ebstein's anomaly. In Stark, J.F., de Leval, M.R. & Tsang, V.S., eds. *Surgery for congenital heart defects*: 3rd edn. Basingstoke: John Wiley & Sons.

Carvalho, J.S., Prefumo, F., Ciardelli, V., Sairam, S., Bhide, A. & Shinebourne, E.A. (2007). Evaluation of fetal arrhythmias from simultaneous pulsed wave Doppler in pulmonary artery and vein. *Heart*, *93*, 1448–1453.

Chung, M.K. (2000). Cardiac surgery: postoperative arrhythmias. *Critical Care Medicine*, *28*(10, Suppl.), 136–144.

Copel, J.A., Pilu, G. & Kleinman, C.S. (1986). Congenital heart disease and extracardiac anomalies: associations and indications for fetal echocardiography. *Am J Obstet Gynecol*, *154*, 1121–1132.

Danford, D.A., Martin, A.B., Fletcher, S.E. & Gumbiner, C.H. (2002). Echocardiographic yield in children when innocent murmur seems likely but doubts linger. *Pediatr Cardiol*, *23*, 410–414.

Deal, B.J., Johnsrude, C.L. & Buck, S.H. (2004). *Pediatric ECG interpretation: An illustrated guide*. Massachusetts: Wiley-Blackwell.

Department of Health (2000). *The NHS plan: a plan for investment; a plan for reform*. London: DH.

Department of Health (2008). *The Child Health Promotion programme: Pregnancy and the first five years of life. Update of Standard One of the National Service Framework for Children, Young People and Maternity Services (2004)*. London: DH.

Einthoven, W. (1901). Un nouveau galvanometre. *Archives Néerlandaises des Sciences Exactes et Naturelles*, *6*, 625.

Elzenga, N.J. (2000). The role of echocardiography in transcatheter closure of atrial septal defects. *Cardiology in the Young*, *10*, 474–483.

Fermont. L., De Geeter, B., Aubry, M.C., Kachener, J. & Sidi, D. (1986). A close collaboration between obstetricians and cardiologists allows antenatal detection of severe cardiac malformations by 2D echocardiography [abstract]. In Doyle, E.F., Engle, M.E., Gersony, W.M. et al, eds. *Pediatric cardiology: Proceedings of the Second World Congress of Paediatric Cardiology)*. New York: Springer, pp. 34–37.

Finkelstein, Y., Nurmohamed, L., Avner, M., Benson, L.N. & Koren, G. (2005). Clopidogrel use in children. *Journal of Pediatrics*, *147*, 657–661.

Fouron, J.C., Fournier, A., Proulx, F., Lamarche, J., Bigras, J.L., Boutin, C. et al. (2003). Management of fetal tachycardia based on superior vena cava/aorta Doppler flow recordings. *Heart*, *89*, 1211–1216.

Frohn-Mulder, I.M., Stewart, P.A., Witsenburg, M., Den Hollander, N.S., Wladimiroff, J.W. & Hess, J. (1995). The efficacy of flecainide versus digoxin in the management of fetal supraventricular tachycardia. *Prenatal Diagnosis*, 15, 1297–1302.

Geva, T., Hegesh, J. & Frand, M. (1988). Reappraisal of the approach to the child with heart murmurs: is echocardiography mandatory? *International Journal of Cardiology*, 19, 107–113.

Gill, H.R., Splitt, M., Sharland, G.K. & Simpson, J.M. (2003). Patterns of recurrence of congenital heart disease: an analysis of 6640 consecutive pregnancies evaluated by detailed fetal echocardiography. *Journal of the American College of Cardiology*, 42, 923–929.

Glatz, J.A., Tabbutt, S., Gaynor, J.W., Rome, J.J., Montenegro, L., Spray, T.L. & Rychik, J. (2007). Hypoplastic left heart syndrome with atrial level restriction in the era of prenatal diagnosis. *Annals of Thoracic Surgery*, 84, 1633–1639.

Gottlieb, L.S. (1961). Willem Einthoven, M.D., Ph.D., 1860–1927. Centenary of the father of electrocardiography. *Archives of Internal Medicine*, 107, 447–449.

Gregoratos, G., Abrams, J., Epstein, A.E., Freedman, R.A., Hayes, D.L., Hlatky, M.A. et al (2002). ACC/AHA/NASPE 2002 guideline update for implantation of cardiac pacemakers and antiarrhythmia devices: summary article: a report of the American College of Cardiology/American Heart Association Task Force on Practice Guidelines (ACC/AHA/NASPE Committee to Update the 1998 Pacemaker Guidelines). *Circulation*, 106, 2145–2161.

Groves, A.M.M., Allan, L.D. & Rosenthal, E. (1996). Outcome of isolated congenital complete heart block diagnosed in utero. *Heart*, 75, 190–194.

Hall, D.M.B. (1999). The role of the routine neonatal examination [editorial]. *British Medical Journal*, 3, 19–20.

Hansmann, M., Gembruch, U., Bald, R., Manz, M. & Redal, D.A. (1991). Fetal tachyarrhythmias: transplacental and direct treatment of the fetus – a report of 60 cases. *Ultrasound in Obstetrics and Gynecology*, 1, 62–70.

Heistein, L.C., Ramaciotti, C., Scott, W.A., Coursey, M., Sheeran, P.W. & Lemler, M.S. (2006). Chloral hydrate sedation for pediatric echocardiography: physiologic responses, adverse events, and risk factors. *Pediatrics*, 117, e434–e441.

Heusch, A., Lawrenz, W., Olivier, M. & Schmidt, K.G. (2006). Transesophageal 3-dimensional versus cross-sectional echocardiographic assessment of the volume of the right ventricle in children with atrial septal defects. *Cardiology in the Young*, 16, 135–140.

Hofbeck, M., Ulmer, H., Beinder, E., Sieber, E. & Singer, H. (1997). Prenatal findings in patients with prolonged QT interval in the neonatal period. *Heart*, 77, 198–204.

Hornberger, L.K., Sanders, S.P., Rein, A.J., Spevak, P.J., Parness, I.A. & Colan, S.D. (1995a). Left heart obstructive lesions and left ventricular growth in the midtrimester fetus: a longitudinal study. *Circulation*, 92, 1531–1538.

Hornberger, L.K., Sanders, S.P., Sahn, D.J., Rice, M.J., Spevak, P.J. & Benacerraf, B.R. (1995b). In utero pulmonary artery and aortic growth and potential for progression of pulmonary outflow tract obstruction in tetralogy of Fallot. *Journal of the American College of Cardiology*, 25, 739–745.

Horrax, F. (2002). *Manual of neonatal and paediatric heart disease*. London: Whurr.

Horvath, K.A., Li, M., Mazilu, D., Guttman, M.A. & McVeigh, E.R. (2007). Real-time magnetic resonance imaging guidance for cardiovascular procedures. *Seminars in Thoracic and Cardiovascular Surgery*, 19, 330–335.

Hyett, J., Perdu, M., Sharland, G., Snijders, R. & Nicolaides, K. (1999). Using fetal nuchal translucency to screen for major congenital cardiac defects at 10–14 weeks of gestation: population based cohort study. *British Medical Journal*, 318, 81–85.

Jaeggi, E.T., Fouron, F.C., Fournier, A., van Doesburg, N., Drblik, S.P. & Proulx, F. (1998). Ventriculo-atrial time interval measured on M-mode echocardiography: a determining element in diagnosis, treatment and prognosis of fetal supraventricular tachycardia. *Heart*, 79, 582–587.

Jaeggi, E.T., Fouron, J.C., Silverman, E.D., Ryan, G., Smallhorn, J. & Hornberger, L.K. (2004). Transplacental fetal treatment improves the outcome of parentally diagnosed complete atrioventricular block without structural heart disease. *Circulation, 110,* 1542–1548.

Jaeggi, E.T., Hornberger, L.K., Smallhorn, J.F. & Fouron, J.C. (2005). Prenatal diagnosis of complete atrioventricular block associated with structural heart disease: combined experience of two tertiary centres ad review of the literature. *Ultrasound in Obstetrics and Gynecology, 26,* 16–21.

Jewkes, F. (2001). Prehospital emergency care for children. *Archives of Disease in Childhood, 84,* 103–105.

Jewkes, F. (2006). Prehospital management of the acutely ill child. *Archives of Disease in Childhood, 91,* 462–464.

Kapusta, L., Thijssen, J.M., Groot-Loonen, J., van Druten, J.A. & Daniels, O. (2001). Discriminative ability of conventional echocardiography and tissue Doppler imaging techniques for the detection of subclinical cardiotoxic effects of treatment with anthracyclines. *Ultrasound in Medicine and Biology, 27,* 1605–1614.

Kirk, J.S., Riggs, T.W., Comstock, C.H., Lee, W., Yang, S.S. & Weinhouse, E. (1994). Prenatal screening for cardiac anomalies: the value of routine addition of the aortic root to the four chamber view. *Obstetrics and Gynecology, 84,* 427–431.

Knilans, T.K. (1995). Cardiac abnormalities associated with hydrops fetalis. *Seminars in Perinatology, 19,* 483–492.

Ko, J.K., Ban, J.E., Kim, Y.H. & Park, I.S. (2004). Long-term efficacy of atenolol for atrioventricular reciprocating tachycardia in children less than 5 years old. *Pediatric Cardiology, 25,* 97–101.

Kohl, T., Sharland, G., Allan, L.D., Gembruch, U., Chaoui, R., Lopes, L.M. et al. (2000). World experience of percutaneous ultrasound guided balloon valvuloplasty in human fetuses with severe aortic valve obstruction. *American Journal of Cardiology, 85,* 1230–1233.

Krapp, M., Kohl, T., Simpson, J.M., Sharland, G.K., Katalinic, A & Gembruch, U. (2003). Review of diagnosis, treatment, and outcome of fetal atrial flutter compared with supraventricular tachycardia. *Heart, 89,* 913–917.

Lee, C. & Mason, L.J. (2001). Paediatric cardiac emergencies. *Anesthesiology Clinics of North America, 19,* 287–308.

Li, J.S., Yow, E., Berezny, K.Y., Bokesch, P.M., Takahashi, M., Graham, T.P. Jr., et al (2008). Dosing of clopidogrel for platelet inhibition in infants and young children: primary results of the Platelet Inhibition in Children On cLOpidogrel (PICOLO) trial. *Circulation, 117,* 553–559.

Lindstrom, K. (1991). Carl Hellmuth Hertz. *Ultrasound in Medicine and Biology, 17,* 421–424.

Machado, M.V., Tynan, M.J., Curry, P.V. & Allan, L.D. (1988). Fetal complete heart block. *British Heart Journal, 60,* 512–515.

Marshall, A.C., van der Velde M.E., Tworetzky, W., Gomez, C.A., Wilkins-Haug, L., Benson, C.B. et al. (2004). Creation of an atrial septal defect in utero for fetuses with hypoplastic left heart syndrome and intact or highly restrictive atrial septum. *Circulation, 110,* 253–8.

Marshall, A.C., Tworetzky, W., Bergersen, L., McElhinney, D.B., Benson, C.B., Jennings, R.W. et al (2005). Aortic valvuloplasty in the fetus: technical characteristics of successful balloon dilation. *Journal of Pediatrics, 147,* 535–539.

Matsui, H. & Gardiner, H. (2007). Fetal cardiac intervention: the cutting edge of perinatal care. *Seminars in Fetal and Neonatal Medicine, 12,* 482–489.

Maxwell, D., Crawford, D., Curry, P., Tynan, M. & Allan, L. (1988). Obstetric importance, diagnosis, and management of fetal tachycardias. *British Medical Journal, 297,* 107–110.

Maxwell, D., Allan, L. & Tynan, M.J. (1991). Balloon dilatation of the aortic valve in the fetus: a report of two cases. *British Heart Journal, 65,* 256–258.

Medforth, J., Battersby, S., Evans, M., Marsh, B. & Walker, A. (2006) *Oxford handbook of midwifery.* Oxford: Oxford University Press.

Mehta, C. & Dhillon, R. (2004). Understanding paediatric ECGs. *Current Paediatrics*, 14, 229–236.

Meyers-Wittkopf, M., Simpson, J.M. & Sharland, G.K. (1996). Incidence of congenital heart disease in fetuses of diabetic mothers - a retrospective study of 326 cases. *Ultrasound in Obstetrics and Gynecology*, 8, 8–10.

National Health Service Quality Improvement Scotland (2008). *Best practice statement* [online]. Available at: http://www.nhshealthquality.org/nhsqis

National Institute for Health and Clinical Excellence (2006a). *Percutaneous fetal balloon valvuloplasty for aortic stenosis*. London: NICE.

National Institute for Health and Clinical Excellence (2006b). *Routine care of women and their babies*. London: NICE.

Newburger, J.W., Rosenthal, A., Williams, R.G., Fellows, K. & Miettinen, O.S. (1983). Noninvasive tests in the initial evaluation of heart murmurs in children. *New England Journal of Medicine, 308*, 61–64.

Nursing and Midwifery Council (2004) *Midwives rules and standards*. London: NMC.

Ochsenschlager, D., Atabaki, S., Holder, M.G. (2005). Could it be cardiac? *Clinical Pediatric Emergency Medicine, 6*, 229–233.

Ou, P., Celermajer, D.S., Calcagni, G., Brunelle, F., Bonnet, D. & Sidi, D. (2007). Three-dimensional CT scanning: a new diagnostic modality in congenital heart disease. *Heart, 93*, 908–913.

Oudijk, M.A., Michon, M.M., Kleinman, C.S., Kapusta, L., Stoutenbeek, P., Visser, G.H. A. & Meijboom, E.J. (2000). Sotalol in the treatment of fetal dysrhythmias. *Circulation, 101*, 2721–2726.

Pandya, P.P., Snijders, R.J.M., Johnson, S.P., De Lourdes Brizot, M. & Nicolaides, K.H. (1995). Screening for fetal trisomies by maternal age and fetal nuchal translucency thickness at 10–14 weeks of gestation. *British Journal of Obstetrics and Gynaecology, 102*, 957–962.

Park, M.K. & Guntheroth, W.G. (2006). *How to read pediatric ECGs*. Mosby/Elsevier.

Paul, T., Bertram, H., Bokenkamp, R. & Hausdorf, G. (2000). Supraventricular tachycardia in infants, children and adolescents: diagnosis, and pharmacological and interventional therapy. *Paediatric Drugs, 2*, 171–181.

Pitetti, R., Glustein J.Z. & Bhende M.S. (2002). Prehospital care and outcome of paediatric out of hospital cardiac arrest. *Prehospital Emergency Care, 6*, 283–290.

Rabi, I. I. (1948). The atomic nucleus: a new world to conquer. *Science, 108*, 673–675.

Rijnbeek, P.R., Witsenburg, M., Schrama, E., Hess, J. & Kors, J.A. (2001). New normal limits for the paediatric electrocardiogram. *European Heart Journal, 22*, 702–711.

Roelandt, J., Kloster, F.E., ten Cate, F. J., van Dorp, W.G., Honkoop, J., Bom, N. & Hugenholtz, P.G. (1974). Multidimensional echocardiography. An appraisal of its clinical usefulness. *British Heart Journal, 36*, 29–43.

Roentgen, W.C. (1959). [On a new kind of ray (first report).] *Münchener medizinische Wochenschrift, 101*, 1237–1239.

Rosenthal, E., Gordon, P.A., Simpson, J.M. & Sharland, G.K. (2005). Letter regarding article by Jaeggi et al 'Transplacental fetal treatment improves the outcome of parentally diagnosed complete atrio-ventricular block without structural heart disease'. *Circulation, 111*, e287–e288.

Ruud, E., Natvig, S., Holmstrom, H. & Wesenberg, F. (2002). Low prevalence of femoral venous thrombosis after cardiac catheterizations in children: a prospective study. *Cardiology in the Young, 12*, 513–518.

Sarubbi, B., Musto, B., Ducceschi, V., D'Onofrio, A., Cavallaro, C., Vecchione, F. et al (2002). Congenital junctional ectopic tachycardia in children and adolescents: a 20 year experience based study. *Heart, 88*, 188–190.

Schindler, M.B., Bohn, D., Cox, P., McCrindle, B.W., Jarvis, A., Edmonds, J. & Barker, G. (1996). Outcome of out of hospital cardiac or respiratory arrest in children. *New England Journal of Medicine, 335*, 1473–1479.

Sharieff, G.Q. & Wylie, T.W. (2003) Paediatric cardiac disorders. *Journal of Emergency Medicine, 26*, 65–79.

Sharland, G. (2001). Fetal cardiology. *Seminars in Neonatology*, 6, 3–15.

Sharland, G.K. & Allan, L.D. (1992). Screening for congenital heart disease prenatally. Results of a 2½ year study in the South East Thames Region. *British Journal of Obstetrics and Gynaecology*, 99, 220–225.

Sharland, G.K., Chita, S.K., Fagg, N., Anderson, R.H., Tynan, M., Cook, A.C. et al (1991). Left ventricular dysfunction in the fetus: relation to aortic valve anomalies and endocardial fibroelastosis. *British Heart Journal*, 66, 219–224.

Simpson, J.M. & Sharland, G.K. (1997). The natural history and outcome of aortic stenosis diagnosed prenatally. *Heart*, 77, 205–210.

Simpson, J. & Sharland, G.K. (1998). Fetal tachyarrhythmias: management and outcome of 127 cases. *Heart*, 79, 576–581.

Simpson, J.M., Yates, R.W. & Sharland, G.K. (1996). Irregular heart rate in the fetus – not always benign. *Cardiology in the Young*, 6, 28–31.

Skoll, M.A., Sharland, G.K. & Allan, L.D. (1991). Is the ultrasound definition of fluid collections in non-immune hydrops fetalis helpful in defining the underlying cause or predicting outcome? *Ultrasound in Obstetrics and Gynecology*, 1, 309–311.

Smythe, J.F., Teixeira, O.H., Vlad, P., Demers, P.P. & Feldman, W. (1990). Initial evaluation of heart murmurs: are laboratory tests necessary? *Pediatrics*, 86, 497–500.

Stasik, C.N., Goldberg, C.S., Bove, E.L., Devaney, E.J. & Ohye, R.G. (2006). Current outcomes and risk factors for the Norwood procedure. *Journal of Thoracic and Cardiovascular Surgery*, 131, 412–417.

Stumper, O., Kaulitz, R., Elzenga, N.J., Bom, N., Roelandt, J.R., Hess, J. & Sutherland, G. R. (1991). The value of transesophageal echocardiography in children with congenital heart disease. *Journal of the American Society of Echocardiography*, 4, 164–176.

Tappero, E.P. & Honeyfield, M.E. (2003). Physical assessment of the newborn – a comprehensive approach to the art of physical examination 3rd edn. California: NICU Ink.

Tegnander, E., Eik-Nes, S.H., Johansen, O.J. & Linker, D.T. (1995). Prenatal detection of heart defects at the routine fetal examination at 18 weeks in a non-selected population. *Ultrasound in Obstetrics and Gynecology*, 5, 372–380.

Tulzer, G., Arzt, W., Franklin, R.C.G., Loughna, P.V., Mair, R. & Gardiner, H.M. (2002). Fetal pulmonary valvoplasty for critical pulmonary stenosis or atresia with intact septum. *Lancet*, 360, 1567–1568.

UK National Screening Committee (2008). *Newborn and infant physical examination – standards and competencies*. London: UK National Screening Committee.

Van Engelen, A.D., Weijtens, O., Brenner, J.I., Kleinman, C.S., Copel, J.A., Stoutenbeek, P. et al. (1994). Management, outcome and follow-up of fetal tachycardia. *Journal of the American College of Cardiology*, 24, 1371–1375.

Vida, V.L., Bacha, E.A., Larrazabel, A., Gauvreau, K., Thiagaragan, R., Fynn-Thompson, F. et al. (2007). Hypoplastic left heart syndrome with intact or highly restrictive atrial septum: surgical experience from a single centre. *Annals of Thoracic Surgery*, 84, 581–586.

Vitiello, R., McCrindle, B.W., Nykanen, D., Freedom, R.M. & Benson, L.N. (1998). Complications associated with pediatric cardiac catheterization. *Journal of the American College of Cardiology*, 32, 1433–1440.

Wakai, R.T., Strasburger, J.F., Li, Z, Deal, B.J, & Gotteiner, N.L. (2003). Magnetocardiographic rhythm patterns at initiation and termination of fetal supraventricular tachycardia. *Circulation*, 107, 307–312.

Walsh, E.P., Saul, J.P. & Triedman, J.K. (2001). *Cardiac arrhythmias in the pediatric patient*. Philadelphia: Lippincott Williams & Wilkins.

Watts, C. (2003). Cardiac screening and the advanced neonatal nurse practitioner: a review of the literature. *Journal of Neonatal Nursing*, 5, 29–34.

Wigton, T.R., Sabbagha, R.E., Tamura, R.K., Cohen, L., Minogue, J.P. & Strasberger, J.F. (1993). Sonographic diagnosis of congenital heart disease: comparison between the four-chamber view and multiple cardiac views. *Obstetrics and Gynecology*, 82, 219–224.

Wolfe, L.T., Rossi, A. & Ritter, S.B. (1993). Transesophageal echocardiography in infants and children: use and importance in the cardiac intensive care unit. *Journal of the American Society of Echocardiography*, 6(3, Pt 1), 286–289.

Wren, C. (1998). Mechanisms of fetal tachycardia. *Heart*, 79, 536–537.

Wren, C., Reinhardt, Z. & Khawaja, K. (2008). Twenty-year trends in diagnosis of life threatening neonatal cardiovascular malformations. *Archives of Disease in Childhood Fetal and Neonatal Edition*, 93, F33–F35.

Yi, M.S., Kimball, T.R., Tsevat, J., Mrus, J.M. & Kotagal, U.R. (2002). Evaluation of heart murmurs in children: cost-effectiveness and practical implications. *Journal of Pediatrics*, 141, 504–511.

Yildirim, S.V., Guc, B.U., Bozdogan, N. & Tokel, K. (2006). Oral versus intranasal midazolam premedication for infants during echocardiographic study. *Advances in Therapy*, 23, 719–724.

Zeigler, V.L. & Gillette, P.C. (2001). *Practical management of pediatric cardiac arrhythmias*. Armonk, NY: Futura.

Websites

Alan E. Lindsay ECG Learning Centre: http://library.med.utah.edu/kw/ecg/image_index/index.html

An Electronic Journal of Cardiac Ultrasound, University of Medicine and Dentistry of New Jersey, Robert Wood Johnson Medical School: http://www2.umdnj.edu/~shindler/index.html

Child Health Promotion Programme: http://www.dh.gov.uk/en/Healthcare/NationalServiceFrameworks/Children/DH_4089111

ECG Library: http://www.ecglibrary.com/ecghome.html

Echo-web (sample fetal echocardiography images): http://www.echo-web.com/asp/samples/sample2.asp

Fetal Echocardiography Library of Images, School of Medicine, University of Pennsylvania: http://www.med.upenn.edu/fetus/

National Child Measurement Programme: http://www.dh.gov.uk/prod_consum_dh/groups/dh_digitalassets/@dh/documents/digitalasset/dh_086725.pdf

Online encyclopaedia of medical images: http://www.images.md/users/explore_chapter.asp?ID=AHD1601%2D06&colID=AHD1601&coltitle=Echocardiography

Paediatric electrocardiogram of the week: http://www.paedcard.com/

School checks: http://www.nhs.uk/Livewell/Screening/Pages/Checkschildhood.aspx

3 Treatment options/management

Tim Jones, Kerry Cook, Richard Crook, Rami Dhillon, Catherine Dunne, Rebecca Hill, Melanie Linzell, Jimmy Montgomerie, Anne Maree Robinson, Douglas Wall

Fifty years ago, there were very few if any treatment options for children born with congenital cardiac problems. The initial attempts at operating on the heart in the 1950s using mechanical circulatory support were initially for the treatment of septal defects. Techniques such as topical hypothermia and cross-circulation, during which the child was supported by the parent's circulation via the parent's femoral vessels, enabled a better understanding of intracardiac anatomy. With the advent of cardiopulmonary bypass (CPB), cardiac surgery became a reality. Improvements in preoperative imaging and our understanding of cardiac morphology, coupled with improved surgical techniques and postoperative support, have made the treatment of complex conditions in neonates possible. Operative mortality has fallen from 90% to 4%. Recent advances in catheter technology and material engineering have enabled the development of interventional cardiology, initially as a diagnostic tool but now as a treatment option for many congenital cardiac conditions. Increasingly, combined approaches using surgery and catheter-based interventions are being used.

The treatment of children and adults with congenital heart disease is frequently complex, and success relies upon an integrated team approach incorporating many disciplines and specialties. For many children and families, it is the beginning of a pathway of care, and the relationship between the clinical team and the patient will be lifelong. The aim of treatment is complete repair, but this may not be possible and palliation via medicine, catheter intervention or surgery may be required.

Admission and preoperative preparation

Orientation to the unit

Admission to hospital has long been recognised as a stressful experience for all family members involved (Hogg & Cooper, 2004; Tromp et al, 2004; Smith & Callery, 2005). This feeling may be ameliorated or aggravated by previous experiences. The position of the family and child along their patient journey can influence the family's coping mechanisms (Spijkerboer et al, 2007). It cannot be assumed that what healthcare professions may see as a routine, lower-risk procedure will necessarily be viewed by the child and family as less stressful. Any surgery, especially that involving the heart, with all the social and emotional significance attached, elicits a stress response (Utens et al, 2001; Wray & Sensky, 2004).

Ensuring that the child and family are introduced to staff and shown around the ward aids the coping process (Hogg & Cooper, 2004; Smith & Callery, 2005). In

> **Box 3.1** Beth's healthcare journey – her parents' experiences following arrival at the cardiac ward
>
> We arrived at the cardiac ward at the children's hospital. It was very scary, and became even more scary when the doctor who had told the GP to send us there had an argument with another doctor who said they were too busy for us. This made me very anxious. But he stood his ground and he became a very big part of Beth's life from that moment. The doctor told us he never turned a child away, especially one with the results he had been told Beth had.
>
> He took us into what is called an echo room and started to do an echocardiogram on Beth. She kept crying, and it took a further 2 hours of perseverance from both him and her before he told us what was wrong. He asked us both to sit down, and then told us Beth had Fallot's tetralogy and she was going to need surgery very soon as her pulmonary artery was already very narrowed. I was speechless, but my husband soon broke the silence as he dropped to the floor in a heap. Beth didn't have to stay in hospital as her body was coping at the moment, but we went back every week for the next 8 weeks, having tests and echos every time.

this way, the ward becomes less of an alien environment. This also holds true for the rest of the hospital, such as the intensive care unit (ICU) if applicable and departments for any necessary investigations, such as the X-ray department (Tromp et al, 2004).

For most families, admission to hospital, for whatever time period, involves organisation. Time off work, child care, finances and transport all need to be addressed (Forister & Blessing, 2002). The potential for planned admissions to be cancelled can also be an added stressor (Utens et al, 2000; Hogg & Cooper, 2004), with families often having to contact the ward either the night before or even on the morning of planned admission to confirm bed availability. The availability of a ward bed does not guarantee that the procedure will not be cancelled. In cases of emergency admissions, this organisation is often on a short-term basis, with these issues having to be read-dressed once the family has been able to gather a better understanding of the situation (Box 3.1).

Preoperative clinic

In many units, patients and families are invited to attend a preoperative clinic. The purpose of the clinic varies between units, but it provides a time when the family can meet with the surgeon to discuss the risks and benefits of surgery and raise questions and concerns. Such a meeting ahead of the planned admission gives the family time to assimilate and reflect on the information discussed. In addition, it provides an opportunity to meet with liaison staff and other members of the team and to visit the wards and paediatric ICU prior to admission. With older children, it gives the team an opportunity to understand the child's perception of the forthcoming surgery and involve play therapists or other specialists as required. If immediately preceding admission, the visit may also be used as a time to repeat investigations such as an electrocardiogram (ECG), chest X-ray and blood tests.

Nursing assessment and preparation

This is the opportunity not only to ensure that the nursing staff have accurate data about the child and family, including contact details and what is 'normal' for that child, but also to build the nurse–child/family relationship (Wilmot, 2007). Integral to this process is the preparation of the child and family for the procedure for which they have been admitted (Hogg & Cooper, 2004). This becomes particularly important when the family have not been able to access a preadmission programme (Tromp et al, 2004).

A major factor of this aspect of the patient's journey is the psychological preparation of both the child and family. Whilst it can be seen as the parents' responsibility to tell their child about the planned hospital admission, they may need help in finding age-appropriate ways of doing this (Hogg & Cooper, 2004; Chessa et al, 2005; Smith & Callery, 2005). Although this is a responsibility of all the team members, play specialists have a particularly important role here and are trained especially for this aspect of care, using a variety of methods to aid the child's assimilation of events (Weaver & Groves, 2007; Wilmot, 2007). They are also seen as a friendly face not associated with anything that hurts!

It is also at this time that pain scores can be introduced and reassurances given that pain will be minimised as much as is possible. Devices such as patient-controlled analgesia pumps can also be explained so that the child and family have an idea of what to expect after the operation and be able to use them more appropriately, optimising effectiveness. Introduction to the pain team may be applicable.

Investigations

The specific investigations that are chosen will differ from unit to unit, between consultant teams and from patient to patient. The investigations are used as an assessment of the patient's current health status and as an aid to decision-making regarding future plans for treatment (Forister & Blessing, 2002). It cannot be assumed that the child or family knows what the investigations are or why they are being done (Jolley, 2007). To ensure informed consent for these procedures, their understanding needs to be ascertained and any necessary information given (National Institute for Health and Clinical Excellence [NICE], 2003; Royal College of Nursing, 2005).

Most patients undergo investigations involving a chest X-ray, ECG, echocardiogram and blood samples (full blood count, urea & electrolytes, clotting, and a group & save or crossmatch) (NICE, 2003). At the time of bloods being taken, an intravenous cannula may be placed. Whilst this may be seen as potentially increasing the infection risk for the patient (Tagalakis et al, 2002), it allows for the child to have to undergo the often distressing venepuncture experience hopefully only once preoperatively. This also allows for intravenous fluids to be given preoperatively if necessary.

All females who are post menarche need to be assessed for the possibility of pregnancy, not only before the procedure but also prior to any necessary X-rays (Kempen, 1997; NICE, 2003). This is a potentially emotive subject and highlights the need for effective communication between the different team members, to limit the number of times this issue needs to be addressed by the child and family.

A more recent addition to the preoperative battery of tests is routinely taking nasal swabs for the screening of meticillin-resistant *Staphylococcus aureus* (MRSA) and other bacteria (Department of Health [DH], 2006). MRSA infections have been on the increase and have been shown to be potentially fatal if introduced into an open wound, and at the very least delay healing (Chief Medical Officer, 2003). Recent policies now consider stopping known MRSA-positive patients from having their elective surgery until they have been treated for the infection and a series of negative swabs has been obtained (DH, 2006).

Whilst the blood test is perhaps seen as the most distressing of the investigations, any of these experiences can be upsetting to the child, family and staff, particularly if the child is uncooperative (Hogg & Cooper, 2004; Wilmot, 2007). Ensuring that the procedure is explained to both family and child in an age-appropriate manner can facilitate this process, helping to decrease the fear of the unknown and enabling consent for the procedure to be gained from the child (Weaver & Groves, 2007).

History-taking and examination

This is essential to ensure that an accurate, up-to-date assessment is made of the child's health and wellbeing, giving a baseline from which to compare future assessments and the effects of any interventions undertaken (Forister & Blessing, 2002).

Although the main body of history-taking and examination is usually undertaken by the nurse practitioner or doctor, the nursing assessment and review by the anaesthetist also contributes to the overall picture. Families have found it easier if repetition of questions is limited. Therefore communication between professionals and accurate record-keeping are vital to improve the child and family's experience (Tromp et al, 2004). The use of a checklist may help to avoid duplication of questions (Hogg & Cooper, 2004; Tromp et al, 2004). This interaction also allows the family another opportunity to ask any further questions they may have.

Consent

Informed consent is required before any procedure can be undertaken (Nursing and Midwifery Council, 2004; Alderson & Goodey, 1998). Depending on the age and competency of the child, this consent may be obtained from the child or from the parents. It is imperative that all are aware of who has the legal responsibility for the child as, with intricate family dynamics, this is not always apparent (Forister & Blessing, 2002). Consent for the procedure should be obtained by the person undertaking the procedure or by a person who fully understands the procedure and the risks involved (Forister & Blessing, 2002).

In providing as much information about the risks and benefits, as well as the technical details, of the procedure, the family can then make an informed decision that they feel is right for them. Whether consent is obtained in a planned or an emergency situation, it has been shown that parents feel happy with their decision-making if they feel fully informed (Hoehn et al, 2004).

Anaesthetics and fasting

Guidelines for fasting have been around for many years, but these are not always strictly adhered to (Crenshaw & Winslow, 2002) and will often depend on the unit or anaesthetist involved. Usually, it is advised that the child has his or her last solids 6 hours prior to the procedure, breastfeeds 4 hours before and has last clear fluids 2 hours before the procedure (Crenshaw & Winslow, 2002; RCN, 2005). Care needs to be taken if the predicted time of the procedure changes, with the potential need to commence intravenous fluids to ensure the child is kept adequately hydrated. This is especially important in those children who are cyanotic and polycythaemic or have a shunt-dependent circulation.

The time when the family see the anaesthetist is also when the child's position on the procedure list is often confirmed, and when the option for a premedication is discussed, as is whether a parent wishes to accompany the child into the anaesthetic room.

Undergoing the procedure

Trying to minimise the time between leaving the ward and going into the anaesthetic room may lessen the stress of the situation as it allows less time for the child and family to be in a state of elevated anxiety – waiting for the procedure and in another strange environment, often with less in the way of distraction than on the ward, especially if they are not in a dedicated children's hospital or unit (Hogg & Cooper, 2004).

Ensuring that the ward has contact details for the parents and that the parents know when they need to be back on the ward helps parents to feel confident that they know what is going on at all times, as well as ensuring that staff can contact the parents if they are needed (Hogg & Cooper, 2004).

Medical/interventional treatment options

Whilst there have been many important therapeutic advances in the field of paediatric cardiac services in recent years, in common with other specialties, many time-honoured therapeutic traditions remain. In this section, we will examine the long-established therapies and those more recently established, as well as previewing some of those with future potential, such as stem cell therapy, currently a topic of considerable interest and research (Schenke-Layland et al, 2008), and newer agents that hold promise in the treatment of heart failure and pulmonary hypertension (Steiropoulos et al, 2008).

Medical therapy

The commonly used medicines in paediatric cardiac practice can conveniently be divided into four major groups:

1. therapies for cardiac failure and systemic hypertension;
2. anticoagulants and antiplatelet agents;
3. pulmonary vasodilators;
4. antiarrhythmics.

The latter group, antiarrhythmics, are considered in some detail in the next section and will not be further considered here.

Therapies for cardiac failure and systemic hypertension

Cardiac failure is the description of a condition in which the function of the heart and circulation is inadequate to meet the metabolic demands of the body's organs and tissues. This broad definition has led some authors to suggest that all children with congenital heart disease that is anything more than 'minor' have a degree of cardiac failure. In practice, cardiac failure in paediatric terms is generally different from that seen in adults and usually describes one or both of two basic pathophysiologies. In cardiac failure arising from either or both of these mechanisms, the child will present with symptoms that usually include breathlessness, poor feeding and sweatiness. In chronic cases, there will be failure to thrive. Easily audible heart murmurs are frequently, but not always, present. There may be a gallop rhythm. Usually, there is hepatic enlargement and the child exhibits increased work of breathing.

The first and most common mechanism of cardiac failure in childhood is pulmonary overcirculation as the result of a large 'left-to-right' shunt between the systemic and pulmonary circulations. A large ventricular septal defect (VSD) or large patent ductus arteriosus (PDA) is a good example. The second pathophysiological mechanism, which may coexist with the first or occur in isolation, is that of impaired pump function of the heart. This is sometimes simplistically described as impaired ventricular function, but it should be remembered that there are many elements that add up to efficient pump function, including systolic and diastolic ventricular function, ventricle–ventricle interaction and atrioventricular transport. These elements are in turn very dependent on changes in preload and afterload on the heart (Suga et al, 1985).

Therapies aimed against systemic hypertension are purposefully included in this section as it has been well demonstrated that in cardiac failure, particularly of the pump failure type, there may be an adverse increase in vasoconstriction, sodium and fluid retention and sympathetic drive (Esler & Kaye, 2000). Hence, therapies that have been used in the treatment of systemic hypertension have also found a place in the treatment of cardiac failure, namely diuretics, angiotensin-converting enzyme inhibitors (ACEIs), beta-blockers and the up-and-coming treatment angiotensin receptor blockers (ARBs) (Ram, 2008).

Diuretics

These are the most widely prescribed medicines in paediatric cardiac practice. The most commonly used substances among them are furosemide (frusemide), amiloride, chlorothiazide and spironolactone. Metolazone, bumetanide and ethacrynic acid are less commonly used. These agents are of great utility in cardiac failure of all types. Their frequency of administration varies. Furosemide has a duration of action of about 6 hours and is therefore used 1–4 times daily. Amiloride, chlorothiazide and spironolactone are usually used once or twice daily. Metolazone, when used, is usually administered once daily. These agents promote a diuresis by increasing the renal excretion of solutes. They thus reduce total body sodium and water, but conversely there is a risk of dehydration, hypovolaemia and significant electrolyte depletion. There have been concerns about a risk of nephrocalcinosis in young, particularly premature, infants treated with furosemide (Hoppe et al, 2002). There is some evidence that spironolactone inhibits cardiac fibrosis (Orea-Tejeda et al, 2007).

Digoxin

Digoxin is a derivative of digitalis, the foxglove (family Plantaginaceae, about 20 different species). The use of extract of digitalis in the treatment of 'dropsy' (heart failure) was first described by William Withering in 1785 (Rahimtoola, 1975). It is a cardiac

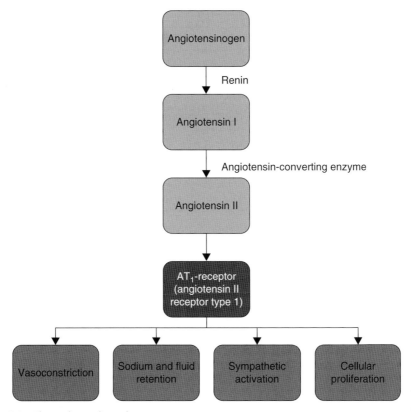

Figure 3.1 The renin–angiotensin system

glycoside and has antiarrhythmic properties as well as having some positive inotropic function. Whilst not as widely used today as it once was, it still has a place in the treatment of cardiac failure, particularly that related to pump impairment. It has a relatively narrow therapeutic window, and its proarrhythmic effects in overdosage are well described. Most practitioners do not routinely measure blood digoxin levels in patients on standard doses who have normal renal function, unless there are additional factors such as the concomitant use of other antiarrhythmics or agents known to affect the bioavailability of digoxin (Staneva-Stoytcheva & Kristeva, 1991; Magro et al, 2008).

ACEIs and ARBs
Via the renin–angiotensin system (Figure 3.1), angiotensinogen is converted to angiotensin II (A2), a powerful vasoconstrictor, also responsible for sodium and fluid retention, increased sympathetic stimulation and vascular cellular proliferation (Heeneman et al, 2007). By reducing the production of A2 or blocking its receptors, ACEIs and ARBs respectively mitigate these influences. At present, there are no published studies of the safety and efficacy of ARBs in cardiac failure in children, and their benefit must at this point be regarded as theoretical. However, the use of ACEIs is well established in paediatric cardiac practice.

As systemic vasodilators, ACEIs are associated with hypotension, and indeed that is part of their anticipated effect. Nevertheless, they must be commenced with caution,

Table 3.1 Properties of commonly used beta-blockers

Beta-blocker	Aqueous solubility	Cardioselectivity	Application
Propranolol	–	–	Antihypertensive Antiarrhythmic Relief of outflow tract obstruction
Atenolol	+	+	Antihypertensive Antiarrhythmic
Nadolol	+	–	Antiarrhythmic
Sotalol	+	–	Antiarrhythmic
Esmolol	–	+	Antiarrhythmic Antihypertensive
Carvedilol	–	Mixed alpha-1-/ beta-blocker	Heart failure
Metoprolol	–	+	Heart failure (adults)
Bisoprolol	–	+	Heart failure (adults)

and it is usual for a small test dose of captopril, which has a relatively short half-life of about 2 hours, to be administered after baseline measurement of blood pressure and heart rate, and for those measures to be repeated half hourly for at least 2 hours after the test dose. Provided the test dose is well tolerated, with no significant symptoms and an acceptable fall in blood pressure, maintenance ACEIs can be initiated. Which ACEI is commenced depends largely on the age of the child, with captopril being favoured for infants and preschool children. It is usually administered three times daily. Lisinopril may be used in school-age children and has the benefit of being required just once daily, best given at bedtime. Whichever ACEI is employed, all have the potential for renal impairment, and it is advisable to check biochemical renal function before the commencement of therapy and about 1–2 weeks after treatment has been established.

Beta-blockers

These agents have a wide range of uses within the practice of paediatric cardiology. In addition to their use as antihypertensives, they have antiarrhythmic properties, of use in both supraventricular and ventricular tachycardias. Propranolol in particular has also been used to relieve the incidence and severity of both right and left ventricular outflow tract obstruction in, for example, tetralogy of Fallot (Garson et al, 1981) and hypertrophic cardiomyopathy (Cabrera-Bueno et al, 2007) respectively. The use of beta-blockers in the treatment of cardiac failure is a relatively new application in paediatric practice, although it was introduced some time earlier in adult practice. The agent most commonly used in this context is carvedilol, which has systemic vasodilatory properties (Bristow, 1998).

In choosing which beta-blocker is most appropriate for a given application, there are several factors that need to be taken into consideration (Table 3.1):

- the availability of a preparation in a particular form for ease of administration, for example suspension or syrup;
- lipid solubility versus water solubility: central nervous system adverse effects (hallucinations, insomnia, nightmares and depression) are more common for agents with greater lipid solubility, which are more readily able to cross the blood–brain barrier;
- cardioselectivity: different agents have variable degrees of beta-2-antagonism. This will have a significant impact on whether a particular beta-blocker is tolerated by

the patient, given the significant incidence and prevalence of asthma in childhood;

■ additional effects, particularly anti/proarrhythmicity. For example, sotalol, as well as being a beta-blocker, has type 3 antiarrhythmic properties;

■ half-life: in many cases, for example for nadolol and atenolol, once-daily preparations are available.

Oral inotropes

Aside from digoxin, these are new arrivals on the therapeutic scene, and at present the only agent used in this context with any regularity is enoximone, a phosphodiesterase inhibitor (Vernon et al, 1991). There are no randomised or controlled studies of its use, and it has been applied in patients with moderate-to-severe impairment of ventricular function, often in patients referred for cardiac transplant assessment. Descriptive studies of its use are in progress, but it will be difficult to draw hard scientific conclusions from these, given the 'rescue' format applied to the use of enoximone and the lack of a control group. In these instances, the intravenous preparation of enoximone is administered orally. It has a rather unpleasant taste, which hampers its tolerability, as does the fact that large volumes are sometimes required.

Anticoagulants and antiplatelet agents

The ability to prevent thrombosis is essential in our daily practice, particularly given the regular use of thrombogenic foreign materials in cardiac surgery and interventional cardiology. These include Gore-tex systemic–pulmonary (e.g. Blalock–Taussig) shunts, prosthetic heart valves, right ventricle–pulmonary artery conduits, extracardiac Fontan conduits, patch material used in pulmonary artery reconstruction, intracardiac occlusive devices and intravascular/intracardiac stents. In addition to these applications is the need to prevent thrombosis in individuals who have demonstrated a tendency towards it, for example those with inherited or acquired prothrombotic tendencies such as protein C or protein S deficiency, or those with previous thrombosis. Furthermore, there are patient groups in which there may be an anatomical substrate for thrombosis (and in which the consequences could be very adverse), for example Kawasaki disease with coronary artery aneurysms.

Warfarin

This is the most commonly used agent for formal long-term anticoagulation. It is a synthetic coumarin and owes its name to the Wisconsin Alumni Research Foundation (WARFarin), with whose funding it was developed (Link, 1959). It works on the extrinsic coagulation pathway by inhibiting the synthesis of vitamin K-dependent clotting factors (II, VII, IX and X). Usually, several doses (at least three) are required for 'loading' before steady-state maintenance doses can be applied. It has a relatively long half-life and is usually given once daily.

There is a relatively narrow therapeutic window, and the International Normalized Ratio (INR) is used to monitor the dose of warfarin. This is derived from the prothrombin ratio and target ranges usually reside within the range 2–4. The actual values, however, vary depending upon the precise application. For example, for Fontan circuits (particularly when fenestrated), a range of 1.5–2.5 (target 2.0) is often used. For prosthetic atrioventricular (e.g. mitral) valves, higher ranges of 3–4 or (even up to 4.5) have been advocated. Practices vary as regards the initiation and control of warfarin therapy, with this being chiefly in the hands of the cardiac department in some centres, whilst being largely overseen by the haematology department in others.

Table 3.2 Drugs affecting the anticoagulant effect of warfarin

Agent	Anticoagulant effect
Alcohol	Possibly ↑
Amiodarone	↑
Barbiturates	↓
Cephalosporins	Possibly ↑
Cranberry juice	Possibly ↑
Ibuprofen	Possibly ↑
Influenza vaccine	Possibly ↑
Macrolide antibiotics	↑
Metronidazole	↑
Non-steroidal anti-inflammatory agents	Possibly ↑
Statins	↑ or ↓ depending on the particular statin

A positive development across the UK has been the provision of home monitoring equipment, which has permitted the fingerprick measurement of INR. This has had a great impact on the lives of many families, particularly those in more remote areas, freeing them of the need to attend the main cardiac centre or another hospital on a very regular basis.

Warfarin unfortunately interacts with many other medicines, affecting levels of the bioavailable drug (chiefly through effects on hepatic metabolism) and hence the anticoagulant effect. A number of botanical and herbal preparations are also thought to interact, and therefore extra care is required to avoid these being used concomitantly with warfarin. If felt to be absolutely essential, such preparations should be used under the advice of the doctors supervising the anticoagulation. Haemorrhage is the most common side-effect, although reduced anticoagulant affect also needs to be considered. Table 3.2 above illustrates some of the more common agents that are known to affect warfarin dosing (Royal College of Paediatrics and Child Health [RCPCH], 2008).

Warfarin is teratogenic, and this is an important factor in females of child-bearing age. Generally, it is not administered in the first trimester, with low molecular weight heparin such as enoxaparin being used instead.

Aspirin
Aspirin (acetylsalicylic acid) is presently the most widely used antiplatelet agent in children. For this application, it is typically used in a once daily dose of 3–5 mg/kg (commonly 5 mg/kg, up to a daily maximum of 75 mg). A link to Reye's syndrome has been well established, and as with the prescription of any medicine, the potential risk–benefit balance must be carefully weighed (Halpin et al, 1982). As a result, aspirin is contraindicated for any use other than as an antiplatelet agent in those aged under 16 years, with the exception of acute Kawasaki disease and rheumatic fever (RCPCH, 2008).

Dipyridamole
This interesting substance, which causes arteriolar smooth muscle relaxation via numerous effects, also importantly inhibits thrombus formation by increasing levels

of extracellular adenosine. That in turn produces increased cyclic adenosine mono-phosphate (cAMP) levels, which inhibit platelet aggregation. It is used alone or in combination with aspirin. In Kawasaki disease, a typical dose would be 1 mg/kg 8-hourly in those up to 12 years of age (RCPCH, 2008).

Heparin

Heparin was discovered in 1916 (Marcum, 2000) and has been in use for many years as an unfractionated intravenous preparation. It is an activator of antithrombin, which in turn inactivates thrombin and other clotting proteases. A loading dose is usually administered, followed by a maintenance infusion of 20–40 units/kg per hour, usually starting at the lower doses. The efficacy/safety of the infusion is then monitored by measuring activated partial thromboplastin (APTT) times. Levels 1.5–2 times the upper limit of normal are usually regarded as therapeutic.

In recent years, low molecular weight heparin (enoxaparin) has emerged as a real alternative to other forms of formal anticoagulation. The mechanism of action is the inhibition of factor Xa activity rather than antithrombin. It is administered subcutane-ously, usually twice daily for 'treatment' and once daily in 'prophylaxis'. Less frequent monitoring is required, and this takes the form of measurement of anti-Xa levels (Ho et al, 2004). Prophylaxis usually requires 1 mg/kg once daily, aiming for anti-Xa levels 3 hours after administration of 0.1–0.3 units. Therapeutic usually means 1 mg/kg twice daily with an anti-Xa level of 0.5–1.0 units.

Clopidogrel and newer antiplatelet agents

Whilst currently unlicensed for use in children, there have recently been a number of promising studies, both published (Li et al, 2008) and as yet unpublished, concerning the safety and efficacy of clopidogrel, which is not linked to Reye's syndrome. Clopidogrel inhibits platelet aggregation by blocking activation of the glycoprotein IIb/IIIa pathway. A number of similar agents are being investigated in adults that hold promise for their applicability in children, pending further research (Frelinger et al, 2008).

Fibrinolytic agents

Whilst not anticoagulants, the fibrinolytic agents tissue plasminogen activator and streptokinase deserve mention in this section. In situations where there is acute thrombosis that is resistant to therapy with anticoagulants, these agents may be required. A good example is arterial thrombosis following cardiac catheterisation that has not resolved following initial therapy with heparin. Both of the above-mentioned fibrinolytics have been used to good effect in this situation. It has to be noted that they both carry a significant risk of bleeding, which can be heavy and/or serious (e.g. intracranial). For this reason, the child must be kept under observation throughout the course of fibrinolysis. End points of therapy are (1) resolution of the thrombus (e.g. return of the arterial pulse), (2) bleeding, and (3) completion of a predetermined time course of infusion. A heparin infusion is usually resumed at the end point of fibrinolysis, usually after a recovery period in the case of (2). Whilst tissue plasmino-gen activator is more expensive than streptokinase, it has a shorter half-life of action and a lower incidence of hypersensitivity reactions. For either therapy, fibrinogen levels need to be within the normal range (>1.5 g/L) during treatment, with levels checked before and 4-hourly during treatment.

Pulmonary vasodilators

Pulmonary hypertension is an issue embedded in the practice of paediatric cardiology. Whilst many practitioners use the term rather loosely to refer to increased pulmonary vascular resistance, in its purest form it simply refers to an increased pressure in the pulmonary arteries. That in turn can be the result of increased pulmonary blood flow, increased pulmonary vascular resistance or a combination of the two. There are situations when it becomes necessary to reduce pulmonary vascular resistance. The following agents are routinely used for this purpose. It should be remembered that oxygen is a potent pulmonary vasodilator, with hypoxia and acidosis promoters of pulmonary vasoconstriction.

Nitric oxide

The discovery of nitric oxide (NO) as the agent previously described as 'endothelium-derived relaxing factor' is one of the major scientific discoveries of the past 20 years (Tare et al, 1990). It is a substance endogenously produced by our vascular endothelium, is a potent vasodilator and, at room temperature and pressure, exists in gaseous form. Administered by inhalation, it has selective pulmonary vasodilatory properties. As in any situation in which we are attempting to achieve pulmonary vasodilatation, careful attention to optimal oxygenation and prevention of acidosis are vital. The NO can then be administered in doses up to 20 parts per million. There is little evidence that doses higher than this are necessary. Treatment in this form has a particular utility following cardiac surgery and has also been employed to good effect in the treatment of newborn babies with persistent pulmonary hypertension of the newborn. It is expensive treatment, however, possibly related to the monopolisation of the provision of NO to the UK market by one company. For practical purposes, the build up of toxic metabolites (particularly NO_2) needs to be monitored during NO usage (Miller et al, 1994).

Sildenafil

This oral agent, famously initially marketed as Viagra by Pfizer, relaxes pulmonary vascular smooth muscle by inhibiting cyclic guanosine monophosphate (cGMP)-binding cGMP-specific phosphodiesterase, which is concentrated in the lungs. Reports of its use have been steadily increasing, and it is now quite commonplace in tertiary and even secondary practice as a pulmonary vasodilator (Carroll & Dhillon, 2003; Shah & Ohlsson, 2007; Tessler et al, 2008). Whilst there is room for more evidence to guide the dosing, it is typically used in maintenance doses of 0.5–1 mg/kg three or four times daily. Doses of up to 2 mg/kg up to 4-hourly have been used. However, there are pitfalls in the use of sildenafil in this context, particularly the failure to recognise haemodynamically significant structural heart disease, especially pulmonary venous occlusive disease. Furthermore, in those patients with pulmonary hypertension secondary to respiratory disease, sildenafil is no substitute for optimisation of respiratory therapy. This focuses on the avoidance of hypoxia, treatment of parenchymal lung and airway disease, avoidance of respiratory infection and optimal nutrition. For these reasons, sildenafil and other specific pulmonary vasodilators are best used in consultation with specialist services, if necessary the regional paediatric pulmonary hypertension centre.

Bosentan

Bosentan is a dual endothelin receptor antagonist, competitively blocking endothelin-1 at the endothelin-A and endothelin-B receptors. As endothelin-1 is a potent vasoconstrictor and is upregulated in sustained pulmonary hypertension, bosentan produces significant pulmonary vasodilatation and is also thought to have potential for vascular remodelling (Giannelli et al, 2005; Liu & Chen, 2006). At present, it is used only under the guidance of regional paediatric pulmonary hypertension centres, which carries the added benefit of supported funding (as it is relatively expensive). Bosentan is teratogenic, and contraception is therefore essential in women of child-bearing age. Known side-effects include hepatotoxicity and anaemia, hence the monthly checks of liver function and haemoglobin.

Prostaglandins
Epoprostenol (prostacyclin) is a prostaglandin that is a potent pulmonary vasodilator administered by continuous intravenous infusion. It is commonly used in idiopathic pulmonary hypertension, delivered through a long-term indwelling central venous line (e.g. Hickman). Typical doses range from 5 to 25ng/kg per minute. It can result in significant systemic hypotension and, through its inhibition of platelet aggregation, significant bleeding. Patients with idiopathic pulmonary hypertension commonly become dependent and later tolerant to epoprostenol, such that the sudden cessation of therapy (e.g. through infusion pump failure) can have dire consequences.

A synthetic analogue of epoprostenol, iloprost has been administered to adults by nebuliser, but experience in children is very limited.

Stem cell therapy
Stem cells are found in most complex organisms and are characterised by *self-renewal*, the ability to repeatedly divide before differentiation, and *potency*, the ability to differentiate into specialised cells. Broadly, there are two types: embryonic and adult stem cells. The potential to culture cells and grow new healthy tissues has sparked the imaginations of clinicians and scientists alike. Naturally, this area is the topic of considerable research. There is also considerable controversy regarding embryonic stem cell research (adult stem cells being less controversial) (Kuflik, 2008).

Adult stem cell therapies are already in use, particularly in haematology (e.g. bone marrow transplants). A number of other therapeutic applications are anticipated. However, we are still many years away from being able to 'grow' entire organs in laboratory conditions, and it remains to be seen what impact such therapy will have on our practice in the near future.

Interventional cardiology

The growth of interventional cardiological techniques has mirrored technological advances, and as these have been rapid, this area of practice has developed at least as briskly as conventional cardiac surgery. Indeed, in many ways, cardiac surgery and interventional cardiology are moving closer together rather than developing in parallel, as demonstrated by recent interest in percutaneous and thoracoscopic cardiac surgical techniques (Jutley et al, 2008; Matsuno et al, 2008).

Balloon valvuloplasty
Balloon pulmonary valvuloplasty
This is one of the most well established cardiac interventions, having first been attempted in the 1950s (Rubio-Alvarez et al, 1953) and established in the 1980s (Kan et al, 1982). It is today generally regarded as the treatment of choice for severe

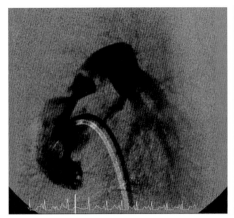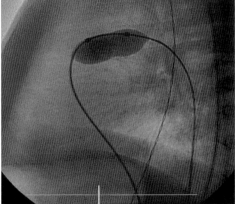

Figure 3.2   Balloon pulmonary valvuloplasty; a) Pre-intervention, b) During intervention

pulmonary valve stenosis, although in very resistant cases surgical relief of pulmo-nary valve narrowing, including transannular patching, may be required. The tech-nique is relatively straightforward. Under anaesthesia, typically general anaesthesia, central venous access is obtained, usually through a femoral vein, although alterna-tives venous routes (e.g. internal jugular or transhepatic) are also technically feasible (Figure 3.2).

A cardiac catheter is then advanced through the systemic vein to the right atrium and then right ventricle. The right ventricular pressure is measured. An angiogram is usually performed in the right ventricle to assess the nature and severity of pulmonary stenosis, to look for additional (e.g. branch pulmonary artery) stenoses and to allow measurement of the valve annulus. A 'soft' (e.g. Terumo) guidewire is then usually advanced across the stenosed pulmonary valve from the catheter in the right ventricle. The catheter is advanced across the guidewire into a distal branch pulmonary artery, although it may also be possible to advance the catheter safely to this location without the use of a guidewire. The pulmonary artery pressure can be measured to establish the stenotic 'gradient'. Peak-to-peak gradients measured in this way that are in excess of 30 mmHg (roughly equivalent to peak instantaneous Doppler-derived gradients in excess of 60 mmHg) would normally qualify for intervention.

Either way, the catheter is replaced with a stiffer guidewire, and a balloon catheter is advanced across that so that it straddles the pulmonary valve. When the balloon is centred on the valve, it is inflated with dilute contrast (in saline) in order to stretch the stenosed valve, and then the balloon is quickly deflated. Great care is taken to size the balloon appropriately, usually to 1.2–1.3 times the diameter of the valve annulus, as determined by echocardiography and/or angiography, and typically the shortest available balloon is used. One balloon inflation is usually all that is required. It is standard to measure a final withdrawal 'gradient' across the valve, and a final right ventricular angiogram is optional.

Whilst the early and late results of this procedure are usually regarded as very good, in a few cases the procedure is insufficient, with conventional cardiac surgery being ultimately required. In some cases, the procedure results in significant pulmonary regurgitation, which rarely may require pulmonary valve replacement in later life (Masura et al, 1993).

Balloon aortic valvuloplasty

This procedure has many similarities to balloon pulmonary valvuloplasty, the important differences being:

- a higher threshold for intervention, given generally slightly less favourable results and the greater clinical significance of producing moderate or greater degrees of valvular regurgitation;
- a retrograde arterial approach to the valve, and hence the routine administration of a bolus dose of intravenous heparin. The limitation of balloon size in relation to the size of the patient (and hence the size of the femoral artery) can be circumvented by the use of two balloon catheters, one introduced through each femoral artery;
- a balloon diameter typically 0.9 times that of the valve annulus;
- the use of longer balloons for stability whilst avoiding impingement on the mitral valve annulus (Brierley et al, 1998);
- the use of techniques to temporarily arrest the heart or greatly reduce the force of ejection in order to achieve a stable balloon position. These include rapid ventricular pacing (David et al, 2007) or the injection of intravenous adenosine (Daehnert et al, 2004).

Mitral (and tricuspid) valvuloplasty

Mitral (and even less commonly tricuspid) balloon valvuloplasty is now infrequently performed in the developed world, although much applied in the developing world. This is largely related to the much higher incidence of rheumatic fever in developing countries and the relative lack of access to conventional cardiac surgery. The procedure follows the same basic principles of valvuloplasty of the semilunar valves, with the balloon catheter being introduced antegradely and rarely, in the case of the mitral valve, retrogradely from the femoral artery. The usual approach to the mitral valve is antegrade (femoral vein–right atrium–left atrium) and relies upon the presence of an atrial septal defect (ASD), either native or created by transseptal puncture. An Inoue-Balloon, which carries a special design, is usually applied (Fawzy, 2007). Whilst this procedure is mainly used in adults, it also has an applicability in carefully selected children with mitral valve stenosis (Kothari et al, 2005).

Balloon angioplasty

Balloon dilatation of stenosed vascular structures has a wide applicability in everyday paediatric cardiac practice. The balloon catheters are introduced to the relevant sites in the standard way, as for balloon valvuloplasty. Amongst the most important considerations with vascular dilatations is that of balloon size, as with balloon valvuloplasty. For most vascular structures (e.g. pulmonary arteries, pulmonary veins and systemic veins), a degree of 'oversizing' of the balloon is required, in terms of the diameter of the stenosis and the adjacent healthy vessel. The exact degree of diameter 'oversizing' depends upon the particular vessel and the clinical context. However, the shortest possible balloons are usually employed in vascular settings.

Vascular stenoses can be very resilient (systemic venous narrowings sometimes surprisingly so) and usually require several atmospheres of pressure (sometimes >10 atmospheres) to provide relief of the stenosis. Complications include aneurysm formation and vessel rupture, which may be fatal. For this reason, the rapid availability of blood and blood products is recommended. Balloon pulmonary angioplasty has one of the narrowest therapeutic windows, and hence highest risks, of the commonly conducted cardiac interventional procedures.

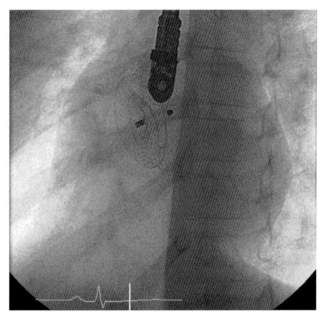

Figure 3.3 Atrial septal defect

There are situations where it is not appropriate to 'oversize' the balloon diameter compared with the adjacent healthy vessel, and this particularly applies to aortic arch narrowings (where one would not normally exceed isthmul diameter) and the diameter of synthetic implants such as Blalock–Taussig shunts.

Device and coil occlusion
In these situations, the cardiac catheter is used to deploy devices, which come in various shapes and sizes and include occlusion coils, to occlude (1) unwanted vascular connections, and (2) intracardiac defects. The former grouping includes PDAs, collateral vessels (e.g. major aortopulmonary collateral arteries [MAPCAs]) and systemic–pulmonary Gore-tex shunts. In these situations, anticoagulants or antiplatelet agents are not usually used after the procedure as the object of the exercise is to abolish flow, not preserve it.

The latter group – (2) – includes interatrial defects (ASDs [Figure 3.3] and patent foramen ovale), VSDs, Fontan fenestrations (often partially occluded) and paraprosthetic valvular leaks. In these situations, anticoagulation, typically intravenous heparin, is usually administered at the time of the procedure and either formal anticoagulation or antiplatelet action continued after the procedure, typically for at least 6 months, depending on the nature of the defect and device deployed.

Stent deployment
This technology, which was initially used in adult cardiological practice for the relief of coronary arterial stenoses (Garratt et al, 1991), found its way into routine paediatric cardiological practice in the early 1990s (O'Laughlin et al, 1991). A stent is a relatively rigid alloy structure that forms a tubular framework when deployed. In this way, it serves to dilate and maintain patency within a stenosed vessel. Before deployment, the stent has a profile thin enough to permit its introduction through a vascular

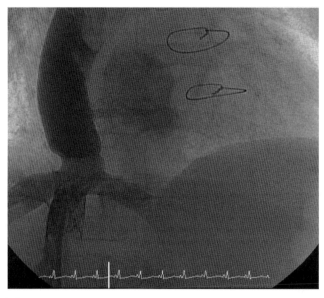

Figure 3.4   Diabolo stent

sheath. Stents, which come in a great range of sizes and materials, are now routinely used in the relief of stenosis of the pulmonary arteries and coarctation of the aorta (including re-coarctation). Less commonly, they are used to relieve pulmonary venous stenosis (with generally short-lived and poor results) and stenosis within synthetic structures (e.g. right ventricle-pulmonary artery conduits after a modified Norwood operation).

Some special applications of stents include stenting of the arterial duct to preserve pulmonary blood flow in neonates with pulmonary atresia, or for systemic blood flow in hypoplastic left heart syndrome (HLHS), the so-described hybrid stage I palliation for HLHS (see below). Stent fenestration is another special application in which a dumbbell-shaped (or diabolo) stent (Figure 3.4) is fashioned to maintain the patency of an existing or specially created fenestration between the atria (or Fontan conduit and atria), hence sacrificing a few per cent of oxygen saturation for improved haemo-dynamics. The dumbbell-shape is produced by limiting the diameter of the waist of the stent-inflating balloon with either surgical suture material or temporary surgical pacing wire (Gewillig et al, 2006; Stumper et al, 2003).

Broadly speaking, stents are either self-expanding or balloon-dilatable, covered or uncovered. They each have their own particular indications, but in paediatric practice perhaps the most important principle is to take account of growth. Whilst some stents can be further dilated some time, often several years after deployment (commonly with associated stent shortening), they may not maintain an adequate diameter over the desired growth period. This factor will usually govern the choice of stent and, indeed, whether a stent can be deployed at all.

Neointimal proliferation and in-stent stenosis are problems that are common to both adult and paediatric practice. Following a degree of success in adult practice, the use of drug-eluting stents is filtering through to paediatric cardiac intervention, although it remains to be seen if this promise will be fulfilled (Munoz-Garcia et al, 2008).

Transcatheter valve replacement

There has been much interest in recent years concerning the use of valves implanted via a catheter. These have chiefly been employed in the right ventricular outflow tract (RVOT) of adult patients with severe pulmonary regurgitation, stenosis or a mixed picture (Khambadkone & Bonhoeffer, 2004). In carefully selected patients, this technique offers an attractive alternative to re-sternotomy in patients who have previously undergone conventional cardiac surgical reconstruction of the RVOT and are quite likely to require further surgical reconstruction.

Even more recently, transcatheter replacement of the aortic valve has been introduced, albeit in an elderly adult age group (Webb et al, 2007). It remains to be seen whether this technique may eventually translate to paediatric practice. The size of the prosthetic valve and hence the arterial delivery sheath, together with the growth of the patient, remain limiting factors.

Cardiac pacing and electrophysiology

Cardiac pacing

The ability to pace the heart electrically is an essential tool in paediatric cardiac practice, both for intrinsic abnormalities of cardiac rhythm and conduction and for those acquired as a result of cardiac surgery. It is standard practice to implant temporary pacing leads for cardiac surgical repairs involving a sternotomy and full exposure of the heart, which nowadays comprise the majority of repairs. By convention, pacing leads are usually implanted on both the atrium and ventricle, to the right and left side respectively of the patient's chest. These are usually removed three or more days after the operation. The usual indication for pacing is a bradyarrhythmia (e.g. sinus node dysfunction) or an abnormality of conduction (e.g. complete heart block), although temporary pacing is sometimes required to restore atrioventricular synchrony in patients with a postoperative tachyarrhythmia (e.g. junctional ectopic tachycardia [JET]).

For 'permanent' pacing, when the indication for pacing is likely to be long term or permanent (Vardas et al, 2007), the pacing system can be implanted through the great veins (transvenous or endocardial) or by a conventional cardiac surgical approach to the surface of the heart (epicardial). In both instances, the pacing lead(s) are tunnelled through and connected to a generator that is implanted subcutaneously or submuscularly in the thorax or abdomen. There are advantages and disadvantages of both approaches to the heart. With improvements in lead and generator technology and a slimming down of both, the transvenous approach is generally favoured in most situations. Transvenous systems avoid the need for a sternotomy, have better lead thresholds and sensitivities (and hence generator longevity) and are thought to have a lower lead fracture rate than epicardial systems. However, transvenous systems leave the legacy of intravenous pacing leads that eventually need extraction, and some practitioners have chosen to opt for an epicardial approach in the very young, replacing the system transvenously when necessary in an older and bigger child.

For a chamber pacing site, there is the option to pace a single chamber (atrium or ventricle) or dual chambers (atrium and ventricle), or use multisite pacing. This latter modality usually involves pacing the right atrium, the right ventricle and the left ventricle through the coronary sinus. It has the benefit of potentially producing a more physiological activation sequence and has been used with considerable success in selected patients with ventricular dysfunction related to ventricular dyssynchrony. This has earned it the name of cardiac resynchronisation therapy (Figure 3.5).

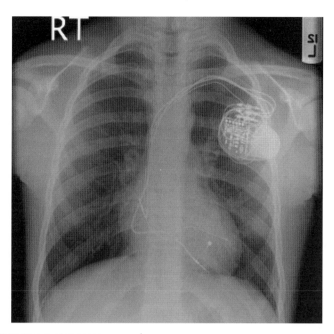

Figure 3.5   Transvenous permanent pacemaker

Table 3.3   The pacemaker code

	Position 1	**Position 2**	**Position 3**	**Position 4**
Significance	Paced chamber(s)	Sensed chamber(s)	Response to sensing	Programmable functions
Options	A = Atrium V = Ventricle D = Dual (A & V) O = None	A = Atrium V = Ventricle D = Dual (A & V) O = None	I = Inhibited T = Triggered D = Dual (triggered & Inhibited) O = None	R = Rate modulation

There is a standard code to denote the mode of pacing, as illustrated in Table 3.3. Whilst a fifth position is sometimes cited to denote antitachycardial functions, the first three positions are the most significant, with an 'R' sometimes added in the fourth position to denote rate modulation. This specifies the ability to sense and respond to increased work of breathing or metabolic demand.

Therefore VVI denotes a single-chamber pacemaker in which the ventricle is both paced and sensed, with a sensed intrinsic impulse inhibiting pacemaker output. The code DDDR applies to a dual-chamber pacemaker that paces and senses both atrium and ventricle and has the capacity to respond to a sensed atrial event by pacing the ventricle, or inhibiting its ventricular output if an intrinsic ventricular event is detected within the predetermined atrioventricular delay interval; rate modulation is also present.

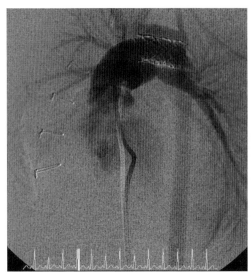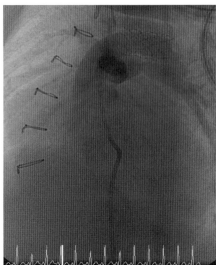

Figure 3.6   Hypoplastic left heart syndrome

Electrophysiology

This terms refers to very specialised techniques used to map the electrical activation pathways within the heart by means of specially designed mapping 'catheters' introduced through the standard vascular routes. The object, apart from diagnostic, is to apply a physical burn to the endocardium in a location that will disrupt an unwanted electrical pathway, and hence remove the substrate for a tachyarrhythmia. With improving technology, these techniques have become established, and as in other areas of paediatric cardiac management, the age/size threshold for treatment has gradually diminished.

Hybrid procedures

These refer to procedures in which interventional cardiologist and cardiac surgeon work even more closely than usual, carrying out a combined operation in which both teams operate on the patient over a short time frame, sometimes in a joint session that relies on skills particular to each. A good example of such an approach is the hybrid stage I palliation for HLHS, when the pulmonary arteries are banded, and either during that procedure or more commonly as a separate procedure soon afterwards, the arterial duct is stented and, if necessary, the atrial septum balloon dilated (Akinturk et al, 2007) (Figure 3.6). Advocates of this approach highlight the avoidance of neonatal CPB, and initial results have proved encouraging. However, there is no doubt that the second stage of surgical palliation is made more complex. It seems likely that such hybrid approaches will gain favour in the future, in the treatment of a variety of lesions.

Anaesthesia

The ideal aim of anaesthesia is to provide an adequate plane of anaesthesia, analgesia and conditions to allow surgery whilst preserving the patient's normal physiological status. Currently, more than 50% of cases undertaken are on children less than 2 years of age, a significant proportion of whom are neonates. In addition to the cardiac lesion, there may be associated with other congenital anomalies or syndromes. It is important for the anaesthetist to have an understanding of the cardiac anomaly, the surgery undertaken and the physiological consequences both before and after surgery, as well as the implications of anaesthetising a child, whether an infant, a neonate or an adolescent.

Conduct of anaesthesia

Provision and planning of anaesthesia begin with the preoperative visit and end with the transfer of care to the ICU following surgery.

During anaesthesia, a combination of technique, appropriate drugs and physiological manipulation are used to achieve stability. As stated previously, different cardiac conditions require different manipulations of the physiological parameters to achieve stability. Examples include avoidance of tachycardia and drops in systemic vascular resistance in cases of aortic or mitral stenosis. Conversely, maintaining or increasing the heart rate and decreasing systemic vascular resistance may be beneficial when aortic regurgitation or mitral regurgitation is the main problem. Manipulation of pulmonary vascular resistance is more frequent in paediatric practice, and balancing both the systemic and pulmonary circulations is important in univentricular circulations.

Pulmonary hypertensive crises are encountered more commonly in paediatric cardiac surgery, particularly in those conditions where there is increased pulmonary blood flow such as large ventricular and atrioventricular septal defects, truncus arteriosus or transposition of the great arteries (TGA). It can also be seen with obstruction of pulmonary blood flow, as seen in cases of total anomalous pulmonary venous drainage. Patients with pulmonary hypertension will be at an increased risk of adverse events perioperatively, and this may alter the decision process when planning the type of surgery undertaken.

The other main general consideration is the physiological difference between adults and children. This is summarised in Box 3.2.

Preoperative visit

The aim of the preoperative visit is to introduce the anaesthetist to the child and parents, and to evaluate the child's cardiac and general condition, the stage of treatment and the preparation for the operation to be performed. The preoperative meeting with the child is also important as it establishes a rapport, especially with adolescents, but equally important is the rapport with the parents as they provide most information and consent. A good preoperative visit can provide a form of anxiolysis.

Gaining a quantitative picture of the child's condition can be difficult, especially if the child is an infant, but simple questions directed at the parents about weight gain, problems with feeding, cyanosis and 'funny turns' may be helpful. The identification of syndromes that may affect anaesthesia (e.g. Pierre Robin syndrome, associated with difficult intubation) and other conditions such as asthma, previous problems with anaesthesia, difficult peripheral and central venous access, difficult intubation and familial problems such as malignant hyperthermia is important in planning.

The clinical notes also allow the analysis of any investigations. These included simple tests such as full blood count, coagulation screen, urea & electrolytes, ECG and chest X-ray, as well as more cardiospecific tests such as recent echocardiography, angiography and 24-hour ECG monitoring and exercise tolerance tests. The results may reveal anaemia or polycythaemia, commonly associated with chronic conditions and cyanosis respectively, coagulation defects or electrolyte disturbances from chronic

Box 3.2 Comparison of neonatal and adult anatomy and physiology

These differences will affect the practical aspects of anaesthesia for a neonate. For example, neonates may be more difficult to intubate and are more prone to desaturation. The dosages, effects and accumulation of drugs differ. Temperature loss is more exaggerated, and glucose levels may need to supplemented. The main changes are highlighted below.

Airway and respiratory
Anterior larynx at the level of the 3rd–4th cervical vertebra
Floppy U-shaped epiglottis
Large tongue compared with oropharynx
Large occiput
Conically shaped glottis (the cricoid ring being the narrowest part)
Trachea length 4 cm (term baby)
Oxygen consumption (8–9 mL/kg per minute) is 2–3 times that of an adult
Deadspace (2–3 mL/kg) and tidal volumes (5–7 mL/kg) are similar to an adult's
Compliant rib cage with horizontal ribs
Closing volume greater than functional residual capacity
Diaphragm is the main source of tidal volume (splinting will significantly decrease respiratory efficiency)
Lungs mature and surfactant production begins at 30–32 weeks' gestational age
Smaller percentage (25%) of type 1 muscle fibres leads to earlier fatigue
Fetal haemoglobin makes up 60% of the total at birth (a shift in the haemoglobin dissociation curve to the left)
Prone to apnoeas and are obligate nasal breathers

Cardiovascular
Rate-dependent cardiac output
Immature neonatal myocardium has a reduced compliance when compared with an adult myocardium, resulting in less of a stroke volume increase with a given increase in preload (contractility sensitive to calcium)
Increased parasympathetic (vagal) compared with sympathetic tone
Transition from fetal to adult circulation (ductus venosus, patent foramen ovale, patient ductus arteriosus). Will revert to a transitional circulation in adverse conditions (hypoxia, hypercapnia, acidosis) and sensitive to changes in systemic or peripheral vascular resistance
80–90 mL/kg circulation volume compared with 70 mL/kg in an adult

Neurological
Myelination not complete
Immature blood–brain barrier
Spinal cord ends at 3rd lumbar vertebrae, dura at the sacral level
Surface anatomy of the iliac crest corresponds to the 5th lumbar – 1st sacral space Epidural space 0.5–1.5 cm deep
Retinopathy of prematurity results from exposure to high oxygen concentrations, especially in premature neonates

Thermoregulation
Immature thermoregulation centre, inability to shiver
Large surface area to body mass ratio (three times that of an adult), underdeveloped insulation
Brown fat (5% adipose tissue) at birth in term neonates but reduced in premature neonates

Metabolism/excretion
Immature liver enzyme system P450 cytochrome
Glucose metabolism (limited glycogen stores) leads to earlier hypoglycaemia
Renal immaturity 33% glomerular filtration rate (adult), reduced concentrating ability and less
    ability to excrete sodium
Extracellular space 45% versus 20% (adult), reduced albumin/alpha-1 acid glycoprotein
Vitamin K required for normal coagulation (levels are low at birth)

diuretic therapy. Cardiac investigations may demonstrate arrythmias and allow an estimation of cardiac function. Results may also reveal difficulties that may be encountered during the operation, such as the close proximity of a pulmonary conduit to the sternum, which may cause a problem when opening the sternum, or evidence of pulmonary hypertension.

An accurate drug history is important as well. ACEIs and phosphodiesterase inhibitors suggest treatment for cardiac failure, sildenafil treats pulmonary hypertension, treatment with aspirin and warfarin may result in more bleeding intraoperatively, and children on steroid therapy may require further replacement perioperatively.

Detailed examination is covered else where, but anaesthetists may focus on factors that predict a difficult intubation such as micrognathia, the state of the peripheral veins for intravenous access, the general condition of the child, heart rate, blood pressure, capillary refill, enlarged liver and ascites, urinary output, respiratory rate, ease of respiration and oxygen saturation, with a note of any additional oxygen requirements.

Another important reason for the preoperative visit is explanation of the anaesthesia to be undertaken and the risks involved, for both the parents and, if appropriate, the child. Procedures such as line placement, the use of blood products and the provision of analgesia are discussed. In addition, a decision is made on whether to include any premedication in the anaesthetic technique.

Premedication is commonly used to provide anxiolysis and sedation, which may help with induction of anaesthesia. Benzodiazepines, normally midazolam, are prescribed. Unfortunately, this may produce an opposite effect with disinhibition, and unless there has been previous history this reaction is unpredictable. Care must be taken when prescribing a sedative premedication if there is a history of airway obstruction or if the child's general condition is unstable as this may worsen the current condition. Other reasons for premedication include the application of topical local anaesthetic cream such as amethocaine gel if intravenous induction is anticipated, giving antisialogogues, the prevention of bradyarrhythmias with glycopyrronium bromide or atropine, and administration of the child's normal medication.

Induction of anaesthesia

Induction is a critical period. It is achieved intravenously or with the inhalation of a volatile anaesthetic such as sevoflurane. Inhalation induction is ideally suited to children who are difficult to cannulate or where a difficult airway or intubation is anticipated, and the preservation of spontaneous breathing until the airway is secure is an advantage. The time taken to achieve an adequate plane of anaesthesia is prolonged when compared with intravenous induction, especially in patients who have a right-to-left shunt. To achieve this plane, a high concentration of volatile anaesthetic is needed, which may adversely affect the child's condition, and intravenous induction is therefore preferable in children whose condition is unstable.

In patients with a fixed cardiac output such as critical aortic stenosis, or other critical obstructive lesions, and in patients with poor ventricular function, anaesthesia needs to be carefully titrated to provide an adequate level of anaesthesia but also prevent the child from decompensating physiologically.

Most cardiac operations will require the patient to be intubated with an endotracheal tube. This allows the ventilation to be controlled and optimised, and provides the conditions essential for intrathoracic operations. Positive-pressure ventilation can be beneficial in cardiac failure as it reduces the work of breathing, preload and afterload of the systemic ventricle. However, the rise in intrathoracic pressure may worsen cardiac output in patients with right ventricular dysfunction or in cases where venous pressure drives the pulmonary blood flow, such as in a Fontan circulation.

Both the nasal and the oral route are used. Commonly, a nasal tube is used in neonates and infants as it is easier to secure and is better tolerated by the child on the ICU when compared with oral tubes. When the child reaches an age where a 6 or 6.5 mm endotracheal tube is the appropriate size, the oral route is more commonly used. Obviously, certain anatomical variants, such as choanal atresia, may make the nasal route impossible, but the main morbidity comes from trauma and bleeding.

Traditionally, in paediatric anaesthetic practice, non-cuffed tubes are used. The main reason is the theoretical advantage that this will reduce the incidence of subglottic stenosis if the appropriately sized tube is used. Cuffed tubes have become more streamlined with emerging technology, and the addition of low-pressure cuffs probably makes this advantage obsolete. Cuffed endotracheal tubes may reduce trauma caused by repeated intubations to find the correct size tube and allow consistent ventilation with changing chest compliance. These benefits may increase the use of cuffed endotracheal tube.

During the operation, two forms of ventilation are commonly used: pressure controlled and volume controlled. Pressure-controlled ventilation sets a constant peak pressure to deliver the required tidal volume. Setting the pressure and the flow characteristics of this mode may lead to a reduction in barotrauma and allow delivery of ventilation in the presence of a significant leak around the endotracheal tube. This is sometimes a problem in paediatric anaesthesia. The main disadvantage is that changes in tidal volume with changes in chest compliance lead to inconsistent ventilation. Kinking in the endotracheal tube, a build-up of secretions and obstruction in the main tracheobronchial tree, or an increase in the pleural space with an effusion or pneumothorax will also reduce ventilation in this mode. It is important to rule these out if ventilation is suddenly reduced during surgery.

Volume-controlled ventilation sets and delivers a constant tidal volume despite changes in chest compliance. The resultant increase in airway pressure associated with decreases in chest compliance may result in barotrauma. Conditions stated above that affect tidal volumes achieved in pressure-controlled ventilation will result in higher airway pressures in volume-controlled ventilation. Again, these need to be ruled out if a sudden increase in airway pressure is encountered in this mode. There are ventilators on which this mode may be pressure limited by setting an upper peak pressure. This allows constant ventilation but will be limited if the upper peak pressure set is reached. This may reduce barotrauma.

There may be times during the operation when hand-ventilation is required. This is particularly the case during thoracotomies in neonates. A Jackson Rees modified T-piece is used. This is the standard circuit used by anaesthetists for both spontaneous and assisted ventilation. It is commonly used in patients weighing less than 20 kg because the high gas flows required make it inefficient in large children. Its design limits deadspace and resistance, which is ideal for neonates. The open-ended bag allows variation in the inspiratory volume when assisting ventilation. The main disadvantages are that peak pressure is not accounted for and that the technique requires a pair of hands that may be needed elsewhere.

The common position is supine for a sternotomy, although operations can be performed through a thoracotomy incision. These include repair of aortic coarctation, ligation of a PDA or a formation of Blalock–Taussig shunt. The side of the incisions depends on the side of the arch of the aorta, and with the arch normally on the left, the first two incisions are performed through a left thoracotomy and the last through a right thoracotomy.

When positioning the patient, care and attention to the pressure areas is important. Operations can last for several hours and perfusion may be suboptimal, so positioning the child in a natural pose with contact areas well padded may prevent nerve damage and skin necrosis. Rolls under the shoulders are used to allow access to the top of the sternum, but care must be taken not to overextend the neck. Care when positioning the neck is especially important when the patient's neck is potentially unstable – for example, children with Down syndrome are prone to atlantoaxial subluxation.

Drugs, equipment and monitoring

A combination of drugs is used to provide anaesthesia. Traditionally, most techniques were based around the use of high doses of opioids. This provided cardiovascular stability and attenuated the stress response. However, it can lead to prolonged recovery and duration of mechanical ventilation, and a more balanced approach is advocated. Opioids are still the mainstay of many techniques, but this is now tailored to the needs of each operation to allow quicker recovery.

Central neuraxial techniques such as epidurals to provide analgesia have advocates. Proposed benefits include a reduction in the stress response, a possible reduction in myocardial ischaemic events and an increased speed of recovery and extubation. In operations where bypass and heparinisation are not required and the child is in a stable condition preoperatively, it may be advantageous.

Below is a summary of the monitoring used during anaesthesia. It is not exhaustive but includes the main components and ones that may become standards of care. Standard minimal monitoring is used as with any anaesthetic. This includes pulse oximetry, end-tidal carbon dioxide, blood pressure, ECG, temperature and inspiratory oxygen concentration. Other simple measures include catheterisation of the bladder for urine output estimation, which indirectly monitors cardiac output and renal function.

Arterial lines are placed to monitor continuous blood pressure and access for arterial gas, electrolyte and metabolic analysis. Common sites are the radial and femoral arteries. Care must be taken when siting them, especially in the brachial artery as this may cause distal limb ischaemia. The site of the surgery is important when placing the arterial line. An arterial line in the right arm will allow the perfusionist to monitor the pressure during aortic arch repair when the right innominate artery is cannulated to perform antegrade cerebral perfusion. Similarly, when a right Blalock–Taussig shunt is fashioned, the continuous arterial trace will be interrupted if the line is in the right arm.

Central venous access is required to measure right atrial pressure and allow the administration of specific drugs. Common sites are the right internal jugular and femoral veins. Less common are the subclavian and left internal jugular veins. Ultrasound rather than the traditional landmark technique is now being used to place these lines as there is greater anatomical variation in children compared with adults, a coagulopathy may be present, and previous access may have resulted in stenosis or thrombosis of the vessel. The placement of these lines and monitoring may vary when considering anatomical variations such as dextrocardia, situs inversus and the presence of bilateral superior venae cavae.

Temperature monitoring and control is essential. Hypothermia is a key method of cerebral and myocardial protection during limited cerebral and coronary perfusion, and various operations are conducted under hypothermic circulatory arrest. Temperature control especially the prevention of hyperthermia postoperatively, may have a bearing on neurological morbidity. In addition, producing a state of mild-to-moderate hypothermia may prevent further neurological morbidity when there is increasing cyanosis or a poor cardiac output state, or in treating resistant tachyarrhythmias. It should be noted that this is not without side-effects: hypothermia below 35 °C may lead to a relative coagulopathy, possible increased susceptibility to infection and a change in the metabolism of drugs used. A combination of these common sites is used to monitor temperature: nasopharynx (cerebral), oesophageal (core) and skin (helpful when rewarming on CPB and an indirect monitor of perfusion).

Pulmonary arterial catheters are rarely used in paediatric cardiac surgery, mainly due to the relative size of the patients compared with the catheters. When operating on conditions that warrant the measurement of left atrial pressure, i.e. TGA, or pulmonary arterial pressure, such as truncus arteriosus or obstructive anomalous pulmonary veins, direct lines are placed during surgery.

Trans-oesophageal echocardiography has increasingly been used to assess the adequacy of the surgical repair as well as the function of the ventricles and regional wall ischaemia. This is particularly useful with operations involving the mitral valve, when views obtained are an improvement on the epicardial view. Again, the size of the probe when compared with the child is a factor. Children weighing less than 5 kg may experience trauma to the oesophagus and obstruction of the trachea.

Activated clotting time is used to assess the heparinisation prior to CPB and its reversal with protamine following its completion. The normal range is 120–140 seconds, with adequate heparinisation for bypass three times the normal value. CPB causes a dilution of coagulation factors, triggering of the coagulation cascade, a fibrinolytic state and a degradation of platelets and their function. The thromboelastograph (TEG) is a dynamic test of coagulation that can help direct protamine and blood product therapy to treat resultant coagulopathies or thrombolytic states. Limiting the exposure of the patient to blood and blood products is of benefit, and the TEG is increasingly being incorporated into management both intraoperatively and subsequently on the ICU.

Glucose monitoring and tight glycaemia control have shown to be of benefit in adult cardiac perioperative care. Whether this has as much significance in paediatric care has yet to be defined, but the prevention of significant hyperglycaemia, relative hypoglycaemia and ketosis as a result of starvation is probably beneficial to the patient.

Near-infrared spectrometry (NIRS) monitors cerebral oxygen saturation. The figures obtained are similar with relation to jugular bulb venous saturation. NIRS gives an indication of cerebral perfusion and the coupling of oxygen delivery and consumption, but it offers the advantage of being less invasive. The monitor can also be used to obtain renal and splanchnic saturation, and gives an indication of cardiac output and oxygen consumption within these regions. It has yet to be decided whether using this can direct cerebral perfusion during CPB and help prevent cerebral morbidity, but increasingly it is being used as an non-invasive monitor of cerebral perfusion and cardiac output, both intraoperatively and on the ICU.

Arterial gas analysis with reference to inspiratory oxygen concentration gives an indication of the adequacy of gas exchange. Electrolytes, acid–base balance and lactate are also measured. Acid–base and electrolyte abnormalities may affect cardiac function, and correction may improve this, as in terms of hypokalaemia and arrhythmias. The process of measuring acid–base balance during CPB and hypothermia has been debated. Two forms are used. One form, pH stat, involves analysis at the actual temperature the blood is taken. Correction of the result may involve the introduction of carbon dioxide into the bypass circuit. Alpha stat analysis takes place at 37 °C regardless of the actual blood temperature. It is suggested that pH stat used during the initial phases of cooling and then continuing an alpha stat strategy for the rest of the cooling phase and rewarming may improve neurological outcomes. Base excess and lactate are commonly used to indicate the state of perfusion. Increases in both these may suggest a reduction in cardiac output. High lactate on admission to intensive care is said to be predictive of poor outcome; but perhaps more useful as a marker is not the absolute value but the trend and rate of change in lactate.

Bispectral analysis is a method of compressing data from electroencephalograph readings to give a figure that correlates to depth of anaesthesia. Readings of 100 correspond to the awake state, less than to 80 sedation and 40–60 to anaesthesia. Using this monitor offers the ability to titrate anaesthesia without fear of awareness. The obvious setting is with an unstable patient where it is advantageous to limit anaesthesia to reduce any side-effects whilst still providing an adequate depth of anaesthesia. However, it has yet to be fully validated in the paediatric population.

Maintenance of anaesthesia

Most operations are performed under CPB, but the same principles apply to operations where bypass is not required.

The surgeon will access the thorax via a sternotomy or thoracotomy. Problems may be encountered at various stages of this process. For example, sternotomy is extremely stimulating, and an adequate level of anaesthesia is required to blunt the sympathetic response. During sternotomy, contact with the mediastinal structures may provoke arrhythmias. Although rare, cardiovascular decompensation can take place with the change in chest compliance once the chest is open. This is particularly true in patients with dilated poorly functioning ventricles. It is common practice to stop ventilation at various times during sternotomy (when using the sternal saw to split the sternum), and sometimes during thoracotomy, to protect the lungs when gaining access.

Conversely, ventilation is maintained during a redo sternotomy. Following previous surgery through a sternotomy, mediastinal structures such as the pulmonary artery, aorta or right ventricle may adhere to the underside of the sternum. Gore-tex pericardial patches are inserted to help prevent this. However, although rare, there is still the potential to damage these structures during the redo sternotomy, and redo operations are set up with the groin or neck exposed to allow cannulation and establish bypass should this happen and the normal sites for bypass cannulation are not accessible. Likewise, the anaesthetist should be ready to provide support in the event; this may be cardiovascular support with fluid, blood and inotropes, defibrillation, superficial cooling with ice to possibly limit cerebral morbidity, and head-down tilt and pressure on the neck if air emboli are likely on the left side of the circulation (paradoxical emboli through a right-to-left shunt may be a possibility with many cardiac defects).

Chest compliance changes during the operation. With a sternotomy, compliance may increase once the chest is open, leading to overventilation if under a pressure-controlled setting, which is common practice in paediatric anaesthesia. Likewise, during a thoracotomy when the lung is retracted, a form of one-lung ventilation takes place. In the lateral position, the compliance of the dependent lung decreases, and it receives less ventilation and more perfusion in contrast to the upper lung, which receives more ventilation and less perfusion. This ventilation–perfusion mismatch can increase when the lung is being retracted, and controlled ventilation and inspiratory oxygen concentration may need to be altered to compensate for this.

Once the site has been exposed and the surgeon starts dissection to expose the areas of interest, various factors may affect anaesthesia. All structures, including the aorta, pulmonary arteries, ductus arteriosus and trachea, can be distorted during the dissection and cannulation of vessels. This can lead to difficulty in ventilation, desaturation, ischaemia, hypotension and hypertension. Communication with the surgeon is important at this point. Changes in ventilation, oxygen concentration, level of anaesthesia and use of inotropes and vasodilators may be required to allow surgery to continue and provide a degree of stability.

Cardiopulmonary bypass

CPB is used to maintain blood flow around the body without using the heart as the pump. It is also, as the name suggests, used to facilitate gas exchange of the blood without involving the lungs. The methods used to accomplish this will be described below, along with associated techniques such as myocardial preservation and haemofiltration.

The heart–lung bypass machine (Figure 3.7) consists of two major components. The first of these is the pump itself. In paediatrics, this is usually a roller pump. The roller pump is essentially a peristaltic pump in which a horseshoe of tubing is compressed by a rotating arm. Different sizes of tubing can be used depending on the size of the patient. A larger size tube will give more blood flow per revolution of the pump head, but will need a larger amount of fluid to fill it. The speed of rotation of the pump is controlled by the perfusionist, and this enables the perfusionist to control the flow rate of blood around the patient's body.

The other type of pump used, usually only in larger paediatric patients and adults, is the centrifugal or constrained vortex pump. These pumps have spinning cones or impellers in a shaped housing that create a vortex. The inlet to the pump is in the centre of the vortex, which has a low pressure, and the outlet of the pump is at the edge, which has a high pressure. In this way, kinetic energy is added to the blood and forward flow is achieved. Once again, the flow rate of the blood is controlled by the perfusionist changing the rate at which the pump revolves. The physical conditions of the vortex mean that these pumps function less well at low flow rates and are therefore not as practical for use on smaller patients. Both types of pump are commonly known as an arterial pump.

We now have a way of replacing the function of the heart, and next we need to replicate the function of the lungs. For this, we use an oxygenator. In the oxygenator is a bundle of hollow fibres. The blood flows around the outside of the fibres, and an air–oxygen mix from a gas blender is passed down the centre of each fibre. The fibres are gas but not fluid permeable, which enables gas transfer to occur across the fibre without any fluid leak. Changes to the amount of oxygen in the blood can be made

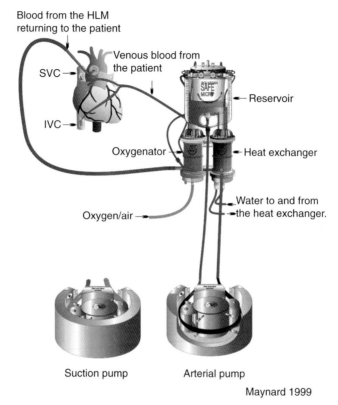

Blood from the HLM
returning to the patient

Venous blood from
the patient

SVC

Reservoir

IVC

Oxygenator

Heat exchanger

Water to and from
the heat exchanger.

Oxygen/air

Suction pump

Arterial pump

Maynard 1999

Figure 3.7 The heart–lung machine (HLM) (from Maynard, 1999, with permission). IVC, inferior vena cava; SVC, superior vena cava

by altering the fraction of inspired oxygen (FiO_2) of the gas, and changes to the amount of carbon dioxide in the blood can be made by altering the flow rate of the gas through the oxygenator. If needed, extra carbon dioxide can be added through the gas blender. For added efficiency, the blood flow and gas flow are usually countercurrent.

Usually within the same housing as the oxygenator is a heat exchanger. This is often made up of stainless steel tubes or plates. The blood flows around the outside of the heat exchanger, with water flowing through the inside. By altering the temperature of the water, it is possible to change the temperature of the blood. Therefore, once that blood is flowing around the patient, the core temperature of that patient can be controlled.

A venous reservoir is connected to the oxygenator/heat exchanger. This is where blood that drains from the patient, usually by gravity alone, is stored prior to being pumped through the oxygenator/heat exchanger and back into the patient. This acts as a capacitance reservoir that allows blood flow to be maintained at a constant rate when small fluctuations in venous drainage occur. It also contains a filter medium to remove any particulate matter, and helps to remove any air that may come down the venous line. These are the basic components of the bypass circuit, but further equipment is also needed to help maintain patient safety and aid the surgeon in the operation.

Any blood that is lost into the surgical field during the bypass run will usually be returned to the venous reservoir and thus the circulation via the pump suckers. The pump suckers are extra pumps that are similar to the main arterial roller pump used to pump the blood around the body. One of these suckers is often placed in the left side of the heart or aorta. This is to prevent any distension and thus damage to the heart that could be caused by blood that may return to the heart, either from the pulmonary veins and the bronchial circulation or from any congenital defects such as ASDs or VSDs. The suckers should also have one-way and pressure relief valves in the tubing to prevent excessive suction or air being pumped into the heart if the tubing is placed in the pump incorrectly.

The basic bypass circuit will perfuse the whole body, but to enable the heart to be opened or operated on without beating, it needs to be artificially arrested. The two most common ways of achieving this are direct application of a low-power electrical current to the heart, causing fibrillation, or using a cardioplegia solution injected into the coronary circulation and causing diastolic arrest. The major advantages of using cardioplegia are twofold. First, it provides a completely bloodless and non-moving heart that is easier to operate on. Second, it also protects the myocardial muscle by providing it with a source of oxygen and other chemicals that prevent damage to the muscle cells.

The method by which cardioplegia arrests the heart is a high dose of potassium (usually 15–20mmol/L) to cause electromechanical diastolic arrest. Often, a much higher concentration of potassium in saline is mixed with blood from the patient, commonly in a 4:1 ratio. This produces a solution with the desired levels of potassium and enough nutrients from the blood to maintain a good level of myocardial protection. The cardioplegia solution is cooled prior to delivery to help stop the heart and reduce its oxygen requirement. The resulting blood cardioplegia solution will also ideally be slightly hyperosmolar and have a high enough colloid osmotic pressure to prevent myocardial oedema.

The cardioplegia solution is usually delivered to the coronary circulation via the aorta. A small cannula is placed in the aorta, and when the heart needs to be stopped a cross-clamp is placed across the aorta, stopping blood flow from the bypass machine entering the coronary circulation. The cardioplegia solution is then pumped through the cardioplegia cannula. The cardioplegia cannula is placed between the aortic root, with the aortic valve closed, preventing flow into the heart, and the cross-clamp so that the cardioplegia solution can only enter the coronary circulation. The effect of the cardioplegia lasts for approximately 20–30 minutes. After this time, further slightly smaller doses can be given if necessary. To restart the heart, the cross-clamp is removed and blood starts to flow through the coronary circulation. As the cardioplegia solution is washed out by the blood, the heart muscle will slowly start to function normally.

A haemoconcentrator is often included in the circuit. This is primarily used to remove water from the circulating blood. It is most commonly situated as an arterio-venous shunt, with the blood flow through the haemoconcentrator controlled by either a physical restriction in the tubing or a pump. When using this system, a small amount of the blood that would normally be returned via the arterial line to the patient is passed through the haemoconcentrator, and water is removed. The concentrated blood is then returned to the venous reservoir and thus into the circulation. The fluid removed also contains electrolytes, which gives the perfusionist a means of altering the electrolyte levels during the bypass run. Increasingly, the filter is also used before the bypass to remove toxins from the priming solution (Table 3.4). The haemoconcentrator can also be used after the bypass to remove excess fluid from the patient.

Table 3.4 Packed red cell/pump blood prime values

	Packed red cells	Pump blood prime
Blood gas values		
pH	6.682	7.378
Partial pressure of CO_2 (kPa)	12.4	5.28
Partial pressure of O_2 (kPa)	6.79	17.9
Acid–base status		
Concentration of bicarbonate ions (mmol/L)	10.4	23
Oximetry values		
Concentration of total haemoglobin (g/dL)	21.2	9.4
Fraction of oxygen in haemoglobin (%)	58.8	97.5
Oxygen saturation (%)	59	99.1
Fraction of carboxyhaemoglobin (%)	0.3	0.3
Fraction of methaemoglobin (%)	0.7	0.7
Calculated values		
Haematocrit (%)	64.5	29.1
Electrolyte values		
Concentration of potassium ions (mmol/L)	17.7	3.8
Concentration of sodium ions (mmol/L)	126	144
Concentration of calcium ions (mmol/L)	0.11	1.04
Concentration of chloride ions (mmol/L)	113	113
Anion gap (mmol/L)	2.5	32.5
Osmolarity (mmol/kg)	275.5	292.3
Metabolite values		
Glucose (mmol/L)	22.9	1.3
Lactate (mmol/L)	18	0.6

This has the beneficial effects of clotting factor concentration as well as haemoconcentration. Along with these benefits, post-bypass ultrafiltration has also been shown to reduce patient oedema by increasing the colloid osmotic pressure of the blood.

In addition to the major components of the circuit, safety and monitoring devices are used. A level detector is placed on the venous reservoir to prevent the level of blood in the reservoir dropping to such a point that air may be introduced into the circuit. An ultrasonic bubble detector is placed, usually in the arterial line leading to the patient, which will stop the pump if air is detected. This should prevent any air being pumped into the patient. The pressure in the arterial side of the circuit is measured to prevent overpressurisation due to kinks in the tubing or obstructions in or caused by the arterial cannula.

The components of the circuit are recognised by the body as being a foreign surface, so the blood will start clot if the patient is not anticoagulated. The most common form of anticoagulation is heparin. Heparin works primarily by increasing the effect of antithrombin III. This stops fibrinogen being turned into fibrin, and prothrombin into thrombin. To check the function of the heparin, blood clotting times are measured throughout the bypass run. If the activated clotting time drops below 480–500 seconds, a further bolus of heparin will be given. Once the CPB run has been completed, the heparin is reversed using protamine. This works by binding to the heparin and rendering it inactive.

It is now common to have continuous in-line blood gas measurement. This gives better control of the blood gases during bypass. In addition, some form of non-invasive cerebral saturation monitoring such as NIRS or transcranial Doppler scans are becoming more common.

The course of a standard bypass run

Prior to the start of the operation, the perfusionist obtains the height and weight of the patient. The body surface area (BSA) is calculated using a nomogram and is checked using the formula:

$$BSA = \frac{\sqrt{Height\ (in\ cm) \times weight\ (in\ kg)}}{3600}$$

This calculation is used to determine the blood flow rate that the patient needs during the time on bypass to maintain good organ function. For a neonate or small paediatric patient, a cardiac index of 2.8–3 L/m^2 is used. This means that a calculated blood flow of 2.8–3.0 L/m^2 is necessary to keep them alive and well perfused whilst on CPB. Using the calculated flow required as a guide, the appropriately sized CPB circuit components are chosen and assembled. The tubing and oxygenators used in CPB come in different sizes. This is to enable the priming volume of the circuit to be kept to a minimum whilst making sure the tubing and oxygenator are large enough to handle the flow rates required.

The oxygenator and circuit are then assembled and primed. The prime constituents are dependent on the patient's size and preoperative blood gases. Assuming a normal haemoglobin level of 12 g/dL in a neonate or small paediatric patient, some blood has to be added to the prime. If blood is not added, the volume of the circuit would mix with the patient's circulating volume when CPB was commenced, to produce a haemoglobin level that would not be high enough to maintain adequate oxygenation.

The priming solution is likely to consist of:

■ crystalloid (Plasmalyte);
■ colloid (albumin or Gelofusine);
■ blood;
■ mannitol;
■ heparin;
■ sodium bicarbonate;
■ calcium chloride;
■ steroids.

The ingredients are mixed so the prime is balanced with no base deficit and the electrolytes are within normal ranges. In addition, the haemoglobin level of the priming solution is such that, when CPB commences, the haemoglobin of the combined patient blood and circuit prime is approximately 10 g/dL.

It is now considered beneficial to wash any blood that is added to the prime as donated bank blood has high levels of potassium, lactate and glucose. If these are not removed prior to commencement of CPB, they can have a detrimental effect. They can be removed either by washing the blood in a cell saver or by adding a large volume of extra crystalloid to the prime and removing the excess through the haemofilter. As the crystalloid is removed by the haemofilter, the excess potassium, lactate and glucose are removed with it.

The patient is then prepared for surgery. The CPB circuit has a sterile portion, which is handed to the surgeons in the sterile surgical field. The lines are then secured to the operating table. Once the chest has been opened, the heart exposed and the major vessels identified, the primed circuit is clamped by the perfusionist, and then clamped and divided at the table by the surgeons.

The patient will then be heparinised by the anaesthetist. Once the heparinisation has been verified by means of an activated clotting time, a cannula will be placed in the patient's ascending aorta and secured using a purse-string suture. This cannula will then be connected to the CPB circuit and its patency checked by the perfusionist. Next, a venous cannula will be placed in the patient's superior vena cava, and this is connected to the venous line of the bypass circuit. A second venous cannula will be placed in the patient's inferior vena cava, which is also connected to the venous line of the bypass circuit. If there is a left superior vena cava, this may require a third cannula. In some cases, it may be possible to just use a single venous cannula placed in the right atrium.

On the surgeons' instruction, CPB is initiated. All the blood that would normally return to the right side of the patient's heart is siphoned down the venous line of the bypass circuit into the venous reservoir. From here, it is pumped through the oxygenator by the arterial pump. Oxygen is added to the blood and carbon dioxide is removed. Once adequate blood flow has been achieved, the ventilation can be turned off. When the blood has passed through the oxygenator and heat exchanger, it goes through the bubble detector. The blood will then pass through the in-line blood gas measuring sensor. From there, it goes up the arterial line, through the arterial cannula and into the aorta.

If the surgeon has decided that the patient needs to be cooled to reduce the metabolic demand, the patient's core temperature can be lowered to the required temperature once CPB has commenced. This process will take between 5 and 25 minutes, depending on the degree of cooling needed. Once the temperature has reached the required level and if the heart needs to be arrested, the cross-clamp is put across the aorta between the heart and the aortic cannula. Once the heart has been stopped and isolated from the rest of the circulation, the surgeon will continue with the operation. Further doses of cardioplegia solution may be given every 20–30 minutes as needed.

Some types of neonatal and paediatric cardiac surgery require a technique known as deep hypothermic circulatory arrest (DHCA). The patient can be cooled to a core temperature of 15–20 °C. Once this temperature has been reached, the circulation can be turned off and the patient drained of blood. This state allows the surgeon to perform extremely complex surgery. As the patient has no blood flowing at all, the cannula can be removed, giving good visibility and access to the heart. This state can be maintained relatively safely for up to 40 minutes.

During the course of the CPB, blood gases are continuously monitored, and electrolytes are measured every 15–20 minutes. Any abnormalities are corrected to maintain normal levels. Haemoglobin levels are also maintained above 10 g/dL, either by adding red cells or by removing water using a haemofilter.

Once the operation is complete, the cross-clamp will be removed and the patient will be slowly rewarmed. With the patient reaching normothermia, the amount of blood returning to the bypass machine will be reduced by partially obstructing the venous line with a clamp. This forces some blood through the right side of the heart and through the lungs. Once this occurs, the patient's heart will start pumping. The ventilation will be recommenced. The amount of blood going to the bypass machine will be gradually reduced until the venous line has been completely occluded and all the blood is being pumped by the heart. The pump will then be turned off. At this stage, post-bypass ultrafiltration will be performed if needed. The patient will then be decannulated and handed back to the care of the anaesthetist.

Anaesthesia and cardiopulmonary bypass

Communication between both the anaesthetist and perfusionist is important as every action taken can have a consequence affecting both of them. Depending on the practice of each individual and unit, the anaesthetist may be involved in the administration of cardioplegia, aid cooling and rewarming with vasodilators such as sodium nitroprusside, and control perfusion pressure with vasopressors such as phenylephrine. Anaesthesia may be maintained with volatile agents or, in older children, with intravenous infusions such as propofol or ketamine. This is supplemented by further doses of opioids, hypnotics and muscle relaxants according to the technique adopted.

Separation from bypass

Separation from bypass following surgery is a critical point, and blood gases, ventilation and cardiac output must be optimised for it to succeed. With regard to the cardiovascular status of the patient, an adequate rate and rhythm need to be established (this can be assisted with sequential pacing of both atrium and ventricle). Inotropes, vasopressors and vasodilators to support cardiac function are commenced based on 'eyeballing' the heart function, haemodynamics numbers and quantitative assessment with echocardiography. Using echocardiography, the adequacy of surgical repair can be ascertained, as can the detection of ischaemia, which is indicated by abnormal regional wall movement. This may correlate with ECG changes. This can be transient, as caused by air in the coronary arteries, or may suggest the need for further surgical intervention before separation from CPB.

Interrelated with cardiovascular status is adequacy of ventilation. The compliance of the lung is decreased during bypass because of increased interstitial fluid, and reduced functional residual capacity associated with anaesthesia will increase the ventilation–perfusion mismatch and necessitate high inspiratory oxygen levels to achieve adequate oxygenation. Surgery, especially operations involving the pulmonary arteries, conditions with high left atrial pressures and recent respiratory chest infections will lead to blood or increased secretions in the bronchial tree. Removal of this, as well as blood or fluid that may have accumulated in the pleural spaces during surgery, will improve ventilation after surgery. Surgical access allows direct vision of the lungs and optimal reinflation of the lungs following surgery.

Balancing adequacy of ventilation and oxygenation can be difficult and alter depending on the situation. A high inspiratory oxygen concentration and low arterial partial pressure of carbon dioxide will reduce pulmonary vascular resistance. This may be beneficial when pulmonary hypertension is encountered. Conversely, in single-ventricle physiology, high pulmonary blood flow and resultant 'stealing' from the systemic circulation can be reduced by raising pulmonary vascular resistance with low inspiratory oxygen concentrations and relative hypoventilation, to raise the arterial partial pressure of carbon dioxide.

Positive-pressure ventilation can produce problems. High intrathoracic pressure may cause barotrauma or contribute to ventilator-induced lung injury. High pressure may also result in cardiovascular instability. This is particularly true when pulmonary blood flow is driven by venous pressure, such as in the Fontan circulation. During positive-pressure ventilation, there is little or no flow into the pulmonary bed during inspiration. It can be difficult in these cases to balance oxygenation, adequacy of ventilation and control of arterial carbon dioxide whilst limiting intrathoracic pressure to improve pulmonary blood flow.

Adequate rewarming to normothermia and correction of acid–base, metabolic and electrolyte abnormalities are also important. Metabolic acidosis and abnormal potassium levels are commonly encountered and must be treated. It is also important to maintain the ionised calcium level, especially in neonates, whose heart contractility is improved with higher calcium levels.

Separation from bypass is a dynamic event and is constantly evolving. All the factors mentioned above will be readdressed throughout this period and acted upon to provide stability. If separation proves difficult or impossible and all factors including surgery have been covered, continuing support with extracorporeal membrane oxygenation may be appropriate. Indications and technical issues are covered elsewhere.

Once the patient has been separated from bypass and is stable, and any surgical bleeding has been addressed, protamine sulphate is used to reverse heparinisation. A dose ratio of between 1:1 and 2:1 is used. Protamine causes a drop in systemic vascular resistance and a possible increase in pulmonary vascular resistance. Slow administration is advised as these actions may lead to a patient decompensating.

Further bleeding may be due to a resultant coagulopathy: platelet function is reduced following CPB, and platelet transfusions are commonly used to treat non-surgical bleeding post CPB. Cryoprecipitate and fresh frozen plasma are also used. Tranexamic acid and aprotinin are used to treat fibrinolytic states. Increasingly, as mentioned above, therapy with protamine and other factors is being directed using results from TEG.

Factor VII has been used as rescue therapy to treat non-surgical bleeding when other methods have been exhausted. It is not used as the mainstay for treating such coagulopathies as little is yet known about possible adverse events such as an increasing incidence of thrombosis.

Closure of the chest and wiring of the sternum have physiological consequences. Chest compliance decreases and may require an altered ventilation strategy to achieve adequate ventilation and oxygenation. Chest closure may also cause physical tamponade of the heart and reduce cardiac output. This is particularly true in neonates and small infants undergoing complex operations, and it is common practice to leave the chest 'open' and to delay closure for 1 or 2 days to allow recovery.

The child is transferred to intensive care to continue recovery once the operation has been completed and the child is stable. Sedation may be required, and analgesia is usually provided by an opioid infusion. Careful conduct is necessary to allow the safe transfer of these patients. It is not uncommon for instability to occur during this stage.

This description is a summary of paediatric cardiac anaesthesia highlighting the various important issues encountered. For further more comprehensive reading on this and other aspects of paediatric anaesthesia, see Lake (1988) and Brown & Fisk (1979).

Introduction to paediatric cardiac surgery

Paediatric cardiac surgery is a relatively young surgical specialty. In recent years, due to improvements in pre-, peri- and postoperative diagnosis and management, overall operative mortality rates have fallen to approximately 4%. This aim of this part of the chapter is to provide an introduction to and overview of the principles of surgical management. Typically, the surgical decisions and management are tailored to the individual patient, particularly for the increasingly more complex work that is being undertaken. A coverage of all aspects of surgical care is outside the scope of this book, and a wider understanding may be obtained by reading Stark et al (2004).

Traditionally, defects have been considered as simple and complex and further divided into:

■ obstructive lesions;
■ left-to-right shunts (acyanotic);
■ right-to-left shunts (cyanotic);
■ complex mixing defects.

An important aspect to consider in each case is whether pulmonary blood flow (Qp) is normal, increased or decreased (see Chapter 2). With this classification in place, it is possible to approach each surgical operation with the object of relieving obstruction, which may occur at the inflow as well as the outflow to a heart chamber, if possible correcting shunts, and balancing pulmonary blood flow against an adequate systemic blood flow (Qs).

The natural history of defects is important with respect to the timing of repair. There has been a gradual move away from early (neonatal) palliation and later repair to single-stage repair, often in the early neonatal period. This shift has been driven by improvements at multiple levels of care in the belief that early definitive repair will provide better outcomes.

The context of any patient presentation is very important to achieve a good outcome. An example is the presentation of a 1.5 kg neonate with cyanosis and tetralogy of Fallot, who will in most centres be treated with an initial systemic-to-pulmonary-artery shunt (to improve pulmonary blood flow) and subsequent full repair. The same defect presenting in a 3.5 kg neonate will for the most part be treated with full repair (VSD closure and reconstruction of the RVOT).

Conduct of paediatric cardiac surgery

The conduct of each operation depends on the nature of the defects to be repaired. An anterior approach via a median sternotomy is the most common approach to the heart, with partial or complete removal of the thymus gland as this is large and obscures the surgical field in children. For some procedures, for example coarctation repair or PDA ligation, a thoracotomy is used. Currently, thoracoscopic techniques have a limited role, used in some centres for clipping a PDA or creation of a pericardial window.

The next consideration is to whether the surgery will require the use of CPB (the 'heart–lung machine' as discussed earlier). Simple lesions not requiring work within the heart, such as pulmonary artery banding and PDA ligation, can usually be performed without CPB. As the surgical complexity increases, CPB is required to give the surgeon maximum control of the operative field without compromising the systemic perfusion. CPB allows the surgeon to provide systemic oxygenated perfusion, control temperature and acid–base/electrolyte balance but allows the heart to beat empty. If an intracardiac procedure is required necessitating a still heart and a bloodless field, cross-clamping the aorta and instilling high-potassium cardioplegia solution into the aortic root results in diastolic cardiac arrest while the repair is undertaken.

Despite these techniques, some complex cases (aortic arch repair) require the circulation to be stopped completely using the technique of DHCA. Many variations exist, but in general temperatures of 15–18 °C are tolerated for periods up to 40 minutes (Wypij et al, 2003). Newer techniques such as selective antegrade cerebral perfusion and intermittent reperfusion are increasingly used to reduce and avoid periods of DHCA.

Surgical repair frequently requires the placement of patches or tubes to either redirect blood flow within the heart or provide flow to structures outside the heart, such as conduits to the pulmonary artery to improve pulmonary blood flow. These conduits can be either autologous tissue (e.g. the patient's own pericardium to close an ASD) or xenografts. Xenografts are either human tissue (homografts – tissue patches and valves) or animal tissue (heterografts – bovine pericardium and porcine or bovine valves). In addition, synthetic patches and tubes may be used constructed from Dacron or Gore-tex. An important aspect of all these tissues is that they do not grow with the patient and, in the case of biological tissues, they undergo time-dependent degeneration, both of which may require reoperation. In addition, foreign tissue may become infected, requiring its removal.

At the closure of most cardiac operations, drains are placed in the pericardial and pleural cavities and temporary pacing wires are placed on the heart to allow postoperative control of the heart rate and rhythm. In patients who will require further operations, a Gore-tex membrane or equivalent may be placed behind the sternum to facilitate safe sternal re-entry.

Pure obstructive lesions

Although obstruction as an isolated defect can occur at any level of the circulation (inflow, within the cardiac mass or outflow), the most common lesions are those of congenital aortic stenosis or pulmonary stenosis as well as the spectrum of coarctation of the aorta, including interrupted aortic arch. In general, the obstructed circulation limits forward flow, which can developmentally result in ventricular hypoplasia or in a hypertrophic ventricular response. A spectrum of obstruction is usually seen, and this determines the age of presentation as well as the urgency with which relief of obstruction is required. An important aspect of obstructive physiology, especially if it is severe, is that the downstream circulations (pulmonary in the case of pulmonary stenosis and systemic in the case of atrial stenosis, coarctation of the aorta and interrupted aortic arch) are *duct dependent*.

This introduces an important physiological consequence of transfer from fetal to neonatal life. The ductus arteriosus, which connects the pulmonary artery to the aortic arch, is a normal fetal structure that allows flow within the high-resistance fetal pulmonary circulation to be directed to the descending thoracic aorta, and hence provides a route to the placenta for deoxygenated blood. Oxygenated blood from the placenta returns to the right atrium via the inferior vena cava and, through the process of streaming, is shunted via the patent foramen ovale at atrial level to the left-sided circulation for flow in the systemic circulation. Transfer from fetal to neonatal life has as an important consequence for these structures, namely duct and patent foramen ovale closure. These events are important as patency of the duct and patent foramen ovale enable mixing at both atrial and ductal levels. In the setting of a *duct-dependent* circulation, the use of intravenous prostaglandin is vital to maintain duct patency prior to surgical or catheter intervention.

Pulmonary stenosis

This group of patients usually has valvular obstruction, but the condition may occur or be associated with dynamic or fixed obstruction at both the subvalvular and/or supravalvular levels, ranging from mild to severe. The presentation of severe pulmonary stenosis is usually in the neonatal period with reduced pulmonary blood flow, a *duct-dependent* pulmonary circulation and variable degrees of right-to-left shunting at atrial level via the foramen ovale (causing cyanosis). The right ventricle is usually thickened (hypertrophied) in response to the obstruction.

Treatment options

Medically, intravenous prostaglandin (E_1) is used to maintain duct-dependent pulmonary blood flow as a temporary measure. The treatment of choice is balloon (performed in the catheter laboratory, see 'Balloon aortic valvuloplasty', above) or open surgical valvotomy to relieve obstruction. A systemic-to-pulmonary shunt (a modified Blalock–Taussig shunt) is indicated in the setting of a small right ventricle/tricuspid valve.

Aortic stenosis

Like pulmonary stenosis, the level of obstruction can be valvular, subvalvular or supravalvular. All result in a restriction to flow from the left ventricle. Critical aortic stenosis presents with a low-cardiac output state and a duct-dependent systemic circulation. Duct closure is an important event in this circulation and, if not corrected with the introduction of prostaglandin E_1, will result in death.

Treatment options

Balloon valvoplasty or surgical valvotomy is needed. In addition, the resection of subvalvular tissue and patch augmentation of supravalvular narrowing may be indicated.

Valve replacement is sometimes required, especially if a large regurgitant component is present, for example after valvotomy. Replacement options in small children are limited because of the limited haemodynamics of currently available commercial valves (bioprosthetic or mechanical), the need for growth and biological tissue degeneration. A useful approach in some children is the use of the patient's own pulmonary valve (pulmonary autograft) as part of the Ross procedure.

Lesser degrees of both pulmonary and aortic stenosis that are not duct dependent have a huge number of possible presentations from the neonatal period to late adult life, including asymptomatic murmur, ventricular failure, angina, syncope, arrhythmias, cyanosis, endocarditis and sudden cardiac death. In general, catheter or surgical intervention is required for all symptomatic patients, patients with increasing gradients and those with complications, for example endocarditis.

Coarctation of the aorta

This is a common obstructive lesion to systemic blood flow at the level of the aortic isthmus (the area of duct insertion distal to the origin of the left subclavian artery).

It may be an isolated defect, but a number of common associations exist, including bicuspid aortic valve disease and VSD. In addition, the aortic arch may be hypoplastic or, in its extreme form, totally interrupted. Once again, the spectrum of disease is such that critical coarctation may present soon after birth with shock and a *duct-dependent* circulation, whilst others may only be appreciated in adult life when 'hypertension' is being investigated. Right-to-left shunting at the ductal level for critical coarctation maintains an important physiological adaptation producing lower limb cyanosis in association with normally saturated upper limbs. In this instance, duct closure may be life threatening.

Treatment options

The obstruction needs to be relieved. In neonates, infants and young children, this is best achieved via surgery, but in older patients balloon dilatation is the intervention of choice (see 'Balloon aortic valvuloplasty', above). An isolated coarctation is approached via a left thoracotomy without using CPB. The narrow section is resected, including all ductal tissue, and the aorta is reconstructed with an end-to-end anastomosis. An alternative in a neonate is to ligate and divide the left subclavian artery and turn down the proximal end of the subclavian artery to widen the narrowed aorta. This is usually well tolerated without any acute or chronic arm ischaemia.

More complex coarctations, particularly those involving hypoplasia of the aortic arch, are dealt with via median sternotomy and patching of the aorta using CPB. Similarly, the treatment of coarctation with associated defects such as VSD requires a median sternotomy and CPB. Arch interruption is managed via median sternotomy, CPB and arch reconstruction, often requiring periods of DHCA with or without selective antegrade cerebral perfusion.

Simple left-to-right shunts

This group of acyanotic conditions is characterised by a left-to-right shunt with increased pulmonary blood flow. It includes ASD, VSD, PDA and atrioventricular septal defects (AVSDs).

A number of common physiological consequences occur as a result of left-to-right shunting, including volume overload and dilatation of both the right and left sides of the heart with increased pulmonary blood flow. If untreated, this may result in arrhythmias, right ventricular dysfunction and pulmonary hypertension. Pulmonary hypertension which if longstanding may become fixed resulting in shunt reversal, i.e. right-to-left shunting, with cyanosis is called Eisenmenger syndrome.

Atrial septal defects

ASD describes a number of defects in the atrial septum, which may occur in isolation or in association with other defects.

Ostium secundum (fossa ovalis defect) is the most common (80%). The treatment of choice is catheter-based closure (see above), but if the lesion is not suitable for this, surgical repair can be undertaken via a sternotomy using CPB with direct or patch closure of the defect.

Ostium primum (partial AVSD) is part of the spectrum of AVSD and is usually associated with a cleft in the left-sided atrioventricular valve. This requires surgical closure via a sternotomy using CPB with patch closure of the defect and repair of the left-sided heart valve.

A sinus venosus defect typically occurs at the junction between the right atrium and the superior vena cava, and is almost always associated with anomalous drainage of the right-sided pulmonary veins. This requires surgical repair as the pulmonary venous blood needs to be redirected, usually through the ASD to the left atrium.

In unroofed coronary sinus, the coronary sinus drains the coronary veins and opens into the right atrium. A communication between the coronary sinus and left atrium will result in a coronary sinus ASD.

Ventricular septal defects

VSDs are a diverse group of defects that can be classified in terms of their location:

- Perimembranous defects border the membranous septum adjacent to the conduction system and are the most common type (75%).
- Muscular defects are usually located in the trabeculated septum and may be single or multiple. In the extreme form, the septum may be called 'Swiss cheese-like'.
- Doubly committed juxta-arterial defects lie immediately beneath the pulmonary valve.

Treatment options

Treatment depends on the size and type of defect, the symptoms and any coexisting cardiac and non-cardiac lesions. Large VSDs ($Qp:Qs > 1.8:1$) usually present with signs of congestive cardiac failure as the pulmonary vascular resistance falls and require closure by 3–6 months of age. Smaller VSDs may be asymptomatic and can be observed and may spontaneously close. This is more likely to occur with muscular defects.

Closure may be surgical or increasingly catheter based (see 'Balloon aortic valvuloplasty', above). Surgery requires a sternotomy, CPB and closure of the defect using a tissue or synthetic patch. A complication of both techniques is complete heart block requiring a pacemaker, due to the proximity of the conduction system, particularly with perimembranous defects.

Atrioventricular septal defect

AVSD is a distinct defect of the endocardial cushions resulting in a VSD beneath a common atrioventricular valve and an ASD immediately above the valve. This morphological defect is strongly associated with Down syndrome, accounting for over 50% of the associated cardiac lesions with a tendency to develop pulmonary hypertensive vascular disease. The size of the ASD, VSD and atrioventricular valve anatomy is variable. The timing of surgery depends upon the symptoms, the size of the VSD and the amount of atrioventricular valve regurgitation. Complete AVSDs require closure by 3–6 months of age. Partial AVSDs without a VSD (see above) are usually closed electively between 2 and 4 years of age.

Treatment options (see also above)

Surgery requires sternotomy, CPB and patch closure of the VSD and ASD with repair and the formation of two competent atrioventricular valves. There is an associated risk of compete heart block and progressive left atrioventricular valve regurgitation requiring further surgery.

If complete repair is not possible for a VSD and AVSD, for example if there are multiple muscular VSDs, coexisting medical problems or prematurity, pulmonary artery banding is undertaken to reduce pulmonary blood flow, protect the pulmonary vascular bed from high blood flow and pulmonary hypertensive disease, and allow later definitive repair if possible. This is an important surgical strategy used to balance Qp:Qs and is useful in many defects of excess pulmonary blood flow.

Right-to-left shunts (cyanotic defects with reduced pulmonary blood flow)

Lesions within this group include:

- tetralogy of Fallot;
- pulmonary atresia (with VSD or intact ventricular septum);
- tricuspid atresia;
- some patients with Ebstein malformation of the tricuspid valve.

The consequence of either functional or anatomical obstruction to flow is reduced pulmonary blood flow, usually with an associated right-to-left shunt (ASD or VSD). At the severe end of the spectrum, pulmonary blood flow and survival are dependent on maintaining ductal blood flow in the immediate postnatal period. Subsequent treatment is aimed at achieving a biventricular (tetralogy of Fallot and pulmonary atresia/VSD) repair, but this may require temporary palliation with the creation of a surgical shunt. For those patients in whom a biventricular repair is not possible (tricuspid atresia), a temporary shunt may be required followed by a more permanent source of pulmonary blood flow.

Surgically created palliative shunts are an important source of pulmonary blood flow. Due to persisting fetal-type physiology, decreasing pulmonary hypertension is present for the first 4–6 weeks of life. To overcome this elevated pressure, systemic-to-pulmonary artery shunts are created, with the most common being the modified Blalock–Taussig shunt. An alternative source of pulmonary blood flow is from the right ventricle either via a right-ventricle-to-pulmonary-artery shunt or conduit, or as part of complete correction with resection and enlargement of the RVOT. Subsequently, in a single-ventricle circulation, a cavopulmonary shunt (joining the superior vena cava to the pulmonary artery) is constructed to achieve longer-term balanced pulmonary and systemic blood flow. These venous shunts require a low pulmonary vascular resistance and are only undertaken after 3–4 months of age.

Tetralogy of Fallot

Tetralogy of Fallot is characterised by the presence of a large VSD, an overriding aorta, RVOT obstruction and secondary right ventricular hypertrophy. The RVOT obstruction usually has a significant infundibular muscular component, and this is responsible for the intermittent cyanotic 'spells' typical of this lesion. The heterogeneity of this congenital lesion is such that it may present in the early neonatal period with severe RVOT obstruction, reduced duct-dependent pulmonary blood flow and cyanosis (right-to-left shunting at the ventricular and atrial level) or late in adulthood with arrhythmias in the context of relatively balanced pulmonary blood flow.

Treatment options

In general, treatment for this condition is surgical, with VSD closure and resection of the RVOT obstruction with reconstruction (patch or homograft) via a sternotomy on CPB. Although many institutions are moving towards early complete repair, an alternative approach is a palliative systemic-to-pulmonary-artery (Blalock–Taussig)

> **Box 3.3** Beth's healthcare journey – surgery for tetralogy of Fallot, her parents' experience
>
> Beth went into theatre at 11 a.m. I just wanted to curl up in a ball. My husband couldn't face it so my good friend came with me. At 3 p.m., I was called to ITU; oh my god, Beth was so tiny, hooked up to all those machines and on a ventilator. Nothing could prepare me for this, but you have to be brave and be there for your child so you are. They kept sending me out as Beth kept dropping her sats. I was so frightened when this happened as you don't know what's going on – all you see are a lot of doctors and nurses rushing to your child, and machines start bleeping everywhere. Thank god my friend is a nurse and could explain it to me.

shunt when the child is a neonate to improve pulmonary blood flow, and repair later at 12–18 months of age.

One parent's experience of surgery is described in Box 3.3.

Pulmonary atresia with intact ventricular septum

This is a rare condition associated with an abnormal, usually small, right ventricle. The pulmonary circulation is duct dependent, and an ASD must be present to enable right-to-left shunting (creating cyanosis).

Treatment options

Medically, intravenous prostaglandin (E₁) is given as a temporary measure to maintain duct-dependent pulmonary blood flow. Adequate pulmonary blood flow is maintained either via a balloon or surgical valvotomy or by creating a systemic-to-pulmonary shunt (modified Blalock–Taussig shunt). Then there may be:

- biventricular repair in patients with an adequately sized right ventricle;
- single-ventricle repair with a cardiopulmonary shunt and ultimately Fontan circulation in patients with a very small right ventricle;
- one and a half ventricle repair for a small right ventricle.

Pulmonary atresia with ventricular septal defect

This is a distinct entity (previously thought to represent the severe end of the tetralogy of Fallot spectrum) where lung development has occurred in the context of limited/absent forward flow from the right ventricle. The right ventricle is usually of adequate size. In the extreme form of this condition, there are very small or no central pulmonary arteries, and MAPCAs have developed. These are vessels that originate from the aorta to provide a source of pulmonary blood flow.

Treatment options

The treatment options for this condition are complex and are made in the context of adequacy of the central pulmonary arteries, the condition of the pulmonary vasculature, the presence or absence of pulmonary hypertension and the extent of MAPCA development. A staged approach is not unusual, with an eventual establishment of central pulmonary arteries (native pulmonary arteries or focalised MAPCAs) fed from the low-pressure right ventricle via a valved conduit. For those patients with pulmonary atresia/VSD, an approach similar to that for tetralogy of Fallot will typically allow biventricular repair but usually requires the reconstruction of the RVOT with a valved conduit.

Tricuspid atresia

Tricuspid atresia is a single-ventricle cardiac congenital defect with atresia of the right atrioventricular junction and an ASD usually associated with hypoplasia of the right ventricle. Unlike most of the previous defects, biventricular repair is usually not possible. In general, this defect is associated with reduced pulmonary blood flow.

Treatment options

A systemic-to-pulmonary-artery (Blalock–Taussig) shunt is set up in the early neonatal period to improve pulmonary blood flow, and staged surgical palliation is then employed using cavopulmonary shunts (bidirectional Glenn and Fontan circulations).

Complex cyanotic defects

Lesions within this group include:

▪ double-outlet right ventricle;
▪ total anomalous pulmonary venous drainage;
▪ TGA;
▪ truncus arteriosus;
▪ HLHS and other single-ventricle congenital anomalies.

This is a diverse group of disorders whose complexities are beyond the scope of this chapter; a wider understating may be obtained by reading the book edited by Stark et al (2004). However, a number of principles apply:

▪ In general, a biventricular repair if possible is preferable to single-ventricle physiology.
▪ A poor biventricular repair with invariably high end-diastolic pressures is not a good end point, and single-ventricle physiology is preferable.
▪ Staged procedures are common in this group.
▪ Obstructive aspects of blood flow within these complex hearts must be relieved whenever possible.
▪ Qp:Qs must be balanced as much as possible to limit volume overload issues, providing for adequate oxygenation of pulmonary blood but in the context of adequate mixing.

Double-outlet right ventricle

This is a complex spectrum of disorders where one of the great arteries and more than 50% of the other great vessel (usually the aorta) are derived from the right ventricle. In addition, there are bilateral muscular infundibula with aortic and pulmonary valves at the same level, with loss of the fibrous continuity between the aortic and mitral valves. A VSD is present in all cases and represents the only outflow of the left ventricle. It is the position of the VSD (subpulmonary [Taussig–Bing anomaly], subaortic, doubly committed or uncommitted) and the presence or absence of pulmonary stenosis (Fallot's type) that determines the flow of blood into the great vessels, with either increased, decreased or relatively well balanced pulmonary blood flow. This determines the nature of the presentation of either congestive heart failure or cyanosis.

Treatment options

Pulmonary artery banding will reduce pulmonary blood flow, and atrial balloon or blade septectomy can be used for some patients with subpulmonary VSD to improve mixing. Systemic-to-pulmonary-artery shunts improve pulmonary blood flow for those with decreased pulmonary blood flow. These options are palliative, and for most patients full correction of the defect is possible using one of the following:

- intracardiac VSD closure that incorporates redirection of the left ventricular outflow to the aorta;
- if left ventricular flow cannot be directed to the aorta but can be reconstructed to the pulmonary artery (hence producing TGA), this can be combined with either an arterial or an atrial switch procedure;
- in the Fallot's type, the procedure must include not only VSD closure, but also relief of the pulmonary stenosis (patch augmentation or placement of a valved conduit);
- in the small group of patients in whom left ventricular flow cannot be redirected to the aorta, a staged single-ventricle/Fontan circulation may be required.

Total anomalous pulmonary venous drainage

This defect is present when all the pulmonary veins that usually drain to the left atrium are connected to the right-sided circulation, thus providing complete mixing at right atrial level. An ASD must be present to allow flow to the left (systemic) side of the heart. The adequacy of the ASD and the presence of pulmonary venous obstruction are important considerations in this defect. Three types are commonly appreciated:

1. *Supracardiac*: drainage is directly into the superior vena cava or vertical vein (which drains into the innominate vein).
2. *Intracardiac*: the common pulmonary vein drains into the coronary sinus or posteriorly into the right atrium.
3. *Infracardiac*: inferior drainage is through the diaphragm to the portal, hepatic or inferior vena caval vein.

The risk of venous obstruction is highest for the infracardiac type as the vein passes through the diaphragm and joins the hepatic circulation. Intracardiac veins are rarely obstructed, and supracardiac veins may become obstructed at the level of the left bronchus/pulmonary artery or on joining the systemic veins.

The degree of obstruction determines the age of presentation with cyanosis and/ or congestive cardiac failure. Patients with obstructed veins require resuscitation and urgent surgery. Patients without obstructions are usually operated on electively.

Treatment options

Supra- and infracardiac types are repaired by anastomosing the confluence of the pulmonary veins directly to the left atrium and closing the ASD. The intracardiac type is repaired by either unroofing the coronary sinus into the left atrium or directing the coronary sinus flow to the left atrium using the ASD (which usually requires ASD enlargement).

Transposition of the great arteries

Although many variations are possible, the most common form, 'simple TGA' (D-TGA), will be discussed here. The defect consists of transposed great vessels with the aorta arising from the right ventricle and the pulmonary artery from the left ventricle. The position of the aorta relative to the pulmonary artery is usually anterior and to the right. About 30% of patients have a VSD, and up to 10% have subpulmonary stenosis.

Adequate mixing of the right and left circulations is required for survival, and this can occur at the atrial, ventricular or ductal level. Balloon atrial septostomy is often undertaken to ensure adequate mixing (see above). Important aspects that determine the treatment option for this condition include age of presentation, pulmonary stenosis, subaortic stenosis, the presence of multiple VSDs and the pattern of the coronary arteries.

Treatment options

The arterial switch operation is currently the operation of choice for most infants with TGA, including those with milder forms of pulmonary stenosis and coronary artery abnormalities. A coexisting VSD can be closed at the same time. TGA and VSD with significant pulmonary stenosis is treated by placement of an intraventricular patch to direct blood from the left ventricle to the aorta and a valved conduit from the right ventricle to the pulmonary artery (Rastelli procedure). The atrial switch using either the Senning or Mustard operation is mainly historical but is still considered in patients with contraindications to an arterial switch.

The group of patients who present late (after 6 weeks of age) with TGA and an intact ventricular septum have usually had significant left ventricular involution. This has occurred because the morphological left ventricle has been working at pulmonary artery pressure and is not sufficiently trained to support the systemic circulation. A pulmonary artery band can be used to train these ventricles in preparation for a second-stage arterial switch operation.

Truncus arteriosus

This is a defect that results from the absence of the aortopulmonary septum. It results in a single great vessel arising from the heart supplying the aorta, pulmonary and coronary arteries, with a VSD underlying a truncal valve. A number of associations are commonly found, including a right aortic arch (30%), various coronary abnormalities and DiGeorge syndrome with associated hypocalcaemia (30%). Various classification systems have been developed, most relating to the pattern of the pulmonary arteries arising from the aorta. The physiological consequences of this defect are excess pulmonary blood flow and intracardiac mixing resulting in cyanosis and congestive heart failure. Repair is indicated for all patients by 2–3 months of life to prevent pulmonary vascular disease (fixed pulmonary hypertension), and sooner in those patients with intractable congestive cardiac failure.

Treatment options

Full repair is with VSD closure, disconnection of the pulmonary arteries from the aorta, central pulmonary artery reconstruction and a right ventricle–pulmonary artery conduit. Pulmonary artery banding is used by some, especially in high-risk small neonates, but mortality with the procedure is high. The functional status of the truncal valve has a significant bearing on outcome, and truncal valve repair for moderate-to-severe regurgitation may also be undertaken at the time of corrective surgery.

Hypoplastic left heart syndrome

This is a complex defect that illustrates many of the diverse aspects of paediatric cardiac surgery. Hypoplasia or underdevelopment of the left-sided heart structures results in a small left ventricle that is not able to support the systemic circulation.

The neonatal circulation is duct dependent, and unrestricted flow across the atrial septum is mandatory for survival. Once universally fatal, this defect can now be palliated using a variety of approaches, with high-volume centres achieving 10% first-stage mortality and survival to 1 year of about 80%. Surgery is palliative with the aim of creating a single-ventricle circulation with the pulmonary and systemic circulations in series. This requires a staged surgical approach with the end point being the Fontan circulation.

Treatment options

Options are:

■ termination of pregnancy;
■ comfort care only;
■ transplantation;
■ staged surgical palliation.

Surgical palliation consists of the Norwood operation to correct outflow tract obstruction (Damus connection and arch reconstruction), allow adequate intracardiac mixing (atrial septectomy) and balance pulmonary blood flow (systemic shunt or right-ventricular-to-pulmonary-artery shunt). Subsequently, a bidirectional Glenn shunt joining the superior vena cava directly to the pulmonary artery is performed at 3–6 months, and a later Fontan completion joining the inferior vena cava to the pulmonary artery at 4–5 years of age completes this three-stage palliation approach. This approach leaves the right ventricle as the systemic ventricle, and the long-term outcome of this is not currently known.

A recent alternative approach is the 'hybrid' procedure, which incorporates ductal stenting and bilateral pulmonary artery bands as the first-stage procedure with deferral of the Damus connection/arch reconstruction, pulmonary artery debanding/reconstruction and bidirectional Glenn shunt to 3–6 months of age.

Postoperative management

This section will concentrate on immediate postoperative care and clinical decision-making, making reference to ongoing patient management and discharge (Box 3.4).

When about to embark on the care of any child following paediatric cardiac surgery, there are some general 'rules' to consider. Most important is to know the type of operation: is it palliative or corrective surgery? And if not corrective, what parameters will be 'normal'? – if in doubt, ask the surgeon. The age of the patient is also important as a determinant of likely postoperative progress – how quickly the child will extubate, the anticipated circulating blood volume, neonatally related complications that are anticipated due to immature immune function, etc. These questions are sound

Box 3.4 Beth's journey – the postoperative experience

The next morning, Beth's sats had settled, but the doctors decided to keep her sedated for another 24 hours. Her consultant was brilliant and called in every day to see us. Once Beth was back on the ward, it was another 2 weeks before we went home as she didn't want to feed, but sadly after only a week home we were back on the ward with RSV virus. Beth was very poorly and we spent our first Christmas and New Year there. Then we were sent home with a feeding tube as she no longer wanted to feed by herself. I had to learn how to replace the tube, which was indeed scary but I got the hang of it.

For the next year and a half, we were in and out of hospital with infections, etc. Beth's immune system wasn't doing so well, and then in March 2004 she passed out in her dad's arms. This happened several times in one week, and her cardiac surgeon decided she needed open heart surgery. On March 23rd, she went down to theatre and came back 6 hours later – she had done well and her surgeon was very happy with her progress. We were home within 10 days, and Beth came on from strength to strength. She still needed her tube, but she started to walk at long last and her hair began to grow!

We have been told that Beth is one of the 15% of children with Fallot's who will need further surgery later in her teens, and it has recently been found through a lung infusion test that the blood flow to her left lung is not good and is going to need some intervention at some point. But at the moment she is coping, so we will see when. All I can say is we have the most brave, caring, funny, loving and determined little girl anyone could wish for and we love her very much.

starting points. Some forethought (and perhaps fore-reading) may streamline what has a high likelihood of becoming a fraught process, depending on how successful the operation has been deemed to be.

The hallmark of streamlining postoperative care is communication. This should include a detailed handover from the anaesthetist (remember that he or she has spent the longest period so far with the patient, and will know all the details regarding pre-, intra- and immediate postoperative management) and will have a good feel for whether or not the child will be imminently extubatable. The patient handover should include all team members, highlight anticipated postoperative problems and discuss targets for management/goal-directed therapy.

All patients should be fully assessed on arrival to intensive care. A comprehensive checklist is provided in Table 3.5. Complications following CPB are generally caused by microemboli, cell damage and dysfunction, surgical nerve damage (phrenic nerve [C3,4,5] palsy) and infection.

Establish monitoring and ventilation as the priority. Once the initial assessment of the patient has occurred, clinical priorities have been dealt with (ventilation adjustment, volume loading, titration of inotropes, sedation, etc.) and investigations (Table 3.6) have been ordered, parental support becomes the next priority. All parents will be spoken to by the surgeon. Enabling parents in their transition to intensive care is the responsibility of both the clinician and nurse looking after the child. Empathic treatment of the parents will go a long way to facilitate this, and initial interaction on the ICU can be a determinant of the success of longer-term therapeutic relationships.

The majority of patients will transit through the ICU without complication. This occurs to such an extent that many institutions are implementing a 'fast-track' system,

Table 3.5 Initial checklist for arrival on the intensive care unit

Respiratory	Pulse oximeter oxygen saturation	Expected value? Pulmonary blood flow adequate or high?
	Endotracheal tube	Check size, evidence of leak, adequacy of taping (especially if oral)
	Check ventilator settings.	Check chest movement, air entry, tidal/minute volume, ventilator alarm settings. Are changes required from blood gas results? Consider monitoring end-tidal carbon dioxide
	If self-ventilating	Adequacy of ventilation, effort and respiratory effort – any signs of airway obstruction?
Cardiovascular	ECG	Heart rate and rhythm – confirm sinus rhythm, rhythm strip as baseline can be useful
	Pressures	Blood, central venous, left atrial and pulmonary artery pressures (mild arterial hypertension may be present due to CPB-induced catecholamine, renin and angiotensin II secretion). Note diastolic pressure in patients with shunts (may be low with large shunt)
	Assess haemodynamics/ adequacy of cardiac output	Is there an immediate need to give colloid or alter inotrope therapy? (refer to low cardiac output section). Check peripheral perfusion (core– peripheral temperature gap/peripheral pulses/ capillary refill time), assess liver size
	Drain losses	Urine output (check whether diuretic was administered in theatre) If >5 mL/kg, perform urgent clotting and TEG. Inform surgeons >10 mL/kg, inform surgeons as re-exploration likely Replace blood loss with appropriate colloid, i.e. packed cells according to haematocrit; fresh frozen plasma or cryoprecipitate according to clotting/TEG results; platelets according to full blood count/TEG (see later section of text) Gelofusine/4.5% human albumin solution should be used to replace drain or other losses in all other circumstances Take note of right and left atrial pressures with blood pressure when determining the rate of fluid replacement. Use small aliquots of fluid (5 mL/kg) With rewarming, systemic vascular resistance falls and fluid will be needed (for bleeding patients refer to Table 3.7)
	Mixed venous gas	A mixed venous O_2 saturation that is 20–25% less than arterial O_2 saturation indicates adequate cardiac output and oxygen delivery

Table 3.5 *Continued*

Gut	Abdominal examination	Liver size, girth, distension – baseline for neonates and possible necrotising enterocolitis, especially in infants with reduced systemic blood flow (e.g. interrupted aortic arch, coarctation of the aorta)
	Renal	Urine output >1 mL/kg per hour
		Evidence of adequate solute excretion (potassium, urea, creatinine within normal limits)
	Fluids	Retention of water and sodium, with depletion of body potassium leading to mild hyponatraemia, hypokalaemia and approximately 5% weight gain are expected. Therefore, intravenous fluids following CPB are restricted, although the extent to which this occurs varies between institutions. Modified ultrafiltration has lessened the severity of fluid restriction, although the duration of CPB will give an indication to the extent of capillary leak/third spacing anticipated.
	Metabolic system	Mild metabolic acidosis is seen early post CPB, with a base deficit of –5. This can be exacerbated by hyperchloraemia following aggressive volume replacement. It usually resolves without treatment within 12–24 hours postoperatively. Hartmann's solution as maintenance fluid can be helpful in these situations.
	Glucose	Maintenance glucose should be guided by blood sugar measurements. Dilution of inotropes in glucose solution is common practice. Hyperglycaemia in neonates can be a problem
	Electrolytes	Potassium and calcium from blood gas (as an immediate guide to replacement). Magnesium from formal urea & electrolytes. Potassium imbalance is the electrolyte abnormality most commonly associated with postoperative arrhythmias
	Nutrition	Feed early, even if only trophic feed volumes
Neurology	Bypass, aortic cross-clamp and circulatory arrest times	Total CPB time gives an indication of the inflammatory response expected, cross-clamp time indicates the extent of myocardial depression anticipated, and circulatory arrest time will give an indication of the risk of cerebral and/or renal ischaemia
	Pupils	Should be equal and responsive to light. Pinpoint usually indicates oversedation.
	Sedation/analgesia	Opiate infusion (fentanyl/morphine) ± sedative (usually midazolam) depending on the expected duration of respiratory support. Paralysis is not normally indicated unless the chest is open, or the child is suspected of/experiencing pulmonary hypertensive crises
	Motor function	Assess motor function when child awake. Watch for deficits (hemiplegia, visual field defects, seizures)

Table 3.5 *Continued*

Sepsis	Fever	Varying degrees of fever (up to 39.5 °C) often present due to CPB, blood product reaction, atelectasis, pleural effusions, low cardiac output syndrome. Persistent pyrexias should be aggressively investigated
	Prophylactic antibiotics	Indicated for between 12 and 24 hours postoperatively depending on agents used (Alphonso et al, 2007). Venous/arterial access sites, drain sites, urinary catheter, etc. are potential sources of infection. C-reactive protein and white cell count will be elevated in the first 48 hours due to a CPB-initiated inflammatory response.
Drug regimes	Routine	Antibiotic prophylaxis, diuretics, intravenous paracetamol, sedative agents
	Lesion specific	Heparinisation may be required prior to establishing aspirin or warfarin (systemic-to-pulmonary-artery shunts, cavopulmonary and Fontan circulations, prosthetic valves)

See text for abbreviations.

of which early extubation (either in the operating room or on immediate return to ICU) and early ICU discharge are features. Obviously, patient selection is paramount, and suitability should be discussed and planned for, ideally at the time the patient is listed.

For other patients, complications will arise. It is useful to anticipate and evaluate immediate postoperative problems in the following way. Determine whether it is a:

- rhythm problem;
- pump/myocardial problem – low cardiac output syndrome;
- structural surgery-related problem;
- 'residual lesion' problem.

Invariably, all the above groups will contribute to haemorrhage, metabolic acidosis and a persistent low cardiac output state. These commonly occurring complications will now be discussed in greater detail.

Rhythm disturbances

These can be common with intracardiac operations performed close to the conduction tissue, either nodal (producing heart block) or damaging the right bundle branch (causing asynchrony of ventricular contraction). Examples of such procedures are repairs for primum ASD, perimembranous VSD, tetralogy of Fallot and arterial valves.

Any child with electrolyte disturbances, especially of potassium, magnesium and calcium, will be prone to arrhythmias. Such electrolyte disturbances are common following CPB, and should be corrected as soon as possible.

In evaluating the ECG, the following questions may assist in both diagnosis and immediate management. The speed with which this is required will depend on whether the child is haemodynamically compromised by the dysrhythmia and, in particular, whether the child's cardiac output is sufficient:

Table 3.6 Investigations required following arrival in the intensive care unit

Laboratory studies	Arterial blood gas and lactate
	Urea & electrolytes + liver function test – correct calcium/magnesium/potassium immediately if low. Don't forget glucose
	Full blood count – haemoglobin, haematocrit, platelet count. Cardiopulmonary bypass will drop platelet levels by 60%. Aim for haemoglobin >10 g/dL in cyanotic lesions and > 8 g/dL in acyanotic lesions
	Clotting screen – APTT and reptilase time are especially important if bleeding
	Thromboelastogram if bleeding will be helpful to distinguish between clotting factor deficiency and surgical bleeding
Chest X-ray	Ascertain: ■ Position of endotracheal tube – the tip should be mid-tracheal, i.e. just below the clavicular heads/1 cm above the carina ■ Mediastinal and chest drain positions ■ Position of nasogastric tube – should be below the left hemidiaphragm ■ Position of central venous catheters (aim for the junction between the superior vena cava and right atrium) ■ Position of the pacing wires ■ Heart size ■ Lung fields: congestion, effusions, pneumothorax, atelectasis ■ Position of the hemidiaphragms (may be the first indication of phrenic nerve palsy) Patients with open chests may have evidence of air within the mediastinum
12-lead ECG	Essential if arrhythmias are evident on arrival. A baseline rhythm strip may indicate subsequent change (e.g. ST depression/elevation). Compare it with the preoperative ECG
	Atrial wires can be used to ascertain P waves in tachyarrhythmias
Postoperative echocardiogram	Often performed on the operating table at the end of/during the operation. Results should be documented
	Repeat echocardiography is indicated if problems are encountered postoperatively and the management outlined below is unsuccessful at establishing stability

- *Onset*: gradual or sudden?
- *QRS complex*: wide or narrow?
- *Rate*: regular or irregular? Fast or slow?
- *P waves visible*: possible supraventricular tachycardia.
- *Atrioventricular dissociation?*: are P waves associated with a corresponding QRS complex? Is this JET?

Management

- Immediate 12-lead ECG and cardiology referral (sinus rhythm is determined by upright P waves occurring prior to every QRS complex in leads I, II and AVF.
- Arterial blood gases to ascertain potassium and ionised calcium levels.
- Check the magnesium level – if the results not yet available, consider administration.

■ Cool the child, particularly if he or she is pyrexial.
■ Overdrive pacing may be useful to 'capture' tachycardia and reduce it if there is JET or supraventricular tachycardia.
■ Amiodarone, especially if there are wide QRS complexes.
■ Adenosine may be useful to terminate supraventricular tachycardia.

In situations of heart block, temporary pacing will be required using the epicardial wires placed at the end of the operation, as these rhythms often result in cardiovascular compromise in most children whose cardiac output is rate dependent. Bradycardia is treated with atrial or ventricular pacing (depending on whether a block is present) or chronotropic agents. A nodal (or atrioventricular junctional rhythm) may reduce cardiac output by 10–15% (Park, 1997), and compromise myocardial oxygen delivery.

Atrial wires will be to the right of the patient's sternum, and ventricular wires to the left, even in the presence of dextrocardia. If there is no heart block, atrial pacing is usually sufficient to initiate sinus rhythm, as long as the atrioventricular delay is set appropriately to allow 1:1 conduction through the atrioventricular node.

Persistent drain losses

This may be due to a variety of aetiologies. In the immediate postoperative period, it will usually be due to bleeding. Chylothoraces may become apparent, especially in univentricular circulations, once full feeding has been re-established. Confirmation of a chylous effusion is considered when fluid sample analysis demonstrates a triglyceride level of over 1.1 mmol/L and the total white cell count is over 1000 cells/mL with more than 80% lymphocytes (Buttiker, 1999). In the absence of adequate fat in the diet, the characteristic milky appearance may not be present, so any drainage persisting longer than 3 days should be investigated.

If a child is bleeding in the immediate postoperative period, ensure there is no element of hypertension as this will exacerbate the problem. Ensure also that the child is warm (36.5 °C) as the clotting cascade will be more efficient within normal temperature ranges.

Drain losses must be calculated and often replaced in mL/kg every 15 minutes in children who are bleeding. Watch for signs of cardiac tamponade, particularly if previously 'brisk' losses via the chest drain suddenly reduce or stop.

Bypass-induced coagulopathy

CPB can cause clinically significant clotting abnormalities due to a number of mechanisms:

■ *Dilution of coagulation factors.* Haemodilution occurs during CPB as fluid in the extracorporeal circuit dilutes the patient's blood. The haematocrit is intentionally reduced to levels between 25% and 35%. Dilutional effects can be especially marked in neonates and infants with total circulating volumes of 80 mL/kg, when circuit prime volumes can reach 500 mL. Despite large relative prime volumes, clinically important dilutional coagulopathy is not seen very often, possibly partly explained by the fact that normal clotting activity is maintained until factor levels fall below 30% of normal.
■ *Deposition on extracorporeal surfaces.* Platelets and coagulation proteins form deposits on the extracorporeal circuit surfaces, reducing their concentrations in circulating blood. Thrombocytopenia and/or qualitative platelet dysfunction is relatively

common after CPB. CPB activates platelets causing them to adhere to the circuit components, change shape, aggregate and release granular and other contents. The net result of CPB is that the patient has fewer platelets, which function less well.

■ *Hypothermia.* Enzyme reactions are slowed approximately 7% for each 1 °C fall in body temperature.
■ *Fibrinolysis.* CPB activates the fibrinolytic pathways, although this does not often reach clinical significance. However, some patients after prolonged bypass exhibit more marked haemostatic consequences – microcapillary bleeding from clot lysis and inhibition of new clot formation.
■ *Consumptive coagulopathy.* Disseminated intravascular coagulation occurs rarely after CPB. Fibrin formation in the bypass circuit during CPB does not cause a disseminated problem because antiplasmins scavenge plasmin re-entering the body from the bypass circuit. Consumptive coagulopathy only occurs if heparin levels are not adequate.
■ *Heparin.* Heparin is used to maintain anticoagulation during CPB and is routinely reversed post bypass. Inadequate reversal or heparin rebound effects are occasionally seen in the first hours after CPB and can be managed by the administration of protamine.

Pre-existing coagulopathy

Patients with cyanotic heart disease, particularly those with a haematocrit of over 60%, frequently have deranged haemostatic function. The cause of this defect is multifactorial and includes reduced plasma volume and disordered platelet function. This may persist into the early postoperative period, despite the haemoglobin returning to 'normal'.

Surgical bleeding

This is often the major concern in the early postoperative period. Surgical bleeding is often relentless or catastrophic in nature, with volumes of over 10 mL/kg per hour. Coagulation parameters are frequently normal or near normal (the TEG may be beneficial in determining this whilst awaiting formal clotting results). As no non-invasive manoeuvre can identify mechanical vascular bleeding with certainty, surgical re-exploration may be required if bleeding continues or there is evidence of cardiac tamponade.

Management of the bleeding patient

Check prothrombin time, APTT, fibrinogen and TEG values, and replace losses (Table 3.7):

■ Aim for a normalised prothrombin time/APPT, fibrinogen ≥ 0.75 g/L and platelets $> 75 \times 10^9$/L.
■ If mainly the prothrombin time and APTT are to be normalised, give fresh frozen plasma.
■ Fresh frozen plasma contains enough fibrinogen to correct mild-to-moderate deficiencies – if mainly fibrinogen is to be normalised, give cryoprecipitate.
■ Cryoprecipitate lacks some coagulation factors and will not reliably correct prothrombin time or APTT.
■ Give products and then recheck clotting immediately; repeat the use of appropriate products on the basis of the most recent result.

Table 3.7 Guidelines for replacement

Postoperative bleeding	Blood component therapy guidelines
Platelets < 100 × 10⁹/L or platelet dysfunction	Platelets 10–15 mL/kg
Prothrombin time and activated partial thromboplastin time to be normalised	Fresh frozen plasma 10–20 mL/kg
Fibrinogen < 1 g/L	Cryoprecipitate 5 mL/kg or 1 bag/5 kg

Table 3.8 Clinical assessment of cardiac output

Physical examination	Low cardiac output	Adequate cardiac output
Peripheral perfusion	Poor capillary refill	Good capillary refill < 3 seconds
Core/peripheral temperature gradient	>3 °C	<3 °C
Pulses	Impalpable or weak	Full peripheral pulses
Urine output	<1 mL/kg per hour	>1 mL/kg per hour
Mental status	Combative, disorientated	Cooperative
Arterial waveform	Small area under the curve. Narrow pulse pressure. Dichrotic notch soon after peak	Large area under curve. Dichrotic notch occurs later
Metabolic acidosis	Base excess > –5 mmol/L	Base excess < –5 mmol/L
Lactate	>4 mmol/L	<2 mmol/L
Blood pressure	Refer to age-related norms	Heart rate
Rhythm	Tachycardic or bradycardic (?sinus rhythm) Arrhythmia	Sinus rhythm; heart rate within normal limits for age

■ If bleeding continues despite relatively normal coagulation results, consider a surgical cause.

Low cardiac output states

Low cardiac output has long been recognised as one of the most important predictors of poor outcome after surgery for congenital heart disease (Parr et al, 1975). However, it is not routinely measured in children undergoing intensive care. For clinical purposes, adequacy of cardiac output status must be inferred from surrogate markers. Table 3.8 lists the main elements that are usually considered when reaching a conclusion as to the adequacy, or otherwise, of cardiac output.

Blood pressure is *not* a reliable indicator of cardiac output in children. Systemic blood pressure is the product of flow (i.e. cardiac output) and resistance (of the systemic circulation):

$$\text{Blood pressure} = \text{cardiac output} \times \text{systemic vascular resistance}$$

Postoperative cardiac patients who are typically vasoconstricted can be normotensive or hypertensive yet have a low cardiac output.

Once a low cardiac output state has been identified in a postoperative cardiac surgical child, it requires prompt treatment and management (Figure 3.8).

Preload
Preload (atrial filling pressures) should be optimised in the first instance with fluid administration. A dynamic assessment of preload can be performed by watching the response of filling pressures to the application of gentle pressure over the child's liver (hepatojugular reflex) or a test bolus of 5 mL/kg of crystalloid fluid. If left atrial pressure or central venous pressure/right atrial pressure increases by more than 3–5 mmHg with minimal improvement in blood pressure or perfusion, hypovolaemia is unlikely to be the predominant problem, and poor ventricular performance should be addressed.
Causes of decreased preload are:

■ intravascular hypovolaemia;
■ vasodilatation associated with rewarming;
■ increased intrathoracic pressure (positive-pressure ventilation);
■ cardiac tamponade.

Causes of increased preload are:

■ volume overload;
■ ventricular dysfunction (especially the right ventricle, e.g. 'stiff' ventricle after Fallot repair).

Myocardial contractility
Myocardial contractility will determine ventricular performance. Inotropes are used to optimise performance but themselves place an increased myocardial oxygen demand on the heart, especially at higher doses. All inotropes will, to differing extents, increase heart rate.

Heart rate
In children, heart rate is the primary mechanism for increasing cardiac output, as they have a relatively fixed stroke volume. Increasing heart rate will increase cardiac output to a certain point, after which extreme tachycardia impairs coronary filing and ventricular performance. It is important to remember that coronary perfusion occurs during diastole; therefore faster heart rates decreasing the diastolic phase will reduce the opportunity for coronary sinus filling.

Afterload
Afterload may become a critical factor determining myocardial function since compensatory changes associated with poor ventricular function tend to increase systemic resistance (the largest component of afterload). Arterial relaxation causes an increase in ejection fraction and a decrease in end-systolic ventricular volume, which becomes very important in children due to a fixed stroke volume. Venous relaxation re-diverts blood to the peripheries, thereby reducing the diastolic volume of both ventricles. Afterload reduction can significantly reduce myocardial work and oxygen requirement.
Milrinone is one of the newer cAMP-specific phosphodiesterase inhibitors, producing both positive inotropic effects and vasodilatation independent of beta-1-adrenergic receptor stimulation in the cardiovascular system, increasing stroke

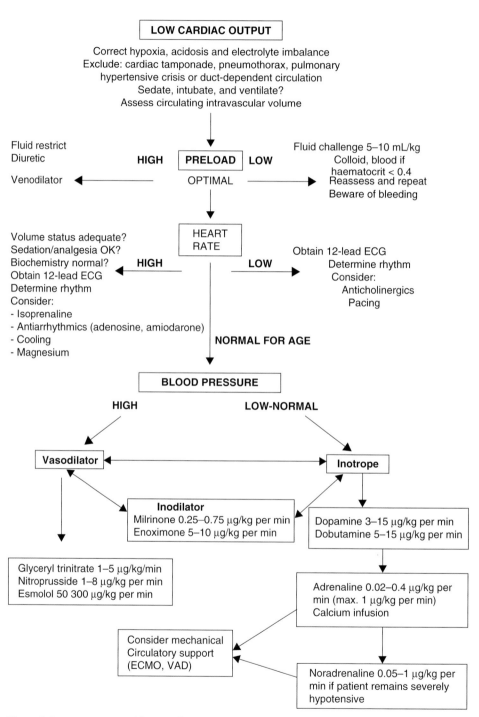

Figure 3.8 Management of low cardiac output. ECMO, extracorporeal membrane oxygenation, VAD, ventricular assist device. (Adapted from Alder Hey Children's NHS Foundation Cardiac Protocol, updated 2005)

volume index and left ventricular contractility, and producing pulmonary vasodi-latation. These qualities have made it a popular choice following paediatric heart surgery.

Pulmonary hypertension

Pulmonary hypertension is characterised by a mean pulmonary artery pressure of greater than 25 mmHg. It should always be expected in lesions with increased pul-monary blood flow (unrestrictive VSD, ASD, complete AVSD, total anomalous pul-monary venous drainage and truncus arteriosus). The management strategy includes inhaled nitric oxide, which is often started in the operating room, with early transition to sildenafil.

If, despite the above assessment and consequent management, inotropic require-ments remain high and serum lactate continues to increase, mechanical support either using ventricular assist devices or extracorporeal membrane oxygenation may become necessary. Before embarking on either of these strategies, it is essential that residual cardiac lesions are excluded, otherwise failure to separate from mechanical support will become the likely scenario.

Residual lesions

These can be identified by a number of means. Heart auscultation can give an indica-tion of residual ASD or VSD following repair. However, the quality of auscultation is often compromised, especially when chest drains are in situ or if the chest is left open following complex surgery.

Echocardiography is the most easily available imaging modality in the ICU. Interob-server variability can be problematic, although it is often the most experienced car-diologist who will provide this service in these situations. Echocardiography is the standard investigation for determining residual lesions or structural complications associated with the surgical repair (valvular incompetence or thromboemboli). Usually, a trans-oesophageal echo examination is performed at the end of surgery, and this can serve to be a useful baseline. Depending on the findings and the aetiol-ogy of the problem, cardiac catheterisation may be required, especially if concerns are raised regarding coronary artery blood supply postoperatively (arterial switch opera-tion and Ross procedure).

Points worth further discussion

Palliation versus total repair

Do not underestimate the unpredictable effects that palliative procedures – pulmonary artery banding and Blalock–Taussig (or other systemic-to-pulmonary artery) shunts – may have on the child's circulation and physiology. Be prepared!

With systemic-to-pulmonary shunts, pulmonary blood flow will be dependent on systemic blood pressure, so avoid hypotension. Systemic arterial oxygen saturation (SaO_2) readings of 70–85% indicate that pulmonary and systemic blood flow is bal-anced. If SaO_2 drops below 70% in the absence of hypotension or abnormal lung function, shunt occlusion should be suspected.

Large shunts resulting in high pulmonary blood flow will result in a high SaO_2, left ventricular failure and pulmonary oedema that may be unilateral on the side of the shunt (usually the right side). This is managed acutely with anti-cardiac failure medi-cations and fluid restriction, but if these measures fail the shunt will need revision.

Low diastolic pressures may impair coronary filling postoperatively due to high pulmonary run-off.

Right ventricular dysfunction is common following a tetralogy of Fallot repair, requiring high filling pressures, particularly if a transannular patch is necessary to relieve RVOT obstruction. Rhythm disturbances are common, especially JET, primarily a result of VSD closure and the close vicinity to conduction tissues. A transatrial approach to VSD closure and infundibular resection has reduced the necessity for right ventriculotomy, reducing both postoperative right ventricular dysfunction and the risk of dysrhythmia. Persistent chest drain losses due to the requirement for high filling pressures can be problematic.

In children who have had cavopulmonary shunts and completion of a Fontan procedure, early extubation is favoured (in the operating room if possible) as pulmonary blood flow is passive and depends on unobstructed venous return. Positive-pressure ventilation will raise intrathoracic pressure and impede venous return to the heart. If ventilation is required, a low positive end-expiratory pressure strategy is used, with pressure support in favour of controlled mandatory breaths. These patients will require diuretic therapy, but this is not usually necessary until postoperative day 1, when drain losses begin to slow and overall fluid balance tends to the positive.

With arterial switch operations, coronary reimplantation is occasionally problematic and heparinisation may be indicated. Problems in these patients generally arise from poor diastolic ventricular function, especially as the left ventricle will require some degree of retraining depending on the age at correction, which means that, immediately postoperatively, volume loading is poorly tolerated in these patients and cardiac output is relatively rate dependent. The aim is to maintain the lowest left atrial pressure (4–8 mmHg) consistent with adequate cardiac output. These neonates will respond well to smaller aliquots of fluid administration (3–5 mL/kg) for this reason.

Dysrhythmias should be aggressively treated (supraventricular tachycardia, JET and heart block may occur), and coronary insufficiency can be anticipated from a variety of sources – myocardial ischaemia from coronary reimplantation, coronary 'stretch' by a dilating left ventricle, and poor left ventricular output failing to perfuse coronary circulation adequately – all of which make regular ECG analysis important. Pulmonary hypertension can be expected with late repair.

Physiotherapy

The aim of respiratory physiotherapy on the paediatric cardiac ICU is to prevent or resolve any respiratory complications and optimise ventilation in order to facilitate extubation and transfer to the ward. The lungs may be affected as a result of the defect, such as increased pulmonary blood flow with a left-to-right shunt, as well as the effect of the anaesthesia, bypass and the surgery itself.

After cardiac surgery, all children admitted to the cardiac ICU will be assessed by a physiotherapist. The assessment includes reviewing the operation report and handover from the surgical team to the ICU staff, the patient charts and the postoperative chest X-ray. If the anaesthetist reports specific respiratory problems in theatre, or there are abnormal findings on either chest X-ray or auscultation, the patient will receive chest physiotherapy. Thereafter all patients, in particular intubated patients, on the cardiac ICU will be assessed on a daily basis.

Following thorough assessment, the physiotherapist will formulate a plan of treatment. The length of treatment may vary according to assessment findings, but sessions should be as quick as possible with minimal handling. The physiotherapist may use several modalities, including positioning, manual hyperinflation (bagging), chest wall vibrations, saline instillation and airway suction. If a change of position is required, it is preferable to limit the number of turns in one treatment session. On occasion, chest clapping may be used, more so in younger extubated patients.

The potential benefits versus risks of physiotherapy treatment must be carefully assessed for patients who are cardiovascularly unstable, for example those who have large or persistent volume losses from their chest drains or those with an untreated pneumothorax. Similarly, special consideration needs to be given to those patients with delayed sternal closure and pulmonary hypertension. The sternum is usually stented open, but on occasion there is no stent. Following assessment, these patients can be turned slightly (a quarter turn from supine) if this is considered beneficial for treatment. Chest wall vibrations in these patients are performed with the hands placed posteriorly on the chest wall and with less force applied.

Young patients (usually those less than 1 year of age who have had excessive pulmonary blood flow, for example from a large VSD) may be at risk of hypertensive crises in the postoperative period. These patients are often kept well sedated and may be pharmacologically paralysed. If there have been episodes of instability, a bolus of fentanyl may be prescribed prior to any handling, including physiotherapy. If the patient is additionally receiving inhaled NO, its delivery must be maintained throughout physiotherapy. The bagging circuit should be set up to deliver the correct dose of inhaled NO depending on the flow of oxygen to the bag. It is preferable to time physiotherapy so the child is not handled continuously.

There is a risk during cardiac surgery (particularly when reoperating) that the phrenic nerve may be damaged. During a respiratory assessment, the chest wall excursion should be assessed. If asymmetry is noted during inspiration, with less outward movement of the abdomen or abdominal wall indrawing on one side, there may be a phrenic nerve injury. A phrenic nerve injury may result in the diaphragm sitting high but immobile, or the diaphragm may move paradoxically on inspiration. The chest X-ray may show an elevated diaphragm and possibly loss of lung volume on the affected side. These changes may not be obvious until ventilatory support is weaned. If a phrenic nerve injury is suspected, it should be investigated as it may delay or even prevent extubation in infants who rely solely on their diaphragm for respiration.

In patients with a Fontan type of circulation (total cavopulmonary pulmonary connection), who rely on passive blood flow to the lungs, special care must be taken when manually hyperinflating these patients. The rise in intrathoracic pressure when positive pressure is applied manually or ventilator hyperinflation may lead to a reduction in antegrade flow to the lungs.

In an infant following a Norwood stage I procedure with a Blalock–Taussig shunt (rather than a Sano modification), it may be necessary to maintain a balance between the systemic and pulmonary circulations. When bagging the patient, care must be taken to bag with an FiO_2 similar to that of the ventilator and to avoid hyperventilation, thereby limiting the oxygen delivered to the patient and avoiding a reduction in carbon dioxide. This will reduce the risk of lowering pulmonary vascular resistance and increasing pulmonary blood flow with the potential for 'stealing' flow from the systemic circulation, most especially the coronary arteries. If the lungs get very wet, this will lead to a reduction in compliance that may adversely affect blood gases, thus making it more difficult to maintain a $Qp:Qs$ of $1:1$.

On occasion, postoperative cardiac function is very poor and the patient may require extracorporeal membrane oxygenation, which supports the function of the heart, allowing it to rest and recover. During physiotherapy, care must be taken not to interfere with the flow in the cannulae, and there is an increased risk of bleeding. It may not be possible to turn the patient for treatment, and care should be taken when using manual techniques for treatment.

When the child has recovered and been extubated, respiratory assessment and treatment may still be needed as indicated. If the child is old enough, he or she will be encouraged to mobilise, gradually increasing in activity. Once children are independently mobile, they can usually be discharged from physiotherapy.

Discharge planning and community support

Planning for discharge should be a normal requirement for all children and young people in hospital (DH, 2004). It may be a simple process if the child has been in hospital only briefly, for example after a cardiac catheterisation, or it may be much more complex following a long hospital stay, where the child has multiple needs that will need continual support at home. In these situations, many more professionals, such as liaison nurses, clinical nurse specialists, community children's nurses, health visitors/school nurses, social workers, occupational therapists, physiotherapists, dietitians and the hospital medical team and GP, are involved in discharge planning to ensure a smooth transition from hospital to home. It is essential that all relevant parties are involved in this discharge planning, both in the hospital and in the community, and that aspects of care such as an adequate supply of drugs and equipment have been organised as well. The outpatient department needs to be involved to make follow-up appointments, and transportation of the child needs to be arranged as appropriate depending on the child's needs. These complex cases require much more thought and time to organise, and therefore the planning process should start as soon as the child is admitted.

Many units provide parental education whilst the child is in hospital, empowering parents (and where appropriate the child/young person) to take over aspects of care that may need to continue at home. This may involve an assessment of competence for the parents as well as for carers who will be involved in the more complex cases in the community. This is supported through the development of a management plan and the provision of leaflets and information booklets that provide parents/carers with relevant information specific to their child's condition or treatment whilst in hospital, and the contact details of relevant professionals if they require any additional advice. Many booklets have also been written in child-friendly language, such that the child/young person is encouraged to take responsibility or have an awareness of their heart problem. These leaflets are generally given to the children and their families as printed documents, but many hospitals have also made this discharge advice and additional information available through their websites, increasing access and knowledge of services once the family are home. Additionally, parental readiness for discharge is improved and readmission rates are reduced if a structured discharge procedure exists (Wesseldine et al, 1999; Weiss et al, 2008).

Specific aspects of care for each child should be detailed within the written discharge leaflet to prevent parents forgetting verbal instructions. Furthermore, general information will be provided depending upon the clinical team's views and the contemporary evidence base (adapted from Birmingham Children's Hospital, 2003, and Horrox, 2002) regarding:

- care of the wound – removal of sutures;
- pain relief;
- safe drug administration – ensuring a suitable supply from the GP;
- fluids and diet – restrictions or special diets;
- dental treatment – the possible need for antibiotic cover;
- immunisations – some are not recommended in certain circumstances;
- signs and symptoms to look out for and when to worry – when to contact staff at the hospital;
- details of follow-up outpatient appointments;
- expected activity level – returning to exercise
- smoking – the effect of passive smoking;
- body piercings – infection risk;
- returning to school/nursery/work;
- wearing car seat belts despite the wound ;
- holidays abroad – notifying the consultant;
- roles of community staff – health visitor/community children's nurse/GP/cardiac liaison nurses/social services;
- concerns about siblings/future babies – genetic screening.

The importance of support groups cannot be excluded here, as many children and young people and their families access the invaluable service that these groups provide, allowing them to communicate with other individuals with similar problems and to support each other too (Chapter 7 highlights this issue further). Generally, parents are given contact details of relevant support groups whilst in hospital, but these can also be found easily via the internet, where many support groups have discussion forums, podcasts and details of other social events for children/young people and their families to take part in.

Summary

The treatment and management of children born with congenital heart disease has undergone major advances in the last three decades. Conditions that were previously not survivable are now associated with a good long-term outcome and quality of life. This has been due to an improvement in our understanding coupled with advances in pharmacology, surgery, cardiology and intensive care medicine.

Many treatment plans are complex, and success relies upon good multidisciplinary teamwork. The active involvement of the patient and family in the care pathway is very important because, for many patients, it is the beginning of a lifelong relationship with the clinical team. Throughout the care process, it is important to address the physiological, physical and psychological needs of the patient and family.

References

Akinturk, H., Michel-Behnke, I., Valeske, K., Mueller, M., Thul, J., Bauer, J. et al (2007). Hybrid transcatheter-surgical palliation: basis for univentricular or biventricular repair: the Giessen experience. *Pediatric Cardiology, 28*, 79–87.

Alderson, P. & Goodey, C. (1998). Theories in health care and research: theories of consent. *British Medical Journal, 317*, 1313–1315.

Alphonso, N., Anagnostopoulous, P.V., Scarpace, S., Weintrub, P., Azakie, A., Raff, G. & Karl, T.R. (2007). Perioperative antibiotic prophylaxis in paediatric cardiac surgery. *Cardiology in the Young*, 17, 12–25.

Birmingham Children's Hospital (2003). *Heart unit discharge advice*. Birmingham: Medical Illustration Department, Birmingham Children's Hospital.

Brierley, J.J., Reddy, T.D., Rigby, M.L., Thanopoulous, V. & Redington, A.N. (1998). Traumatic damage to the mitral valve during percutaneous balloon valvotomy for critical aortic stenosis. *Heart*, 79, 200–202.

Bristow, M. (1998). Carvedilol treatment of chronic heart failure: a new era. *Heart*, 79(Suppl. 2), S31–S34.

Brown, T.C.K. & Fisk, G.C. (1979). *Anaesthesia for children: including aspects of intensive care*. Oxford: Blackwell Scientific.

Buttiker, V., Fanconi, S. & Burger, R. (1999). Chylothorax in children: guidelines for diagnosis and management. *Chest*, 116, 682–687.

Cabrera-Bueno, F., Garcia-Pinilla, J.M., Gomez-Doblas, J.J., Montiel-Trujillo, A., Rodriguez-Bailon, I. & de Teresa-Galvan, E. (2007) Beta-blocker therapy for dynamic left ventricular outflow tract obstruction induced by exercise. *International Journal of Cardiology*, 117, 222–226.

Carroll, W.D. & Dhillon, R. (2003). Sildenafil as a treatment for pulmonary hypertension. *Archives of Disease in Childhood*, 88, 827–828.

Chessa, M., De Rosa, G., Pardeo, M., Negura, D.G., Butero, G., Giamberti, A. et al (2005). What do parents know about the malformations afflicting the hearts of their children? *Cardiology in the Young*, 15, 125–129.

Chief Medical Officer (2003). *Winning ways: working together to reduce healthcare associated infection in England*. London: DH.

Crenshaw, J.T. & Winslow, E.H. (2002). Preoperative fasting: old habits die hard. Research and published guidelines no longer support the routine use of 'NPO after midnight', but the practice persists. *American Journal of Nursing*, 102, 36–44.

Daehnert, I., Rotzsch, C., Wiener, M. & Schneider, P. (2004). Rapid right ventricular pacing is an alternative to adenosine in catheter interventional procedures for congenital heart disease. *Heart*, 90, 1047–1050.

David, F., Sanchez, A., Yanez, L., Velasquez, E., Jimenez, S., Martinez, A. & Alva, C. (2007). Cardiac pacing in balloon aortic valvuloplasty. *International Journal of Cardiology*, 116, 327–330.

Department of Health (2004). *National Service Framework for children, young people and maternity services*. London: DH.

Department of Health (2006). *Screening for meticillin-resistant* Staphylococcus aureus *(MRSA) colonisation: a strategy for NHS trusts – a summary of best practice*. London: DH.

Esler, M. & Kaye, D. (2000) Measurement of sympathetic nervous system activity in heart failure: the role of norepinephrine kinetics. *Heart Failure Review*, 5, 17–25.

Fawzy, M.E. (2007). Percutaneous mitral balloon valvotomy. *Catheterization and Cardiovascular Interventions*, 69, 313–321.

Forister, J.G. & Blessing, J.D. (2002). Considerations in preoperative evaluation. *Physician Assistant*, 26, 36–45.

Frelinger, A.L. III, Jakubowski, J.A., Li, Y., Barnard, M.R., Linden, M.D., Tarnow, I. et al (2008). The active metabolite of prasugrel inhibits adenosine diphosphate- and collagen-stimulated platelet procoagulant activities. *Journal of Thrombosis and Haemostasis*, 6, 359–365.

Garratt, K.N., Holmes, D.R. Jr. & Roubin, G.S. (1991). Early outcome after placement of a metallic intracoronary stent: initial Mayo Clinic experience. *Mayo Clinic Proceedings*, 66, 268–275.

Garson, A. Jr., Gillette, P.C. & McNamara, D.G. (1981). Propranolol: the preferred palliation for tetralogy of Fallot. *American Journal of Cardiology*, 47, 1098–1104.

Gewillig, M., Boshoff, D. & Delhaas, T. (2006). Late fenestration of the extracardiac conduit in a Fontan circuit by sequential stent flaring. *Catheterization and Cardiovascular Interventions*, 67, 298–301.

Giannelli, G., Iannone, F., Marinosci, F., Lapadula, G. & Antonaci, S. (2005). The effect of bosentan on matrix metalloproteinase-9 levels in patients with systemic sclerosis-induced pulmonary hypertension. *Current Medical Research and Opinion*, 21, 327–332.

Halpin, T.J., Holtzhauer, F.J., Campbell, R.J., Hall, L.J., Correa-Villasenor, A., Lanese, R. et al (1982). Reye's syndrome and medication use. *Journal of the American Medical Association*, 248, 687–691.

Heeneman, S., Sluimer, J.C. & Daemen, M.J. (2007). Angiotensin-converting enzyme and vascular remodeling. *Circulation Research*, 101, 441–454.

Ho, S.H., Wu, J.K., Hamilton, D.P., Dix, D.B. & Wadsworth, L.D. (2004). An assessment of published pediatric dosage guidelines for enoxaparin: a retrospective review. *Journal of Pediatric Hematology and Oncology*, 26, 561–566.

Hoehn, K.M., Wernovsky, G., Rychik, J., Tian, Z., Donaghue, D., Alderfer, M.A. et al (2004). Parental decision-making in congenital heart disease. *Cardiology in the Young*, 14, 309–314.

Hogg, C. & Cooper, C. (2004). *Meeting the needs of children and young people undergoing surgery*. London: Action for Sick Children.

Hoppe, B., Duran, I., Martin, A., Kribs, A., Benz-Bohm, G., Michalk, D.V. & Roth, B. (2002). Nephrocalcinosis in preterm infants: a single center experience. *Pediatric Nephrology*, 17, 264–268.

Horrox, F. (2002). *Manual of neonatal and paediatric heart disease*. London: Whurr.

Jolley, S. (2007). An audit of patients' understanding of routine preoperative investigations. *Nursing Standard*, 21, 35–39.

Jutley, R.S., Waller, D.A., Loke, I., Skehan, D., Ng, A., Stafford, P. et al (2008). Video-assisted thoracoscopic implantation of the left ventricular pacing lead for cardiac resynchronization therapy. *Pacing and Clinical Electrophysiology*, 31, 812–818.

Kan, J.S., White, R.I. Jr., Mitchell, S.E. & Gardner, T.J. (1982). Percutaneous balloon valvuloplasty: a new method for treating congenital pulmonary-valve stenosis. *New England Journal of Medicine*, 307, 540–542.

Kempen, P.M. (1997). Preoperative pregnancy testing: a survey of current practice. *Journal of Anaesthesia*, 9, 546–550.

Khambadkone, S. & Bonhoeffer, P. (2004). Nonsurgical pulmonary valve replacement: why, when, and how? *Catheterization and Cardiovascular Intervention*, 62, 401–408.

Kothari, S.S., Ramakrishnan, S., Kumar, C.K., Juneja, R. & Yadav, R. (2005). Intermediate-term results of percutaneous transvenous mitral commissurotomy in children less than 12 years of age. *Catheterization and Cardiovascular Intervention*, 64, 487–490.

Kuflik, A. (2008). The "future like ours" argument and human embryonic stem cell research. *Journal of Medical Ethics*, 34, 417–421.

Lake, C.L. (1988). *Pediatric cardiac anaesthesia*. Stamford, CT: Appleton & Lange.

Li, J.S., Yow, E., Berezny, K.Y., Bokesch, P.M., Takahashi, M., Graham, T.P. Jr. et al (2008). Dosing of clopidogrel for platelet inhibition in infants and young children: primary results of the Platelet Inhibition in Children On cLOpidogrel (PICOLO) trial. *Circulation*, 117, 553–559.

Link, K.P. (1959). The discovery of dicumarol and its sequels. *Circulation*, 19, 97–107.

Liu, C. & Chen, J. (2006) Endothelin receptor antagonists for pulmonary arterial hypertension. *Cochrane Database of Systematic Reviews*, (3), CD004434.

Magro, L., Conforti, A., Del, Z.F., Leone, R., Iorio, M.L., Meneghelli, I. et al (2008). Identification of severe potential drug–drug interactions using an Italian general-practitioner database. *European Journal of Pharmacology*, 64, 303–309.

Marcum, J.A. (2000) The origin of the dispute over the discovery of heparin. *Journal of the History of Medicine and Allied Sciences*, 55, 37–66.

Masura, J., Burch, M., Deanfield, J.E. & Sullivan, I.D. (1993) Five-year follow-up after balloon pulmonary valvuloplasty. *Journal of the American College of Cardiology*, *21*, 132–136.

Matsuno, Y., Mori, Y., Umeda, Y., Imaizumi, M. & Takiya, H. (2008) Minimally invasive video-assisted thoracoscopic left ventricular epicardial lead implantation for biventricular pacing in a patient with persistent left superior vena cava. *Heart and Vessels*, *23*, 289–292.

Maynard, R. (1999) The Cardiopulmonary Bypass Machine, Unpublished Trust Literature.

Miller, O.I., Celermajer, D.S., Deanfield, J.E. & Macrae, D.J. (1994). Guidelines for the safe administration of inhaled nitric oxide. *Archives of Disease in Childhood Fetal and Neonatal Edition*, *70*, F47–F49.

Munoz-Garcia, A.J., Dominguez-Franco, A.J., Alonso-Briales, J.H., Jimenez-Navarro, M.F., Hernandez-Garcia, J.M. & de Teresa-Galvan, E. (2008). Comparison of incidence and angiography patterns in definite thrombosis between drug-eluting and bare-metal stents. *International Journal of Cardiology*, July 30 [Epub ahead of print].

National Institute for Clinical Excellence (2003). *Preoperative tests: The use of routine preoperative tests for elective surgery*. Clinical Guideline 3. London: National Collaborating Centre for Acute Care.

Nursing and Midwifery Council (2004). *The NMC code of professional conduct: Standard for conduct, performance and ethics*. London: NMC.

O'Laughlin, M.P., Perry, S.B., Lock, J.E. & Mullins, C.E. (1991) Use of endovascular stents in congenital heart disease. *Circulation*, *83*, 1923–1939.

Orea-Tejeda, A., Colin-Ramirez, E., Castillo-Martinez, L., Sensio-Lafuente, E., Corzo-Leon, D., Gonzalez-Toledo, R. et al (2007). Aldosterone receptor antagonists induce favorable cardiac remodeling in diastolic heart failure patients. *Revista de investigación clínica*, *59*, 103–107.

Park, G. (1977). Controlled trials in the critically ill. *Care of the Critically Ill*, *13*, 6.

Parr, G.V., Blackstone, E.H. & Kirklin, J.W. (1975). Cardiac performance and mortality early after intracardiac surgery in infants and young children. *Circulation*, *51*, 867–874.

Rahimtoola, S.H. (1975). Digitalis and William Withering, the clinical investigator. *Circulation*, *52*, 969–971.

Ram, C.V. (2008). Angiotensin receptor blockers: current status and future prospects. *American Journal of Medicine*, *121*, 656–663.

Royal College of Nursing (2005). *Perioperative fasting in adults and children: An RCN guideline for the multidisciplinary team*. London: RCN.

Royal College of Paediatrics and Child Health (2008). *British national formulary for children*. 4th edn. London: BMJ Group/RPS Publishing/RCPCH Publications.

Royal Liverpool Children's Hospital (2005). *Protocols for cardiac patients on the PICU*. Alder Hey: RLCH (unpublished).

Rubio-Alvarez, V., Limon, R. & Soni, J. (1953). [Intracardiac valvulotomy by means of a catheter]. *Archivos del Instituto de Cardiología de México*, *23*, 183–192.

Schenke-Layland, K., Strem, B.M., Jordan, M.C., Deemedio, M.T., Hedrick, M.H., Roos, K.P. et al (2008). Adipose tissue-derived cells improve cardiac function following myocardial infarction. *Journal of Surgical Research*, April 10 [Epub ahead of print].

Shah, P.S. & Ohlsson, A. (2007). Sildenafil for pulmonary hypertension in neonates. *Cochrane Database of Systemic Reviews*, (3), CD005494.

Smith, L. & Callery, P. (2005). Children's accounts of their preoperative information needs. *Journal of Clinical Nursing*, *14*, 230–238.

Spijkerboer, A.W., Helbing, W.A., Bogers, A.J.J.C., Van Domburg, R.T., Verhilst, F.C. & Utens, E.M.W.J. (2007). Long-term psychological distress, and styles of coping, in parents of children and adolescents who underwent invasive treatment for congenital cardiac treatment for congenital cardiac disease. *Cardiology in the Young*, *17*, 638–645.

Staneva-Stoytcheva, D. & Kristeva, E. (1991). Effects of amiodarone on the pharmacokinetics and toxicity of digoxin in laboratory animals. *Acta Physiologica et Pharmacologica Bulgarica*, *17*, 37–42.

Stark, J., de Leval, M. & Tsang, V., eds. (2004). *Surgery for congenital heart defects.* 2nd edn. New York: Wiley & Sons.

Steiropoulos, P., Trakada, G. & Bouros, D. (2008). Current pharmacological treatment of pulmonary arterial hypertension. *Current Clinical Pharmacology, 3*, 11–19.

Stumper, O., Gewillig, M., Vettukattil, J., Budts, W., Chessa, M., Chaudhari, M. & Wright, J.G. (2003). Modified technique of stent fenestration of the atrial septum. *Heart, 89*, 1227–1230.

Suga, H., Igarashi, Y., Yamada, O. & Goto, Y. (1985). Mechanical efficiency of the left ventricle as a function of preload, afterload, and contractility. *Heart and Vessels, 1*, 3–8.

Tagalakis, V., Kahn, S.R., Libman, M. & Bostein, M. (2002). The epidemiology of peripheral vein infusion thrombophlebitis: a critical review. *American Journal of Medicine, 113*, 146–51.

Tare, M., Parkington, H.C., Coleman, H.A., Neild, T.O. & Dusting, G.J. (1990). Hyperpolarization and relaxation of arterial smooth muscle caused by nitric oxide derived from the endothelium. *Nature, 346*, 69–71.

Tessler, R., Wu, S., Fiori, R., Macgowan, C.K. & Belik, J. (2008). Sildenafil acutely reverses the hypoxic pulmonary vasoconstriction response of the newborn pig. *Pediatric Research, 64*, 251–255.

Tromp, F., van Dulmen, S. & van Weert, J. (2004). Interdisciplinary preoperative patient education in cardiac surgery. *Journal of Advanced Nursing, 47*, 212–222.

Utens, E.M.W.J., Verslius-Den Bieman, H.J., Witsenburg, M., Bogers, A.J.J.C., Vandvik, I.H. & Forde, R. (2000). Ethical issues in parental decision-making. An interview study of mothers with hypoplastic left heart syndrome. *Acta Paediatrica, 89*, 1129–1133.

Utens, E.M.W.J., Verslius-Den Bieman, H.J., Verhulst, F.C., Witsenburg, M., Bogers, A.J.J.C. & Hess, J. (2001). Psychological distress and styles of coping in parents of children awaiting elective cardiac surgery. *Cardiology in the Young, 10*, 239–244.

Vardas, P.E., Auricchio, A., Blanc, J.J., Daubert, J.C., Drexler, H., Ector, H. et al (2007). Guidelines for cardiac pacing and cardiac resynchronization therapy. The Task Force for Cardiac Pacing and Cardiac Resynchronization Therapy of the European Society of Cardiology. Developed in collaboration with the European Heart Rhythm Association. *Europace, 9*, 959–998.

Vernon, M.W., Heel, R.C. & Brogden, R.N. (1991). Enoximone. A review of its pharmacological properties and therapeutic potential. *Drugs, 42*, 997–1017.

Weaver, K. & Groves, J. (2007). Fundamental aspects of play in hospital. In Glasper, A., Aylott, M. & Prudhoe, G., eds. *Fundamental aspects of children's and young people's nursing procedures.* Gateshead: MA Healthcare. Ch. 5.

Webb, J.G., Pasupati, S., Humphries, K., Thompson, C., Altwegg, L., Moss, R. et al (2007). Percutaneous transarterial aortic valve replacement in selected high-risk patients with aortic stenosis. *Circulation, 116*, 755–763.

Weiss, M., Johnson, N.L., Malin, S., Jerofke, T., Lang, C. & Sherburne, E. (2008). Readiness for discharge in parents of hospitalized children. *Journal of Pediatric Nursing, 23*, 282–295.

Wesseldine, L.J., McCarthy, P. & Silverman, M. (1999). Structured discharge procedure for children admitted to hospital with acute asthma: a randomised controlled trial of nursing practice. *Archives of Disease in Children, 80*, 110–114.

Wilmot, M. (2007). The specialised play specialist. *Paediatric Nursing, 10*, 33.

Wray, J. & Sensky, T. (2004). Psychological functioning in parents of children undergoing elective cardiac surgery. *Cardiology in the Young, 14*, 131–139.

Wypij, D., Newburger, J.W., Rappaport, L.A., duPlessis, A.J., Jonas, R.A., Wernovsky, G. et al (2003). The effect of duration of deep hypothermic circulatory arrest in infant heart surgery on late neurodevelopment: The Boston Circulatory Arrest Trial, *J Thorac Cardiovasc Surg, 126*, 1397–1403.

4 Impact of heart disease on young people and their families: an introduction

Jo Wray, Caroline Green, Fiona Kennedy

Cardiac disease is the most common congenital defect in children, with an incidence, which has remained stable, of 8 per 1000 live births (Behrman et al, 1992). Cardiac defects are distributed throughout the entire population, with no distinction on the basis of socio-economic status or race (Fixler et al, 1993), and approximately one million children are born worldwide each year with heart disease. Significant improvements in the surgical and medical management of children with congenital heart disease (CHD) have resulted in a dramatic reduction in mortality, such that 80–85% of children born today with CHD are now expected to live to adulthood (British Cardiac Society, 2002). Similarly, children and young people who develop acquired heart disease are likely to be offered previously unavailable treatment options to prolong their life, in contrast to several decades ago. However, despite improvements in all aspects of diagnosis, treatment and care, morbidity remains a concern as an increasing population of children and young people are living with heart disease and its impact on their everyday life.

This chapter will focus on the impact of heart disease for children/young people and their families, from the time of diagnosis through the period of transition into adult services.

How are 'outcomes' measured?

The paradigm shift from mortality to morbidity has resulted in a corresponding shift in the way outcomes are assessed. Early studies focused primarily on survival rates, but today a whole plethora of physical and psychological outcomes are evaluated as part of the care of children and young people with CHD. Factors such as functional ability, exercise testing (typically using a treadmill or cycle ergometer) and cardiopulmonary function are often assessed as measures of physical outcome alongside the routine cardiac and medical parameters, whilst domains such as neurodevelopmental functioning, cognitive and academic abilities, behaviour, emotional functioning, self-perception and parental adjustment are increasingly being evaluated to determine the psychosocial impact on children and their families.

Neurodevelopmental and cognitive abilities are assessed with the use of specific psychometric tests administered to the child (such as the Weschsler Intelligence

Scales, NEPSY, Bayley Scales of Infant Development, McCarthy Scales of Children's Abilities, Wide Range Achievement Test and Kaufman Assessment Battery for Children). With the development and increased accessibility of technologies such as magnetic resonance imaging and near-infrared spectroscopy, researchers are now studying brain structure and factors such as cerebral blood flow, and relating these to the results of psychometric testing in order to understand the mechanisms resulting in impaired function and ultimately to intervene to improve outcome.

Questionnaires are widely used to gather information about aspects such as behaviour, self-esteem and mood; these are more usually completed by parents or other caregivers, and it is only in more recent years that researchers have actually asked children themselves to complete such measures. It still remains relatively uncommon for a qualitative methodology, rather than a hypothesis-driven quantitative approach, to be utilised to understand the day-to-day experience of life with CHD. More recently, attention has focused on the global concept of quality of life (QoL), from both an individual and an economic perspective, and there is a new emphasis on trying to identify how physical and psychological concomitants of CHD relate to the 'lived experience' and what this actually means in terms of everyday life.

Quality of life – measurement issues

The concept of QoL is an integral constituent of modern life, although as a concept it is nebulous, subjective and therefore difficult to define. In 1993, the World Health Organization defined QoL as:

> an individual's perception of their position in life in the context of the culture and value systems in which they live and in relation to their goals, expectations, standards and concerns. It is a broad-ranging concept, incorporating in a complex way the person's physical health, psychological state, level of independence, social relationships, and their relationship to salient features of their environment. (WHOQOL Group, 1993, p. 153)

A further concept of health-related QoL (HRQoL), encompassing the domains of disease state and physical functioning, functional status, psychological functioning and social functioning, has also been developed to address issues of QoL associated with illness. How to measure QoL is another contentious topic, and within chronic illness researchers have tended to utilise either generic or disease-specific measures, both of which have advantages and disadvantages. Generic measures enable comparisons to be made with the healthy population as well as with other illness groups, but they may not be sensitive to changes in condition or function and may overlook clinically relevant aspects of a person's life related to their condition. Disease-specific measures, which assess QoL in a particular condition or disease, may be more comprehensive for a specific disease, more sensitive to change in condition or status over time or following a specific treatment, and better for discriminating between subgroups within a disease category. However, disease-specific measures do not allow for a comparison with either healthy or other disease groups. Given the strengths and weaknesses of the two approaches, using both a disease-specific and a generic measure would seem to be the optimum way of comprehensively assessing QoL within illness.

Assessing HRQoL in the pediatric population is challenging due to the wide age range and developmental spectrum of the population being studied, and within CHD it is further complicated by the variety of congenital and acquired diseases, the range of medical, surgical and interventional therapeutic modalities and the spectrum of outcomes. A further crucial factor within paediatrics is the nature of patient–family interactions and the role of parent–proxy reporting. Cross-informant variance has been widely debated, and within other chronic illnesses children and their parents have demonstrated varying levels of agreement on parameters of psychological functioning and QoL assessment, highlighting the importance of seeking information from both patients and their parents.

The infant and toddler with congenital heart disease

Within the general population, chronic illness in infancy may compromise development (Eiser, 1981; So et al, 1987; Stewart et al, 1987; Davis et al, 1990; Wayman et al, 1997), with gross motor and language development in particular being affected (Polinsky et al, 1987). In the population of children with CHD the majority of work addressing the impact of CHD on the infant and preschool-aged child has addressed neuropsychological and developmental function both before and after surgery; overall, children with CHD, particularly those with cyanotic lesions, have been found to be at increased risk of developmental and cognitive impairment. Abnormal neurological findings (such as hypotonia, hypertonia, jitteriness and absent suck) were identified in 50% of newborn babies with CHD prior to surgery (Limperopoulos et al, 1999), and a third have been reported to have microcephaly (Limperopoulos et al, 1999, 2002), which has been attributed to factors such as low cerebral blood flow both in utero (Kochilas et al, 2001) and in the postnatal period (van Houten et al, 1996). A prospective study of 131 infants who were less than 2 years old at the time of surgery found that preoperative microcephaly was associated with developmental delay 12–18 months after surgery (Limperopoulos et al, 2002), indicating the importance of risk factors in the prenatal and neonatal periods for later development.

A significant amount of work has looked at intraoperative factors and subsequent developmental and cognitive function. It has been estimated that postoperative neurological dysfunction, including seizures, learning and communication problems and motor deficits, occurs in up to 25% of infants (Ferry, 1987a, 1987b), resulting in a sizeable population of children with successfully repaired CHD but with the chronic sequelae of acquired brain injury (DuPlessis, 1997). Studies have specifically focused on the risks and benefits of the intraoperative support mechanisms of cardiopulmonary bypass (CPB) and deep hypothermic circulatory arrest (DHCA). In the largest prospective randomised control trial to date, the Boston Circulatory Arrest Trial, 171 infants with transposition of the great arteries (TGA) were assigned to undergo arterial switch surgery with either predominantly low-flow CPB or predominantly DHCA. Early postoperative findings indicated that infants assigned to DHCA had a higher incidence of neurological morbidity and developmental impairment than those assigned to low-flow CPB (Newburger et al, 1993; Bellinger et al, 1995, 1997), and at 1 year after surgery infants in the DHCA group had a lower score on the psychomotor development index on the Bayley Scales than those in the low-flow CPB group.

A number of other studies of development after cardiac surgery report that infants and preschool children with cyanotic lesions have mean IQ or developmental scores that are within the normal range but at lower levels than expected for population norms, with some studies also identifying specific areas of deficit (Rogers et al, 1995; Bellinger et al, 1997; Kern et al, 1998; Wray & Sensky, 1999; Hovels-Gurich et al, 2001; Tabbutt et al, 2008). In particular, problems have been identified with different aspects of language development, gross and fine motor skills and general locomotor development. The duration of hypoxia and its relationship to developmental outcome has also been investigated, and in a study of 38 children with TGA who had undergone the Mustard procedure, older age at repair (and therefore longer duration of hypoxia) was associated with lower scores on standardised developmental testing (Newburger et al, 1984). Other researchers, however, have failed to find an association between duration of cyanosis and subsequent developmental scores in other lesions (Oates et al, 1995; Uzark et al, 1998; Wernovsky, et al, 2000; Wray & Sensky, 2001).

With the introduction and increased use of treatment options such as transplantation for children with end-stage heart disease, a number of studies have specifically addressed neurodevelopmental and behavioural functioning in this group of patients. Overall, for infants and preschool-aged children, the results of testing suggest that development is within the normal range but at a lower level than that of healthy children (Wray et al, 1992; Baum et al, 1993; Eke et al, 1996; Suddaby et al, 1996). In an evaluation of 48 infants transplanted before the age of 6 months for hypoplastic left heart syndrome, mean scores on both the mental development index and psycho-motor development index of the Bayley Scales were within the normal range, with two-thirds of the children obtaining scores in that range (Baum et al, 1993). In a further longitudinal assessment of neurodevelopmental outcome in 39 children transplanted in infancy, motor development was consistently mildly delayed, and there was an age-dependent variability in cognitive function, with a decrease in performance at 18 months and again at between 28 and 36 months of age (Freier et al, 2004). In a study of children under the age of three and a half years who were assessed for transplant, children with a diagnosis of CHD performed significantly less well than those with cardiomyopathy on a number of parameters, including locomotor abilities, speech and hearing, eye–hand coordination and performance. The children with CHD had been diagnosed for longer, spent longer in hospital, were more likely to have been admitted to a special care baby unit at birth and had undergone more previous procedures under general anaesthetic than those with cardiomyopathy, all of which may have contributed to poorer developmental functioning (Wray & Radley-Smith, 2004).

There are a number of other factors that may have an impact on the development of the infant with CHD, including embolic events, congestive heart failure, episodes of arrhythmias or cardiac arrest, chromosomal abnormalities and poor nutrition. Children with CHD can be difficult to feed because of, for example, fatigue, breathlessness and other symptoms of heart failure, and this can result in poor weight gain and impaired nutritional status. As 50% of the normal postnatal brain growth occurs during the first year of life, poor growth and nutrition during this period can put the infant at risk. Congestive heart failure may also contribute to poor neurodevelopmental outcome due to enforced physical inactivity and failure to thrive (Silbert et al, 1969). Developmental tests for infants and toddlers depend to a significant extent on physical activity, therefore disadvantaging some children with CHD. Furthermore, impaired physical abilities have a detrimental impact on the development of other skills, such as exploratory behaviour, all of which can contribute to poorer performance on psychometric tests.

For many children with CHD, hospitalisation during the first 4 years of life is likely to be a reality, and this in itself can further impact on development. It is well documented that there is a critical period between 6 months and 4 years of age during which hospitalisation can have a particularly detrimental psychological effect on the child (Vernon et al, 1966; Goslin, 1978) due to factors such as the physical environment and the number of different people involved in caring for the child, as well as factors related to the illness and treatment. Overall, for infants or toddlers with CHD, there are a number of factors that put them at increased risk of impaired development, and it is important that all of these are given consideration so as to minimise the risk to the individual patient.

When considering the behavioural and emotional development of young children with CHD there are a number of issues that need to be taken into account. Repeated hospitalisation, the need for intrusive treatments or frequent blood tests, separation from family members and disruption to normal routines can have a potentially traumatic impact on the young child. For some children it is physically impossible for them to engage with healthy children in normal play, whilst for others parental anxiety and overprotectiveness may result in the children being hindered in peer group interactions. It is perhaps not surprising, therefore, that an increased prevalence of social isolation and depression has been identified in young children with end-stage heart disease who were listed for heart transplant (Wray & Radley-Smith, 2004), although in children with less severe heart defects internalising and externalising behaviours were found to be equally prevalent in this age group (Utens et al, 2001). However, studies evaluating the behaviour of young children with CHD are few in number and are largely assessed by questioning parents. It is acknowledged that maternal mental health influences the way in which mothers perceive their child's behaviour (Angold et al, 1987; Webster-Stratton, 1990; Mulhern et al, 1992), thus making it difficult to determine, in the absence of observational studies, how CHD actually impacts on the behaviour of young children.

School-age children

Studies of physical and psychological functioning in school-aged children with CHD have assessed a number of areas of adjustment, including physical activity, cognitive and academic abilities, behaviour, self-esteem, social competence, adherence and QoL.

Physical impact of CHD

For children and young people with less severe congenital heart defects, there may be very little or no residual physical impairment and they are, in effect, able to lead normal lives with no restrictions in terms of physical or social activities. Such young people do not need medication, and many will only require annual or less frequent hospital check-ups. In contrast, some children and young people with congenital heart defects at the severe end of the spectrum may have significant restrictions, including very limited exercise tolerance, cyanosis at rest and short stature. Life for such patients may involve demanding medical regimens, including multiple daily medications, regular hospital check-ups, repeated medical or surgical interventions and, in some cases, the development of life-threatening cardiac problems such as arrhythmias or ventricular dysfunction. They may be unable to attend full-time school or participate in physical activities, and their longer-term prospects in terms of employment may be severely limited.

Participation in physical activities and sports is part of the everyday experience of healthy children and young people, and the benefits of regular activity are well documented (Fletcher, 1996; Thompson et al, 2003; Marcus et al, 2006). An inability to take part in sports and physical activity can have a negative impact on perceived QoL as well as on other aspects of physical health, and encouraging children with CHD to exercise safely but at the same time optimising their exercise ability is therefore an important component of their long-term care. The results of exercise testing are increasingly being reported in the literature as outcome measures and indicators of physical status, particularly in children with specific diagnoses such as tetralogy of Fallot, TGA or single-ventricle physiology. Evaluation of school-aged children after repair of congenital lesions in infancy found that those with simple lesions have normal exercise ability (Norozi et al, 2005), and excellent exercise capacity has also been reported after procedures such as neonatal repair of TGA (Hovels-Gurich et al, 2003) and the Ross procedure (Marino et al, 2006), but children with other diagnoses may have varying degrees of exercise impairment. There is evidence that such impairment is mild for those who have had repair of a total anomalous venous connection (McBride et al, 2007), for example, whereas for those who have undergone a Fontan procedure, exercise limitations are more severe (Takken et al, 2007).

Whilst limitations in exercise capacity are often attributable to the abnormal hemodynamics and physiology associated with the congenital heart defect, a further contributing factor may be a low level of daily physical activity (Fredriksen et al, 2001; Reybrouck & Mertens, 2005; Dua, 2007). Parental overprotection has been suggested as a mechanism in this (Reybrouck & Mertens, 2005), although other research suggests that it is physicians who have been reluctant to encourage physical activity, and have either imposed unnecessary restrictions even in those with mild CHD or have failed to give specific advice regarding appropriate exercise (Swan & Hillis, 2000; Fekkes et al, 2001; Therrien et al, 2003). A recent study of 147 patients aged 7–18 years who had undergone the Fontan procedure at a median of 8.1 years previously found that physical activity levels were reduced, irrespective of exercise capacity, and were associated with lower perceived general health but not with other aspects of functional status (McCrindle et al, 2007).

Misconceptions regarding exercise also appear to be prevalent, with parents, teachers and children underestimating exercise ability or, through lack of information, imposing unnecessary restrictions (Casey et al, 1994; Rogers et al, 1994). Conversely, some patients have been found to overestimate their ability to exercise, to the extent that they have exercised at dangerous levels (Swan & Hillis, 2000; Kendall et al, 2007), indicating the need for education about appropriate exercise and its importance.

A number of researchers have evaluated the efficacy of exercise and rehabilitation programmes for young people with CHD (Fredriksen et al, 2000; Rhodes et al, 2005) and found that, in the short term, exercise ability has been improved by participation in such schemes, although whether such benefits are maintained in the longer term requires further evaluation. However, it is also clear that recruiting young people into these programmes, retaining them once started and sustaining their motivation once the programme has finished are areas of difficulty (Marcus et al, 2006), indicating that structured activity programmes are not appropriate for all young people. Another approach has been that of sports camps, and in an evaluation of 31 children with CHD who attended a 3-day camp, there was a significant improvement in the children's perceptions of their physical functioning, self-esteem and other aspects of subjective health status (Moons et al, 2006a). At a 3-month follow-up improvements in perceived health status were still evident (Moons et al, 2006b), although it is not yet known whether such benefits are maintained in the longer term.

Cognitive and academic abilities

Assessing cognitive and academic abilities in children with CHD has been the focus of many studies, and overall the research to date indicates that CHD does not have an adverse impact on cognitive functioning for all children and adolescents, although children with cyanotic lesions have been identified as being at greater risk of impaired cognitive functioning (McCusker et al, 2007). A recent meta-analysis suggested that there are some groups of children who are at specific risk, with disease severity being related to overall cognitive functioning (Karsdorp et al, 2007). Children with a diagnosis of hypoplastic left heart syndrome and TGA have been found to demonstrate decreased cognitive functioning compared with normative data and study-recruited control groups in some studies, with deficits being particularly evident in the domain of perceptual organisational abilities (Karsdorp et al, 2007).

In a follow-up of the infants recruited to the Boston Circulatory Arrest Trial, at both 4 years and 8 years the cognitive differences between the groups assigned to either low-flow CPB or DHCA were minimised, and were limited primarily to abnormalities of executive planning, visual–motor integration, behaviour and speech (Bellinger et al, 1999, 2003a). Testing of the whole cohort at 4 years indicated that overall IQ scores were slightly worse than those of the normative population, but by 8 years scores were essentially normal, contradicting some other studies of patients with TGA. In contrast, an increased risk of deficits in visual–spatial skills was seen at 8 years in the whole cohort (Bellinger et al, 2003b). Interestingly, a longer duration of time spent in hospital and intensive care in the neonatal period was associated with worse cognitive function at 8 years, even when controlling for perioperative events, perfusion times and socio-economic variables (Newburger et al, 2003).

Studies of motor competence in school-aged children suggest a higher prevalence of gross and/or fine motor delay compared with healthy children (Holm et al, 2007; Hovels-Gurich et al, 1997; Majnemer et al, 2006a). In a study of 90 4-year-old children with CHD (McCusker et al, 2007), all children with severe CHD, regardless of cyanotic status or surgical procedure, were found to be at risk of sensorimotor problems. Impaired motor functioning may affect aspects of daily living such as self-care activities, participation in sports and other social activities, which can result in a more inactive lifestyle, lower self-esteem and poor academic achievement, and affect a child's status within a peer group. It has been suggested that some form of movement treatment or sensory integration (Vargas & Camill, 1999) or rehabilitation programmes may be useful to ameliorate some of the observed deficits.

Results are mixed concerning other aspects of cognitive and neuropsychological functioning in the school-aged child. Several studies of memory functioning suggest that some groups of children with CHD perform within the normal range on memory tasks (Wright & Nolan, 1994; Oates et al, 1995; Hovels-Gurich et al, 2001), whereas other studies have identified some groups of children with CHD to be at increased risk of impaired memory functioning (Bellinger et al, 2003a; Miatton et al, 2007a), particularly those with single-ventricle physiology (Forbess et al, 2002). In contrast, studies of language development suggest more widespread deficits (Hovels-Gurich et al, 2006, 2008), with about one-fifth of children with TGA, for example, demonstrating deficits in receptive and/or expressive language tasks (Hovels-Gurich et al, 2002a). Attention and executive function also appear to be impaired in some children with CHD (Hovels-Gurich et al, 2007; Miatton et al, 2007b), although this is not an area that has been comprehensively studied. As with other domains of cognitive and neuropsychological functioning, socio-economic status, age at testing and intra-operative factors are important determinants of outcome.

Academic functioning has also been studied in children with CHD, and again those with cyanotic lesions appear to fare worse on academic parameters of arithmetics, reading and spelling (Wright & Nolan, 1994; Mahle et al, 2000; Wernovsky et al, 2000; Wray & Sensky, 2001; Hovels-Gurich et al, 2002b). In a longitudinal evaluation of school-aged children who had undergone neonatal surgery for TGA, there was a significant reduction over time in mean scores on measures of learning and academic abilities, indicating that the children were failing to keep up with age-normative data (Hovels-Gurich et al, 1997, 2002b). Whilst the vast majority of children will be able to attend mainstream school, studies suggest that some children will be restricted at school, most commonly in the areas of physical activities, play-time and school trips. From an academic perspective, some children will require extra learning support and may be restricted in terms of their ability to follow the normal curriculum, but for these children in particular it is important that an alternative curriculum is followed that meets their specific needs and helps them to fulfil their academic potential.

In patients who have undergone transplantation, performance on both cognitive and academic parameters is within the normal range (Wray et al, 1994; Baum et al, 2004; Wray & Radley-Smith, 2005), but those with a pretransplant diagnosis of CHD perform significantly less well than those with a pretransplant diagnosis of cardio-myopathy. Almost half of all the children who had been transplanted were found to be underachieving on academic parameters at 2 years post transplant (Wray & Radley-Smith, 2005), which, although not significantly different from that seen in the comparison group of healthy children, was largely attributed to missed schooling. There are clearly implications for the delivery of school services to children who are absent from school for prolonged or repeated episodes in order to try and minimise the impact of lost time at school.

It is evident from the research literature that, whilst there are risk factors for poorer cognitive and academic functioning in children and adolescents with CHD, the findings are not clear cut. More important, perhaps, is whether statistically significant findings are of clinical significance and, if so, what interventions can be implemented to assist those children at greatest risk.

Behavioural and emotional functioning

A meta-analysis addressing psychopathology in children with CHD found that they exhibited more overall, internalising (e.g. anxiety, depression and withdrawal) and externalising (e.g. hyperactivity and aggression) behaviour problems than controls (Karsdorp et al, 2007). However, when potential moderating factors were taken into account, it was only older children and adolescents who demonstrated an increased risk of overall, internalising and, to a lesser extent, externalising behaviour problems.

A number of studies have suggested that children with cyanotic lesions have more behavioural and attention problems than children with acyanotic lesions (Dunbar-Masterson et al, 2001; Kirshbom et al, 2005), which has been attributed, at least in part, to hypoxia. In their study of 31 school-aged children aged 5.6–13.0 years with repaired TGA, O'Dougherty and colleagues (1985) found that, when compared with healthy children, children in the CHD group were rated as significantly more dependent, passive and hypoactive and less attentive, task oriented and self-confident. They suggest that some children who endure a period of chronic hypoxia have an attention deficit disorder with hypoactivity.

In a longer term follow-up study of children with TGA who were assessed 6.3–17.9 years after surgery, the population of children who met the American Psychiatric Association Diagnostic and Statistical Manual of Mental Disorders IV criteria for a psychiatric diagnosis was slightly higher than expected, with an internalising pattern of behaviour predominating (Alden et al, 1998). However, psychological problems were more prevalent in those with poorer cardiac status, making it difficult to separate out the possible effects of early chronic hypoxia from other medical factors on later behaviour. A further long-term evaluation of 60 children who underwent a neonatal repair for TGA found that, in multivariate analysis, severe preoperative hypoxia predicted social problems and deficits in social involvement, as measured on the Child Behavior Checklist (Hovels-Gurich et al, 2002a). Perioperative and postoperative cardiac insufficiency also predicted internalising and externalising behaviour problems and attention deficits. The authors suggest that this can be attributed to deficits in cerebral perfusion having a detrimental impact on vulnerable regions of the brain, such as the frontal lobes, hippocampus and cerebellum, although magnetic resonance imaging studies were not conducted to confirm this.

In contrast, more recent research has suggested that it is only those children who have undergone palliative interventions or who have more severe disease who are at risk of poor behavioural outcomes (McCusker et al, 2007), rather than cyanosis itself being associated with poorer outcomes. Furthermore, in their study of 90 children with a range of acyanotic and cyanotic conditions, the authors found that parenting style, marital status, maternal worry and maternal mental health difficulties were more important for predicting behavioural outcomes than cyanosis or surgical factors.

Children with hypoplastic left heart syndrome have an increased incidence of attention deficit hyperactivity disorder (Hagemo et al, 1997; Mahle et al, 2000). Although this has not been specifically attributed to hypoxia, studies of children with sleep-disordered breathing have established a link between attention deficit hyperactivity disorder and hypoxia (Chervin et al, 1997, 2002; O'Brien et al, 2003), even in children who exhibit milder (90–95%) levels of oxygen desaturation. The results obtained from children with hypoplastic left heart syndrome are in contrast to some findings from other groups of children with cyanotic heart disease, in which behaviour is characterised by attention problems with hypoactivity. The reasons for such discrepancies are not clear but may be related to factors such as study design and methods of assessment, together with patient factors such as cardiac status.

The effects of cardiac arrest on later behaviour are also important for children with CHD. In a follow-up study of 25 children who survived a cardiac arrest (20 of whom had CHD), scores on measures of adaptive behaviour were lower than normal, particularly for children in whom the arrest period was more than 15 minutes (Morris et al, 1993). Internalising behaviour problems and hyperactivity were also more prevalent in children who had longer arrest periods and more medical risk factors. In an effort to assess the additive impact of cardiac arrest on children with CHD, Bloom and colleagues compared children with CHD who had sustained an in-hospital arrest with a group of medically similar children with CHD who had not incurred a cardiac arrest (Bloom et al, 1997). Children in the arrest group, particularly those who had more severe disease, demonstrated impairment in adaptive behaviour.

Relatively few investigators have actually asked children and adolescents how they feel about having CHD and what their experiences are of living with a heart condition. A qualitative study with 35 children and young people aged 8–19 years with a variety of heart lesions identified that whilst many believed that they coped well with their condition, for others there was a significant impact on everyday life. Particular themes identified included the physical restrictions associated with their condition, others' attitudes, feeling different from their peers, aspects related to information about their condition and factors related to privacy, both in the hospital setting and at home (Birks et al, 2007).

Early work addressing self-perception in children and teenagers produced conflicting results. Children with CHD were found to have a constricted body image compared with healthy children (Green & Levitt, 1962), and young people with CHD reported more feelings of inferiority (Kramer et al, 1989). In contrast, a study of adolescents found that, overall, they differed little from their healthy peers, although those with more severe disease had a more negative self-concept (Uzark et al, 1989). In a prospective evaluation of children undergoing cardiac surgery, children rated themselves preoperatively as weaker (poorer body image), more frightened and more ill than a healthy comparison group, but a year after surgery there were no differences between the two groups, with those in the CHD group rating themselves as less ill after surgery compared with beforehand (Wray & Sensky, 1998).

More recent research has suggested that adolescent boys have a more negative self-concept than girls, which has been partly attributed to reduced physical abilities interfering with peer relationships (Salzer-Muhar et al, 2002), and those with severe heart disease report lower self-esteem than adolescents with moderate or mild disease (Cohen et al, 2007).

Social competence, which encompasses functioning at school, peer relationships and participation in sports and activities both within and outside the home, has not been widely studied in children with CHD. However, in a recent study of 43 children, parents' ratings of their children's social functioning and participation in activities did not differ from parental ratings of a healthy control group, but children with CHD were rated as having poorer functioning in the domain of school competence (Miatton et al, 2007c). In contrast, the children's self-reports on perceived competence at school did not differ from those of the healthy group. In studies of transplantation, poor social competence has been identified in up to 50% of heart and/or lung transplant patients (Uzark et al, 1992; Wray & Radley-Smith, 2006), with those who had poorer functioning also rating themselves as more anxious and/or depressed.

Some authors have also looked at behaviour and adjustment within the school environment. In an evaluation of 168 children who had undergone cardiac surgery 4–8 years previously, teachers did not rate their behaviour any differently from that of healthy children (Oates et al, 1994). In contrast, in a study of children who had undergone heart transplantation, those with a pretransplant diagnosis of CHD had a higher prevalence of behaviour problems at school than those transplanted for cardiomyopathy and than healthy children (Wray et al, 2001). However it is important to take into account how the school life of children with CHD may be affected by their condition. Children with CHD are more likely than healthy children to have to repeat an academic year (Miatton et al, 2007c), to miss school to attend hospital appointments and to be unable to participate in physical activities, which can result in lower self-esteem and difficulties in a number of areas of school life, including peer relationships. It is therefore essential that appropriate support is put in place on an individualised basis to enable children to maximise their potential within the school environment, from both an academic and a social perspective.

Adherence

Evaluation of adherence in chronically ill populations has typically focused on the adolescent age range, with estimates that approximately 50% of adolescents with chronic illness are non-adherent to some aspect of the treatment regimen (La Greca & Schuman, 1995). Risk-taking is one of the normal and adaptive behaviours used by adolescents to accomplish the developmental tasks of separation–individuation, identity formation and establishing relationships outside the family (Ponton, 1997). There is a spectrum of risk-taking behaviours from benign, age-appropriate activities to high-risk behaviours such as substance abuse, and non-adherence to certain aspects of the medical regimen has been conceptualised as part of this spectrum (Shaw, 2001). Within the CHD population, there is surprisingly little information on this topic, but adherence to antibiotic prophylaxis is one area that has been investigated. Knowledge of the need for antibiotic prophylaxis has been found to be relatively poor amongst both caregivers and young people with CHD (Cetta et al, 1993; Knirsch et al, 2003; Wray et al, 2004), resulting in poor adherence to appropriate treatment protocols. Good communication between health professionals, young people with CHD and their carers about the risks of endocarditis and appropriate antibiotic prophylaxis is therefore of paramount importance.

Adherence following heart transplantation has been flagged up as a major area of concern, and some who have a very rigid definition of adherence would say that non-adherence is an inevitable consequence of transplantation. A recent study found that about one-third of adolescent and young adult recipients were non-adherent to their immunosuppression, with the majority of these being unintentionally non-adherent (i.e. forgetting to take their medication on occasion) (Wray et al, 2006). With the necessity for immunosuppression to be taken regularly, practical strategies for helping young people to remember and take their medications need to be identified and implemented into their daily routine. As with any children or young people who have to adhere to a treatment protocol, strategies to improve knowledge and under-standing and empowering young people to take responsibility for their condition and its management need to be devised and implemented as part of the routine care of patients and families.

Quality of life

Whilst there are numerous reports in the literature about aspects of physical and psychological functioning in children and young people with CHD, it is still not clear how such factors impact on QoL. Quantitative assessment of QoL in children with congenital and acquired heart disease is very limited, unlike other paediatric conditions such as cancer and asthma, although a number of studies claim to measure QoL. A recent evaluation of 70 studies purporting to measure QoL in patients with CHD found that only one study asked patients to rate their perceived QoL (Moons et al, 2004), and furthermore a number of studies assessed factors such as functional status or behaviour, rather than QoL.

The first systematic attempt to look at QoL in patients with CHD was in 1993 (Gersony et al, 1993), when information was collected on 2401 patients relating to their personal perception of their health, marital and employment status, educational attainment, health and life insurance coverage and New York Heart Association (NYHA) status. Since that time, particular groups of children with CHD have been studied, mainly using generic measures completed by parents. Some studies have reported excellent QoL for children and young people with CHD that does not differ significantly from that of their peers (Moyen Laane et al, 1997; Culbert et al, 2003; Dunbar-Masterson et al, 2001; Walker et al, 2004), whilst others have reported QoL to be significantly poorer than that of healthy controls, particularly in the areas of physical and social QoL and overall functioning (Uzark et al, 2003; Mussatto & Tweddell, 2005; Landolt et al, 2008). In one of the few studies to look at QoL and psychological functioning in children with an implantable cardioverter–defibrillator, parental perceptions of QoL were poorer than scores for healthy children, with QoL scores being more highly correlated with levels of anxiety and depression and parameters of family functioning than with the severity of the cardiac condition (DeMaso et al, 2004).

Overall, results are mixed about QoL for children and young people with CHD. One difficulty is that many of the studies rely solely on parental reporting and do not report patients' own perceptions of their QoL, and within some other illness groups parents' ratings of their child's QoL have been found to differ significantly from the children's own ratings (Parsons et al, 1999; White-Koning et al, 2007). In particular, it has been hypothesised that for less observable aspects of QoL, such as emotional functioning, parent–child agreement is weaker (Eiser & Morse, 2001; Krol et al, 2003). However, whilst there are clearly some children who have impaired QoL, with some specific diagnostic subgroups being at greater risk of poorer functioning, many children and young people with CHD are reported to have an excellent QoL and demonstrate resiliency and adaptive coping mechanisms in their everyday life.

Working with and caring for children and young people with CHD and mental health disorders

It is estimated that 1 in 6 children and young people with a chronic or life-limiting disorder also has a diagnosable mental health disorder (Meltzer et al, 2004). Children and young people who have cardiac conditions fit into this group, and it is likely that their illness will have some impact on their emotional, psychological and mental health state. This can vary and may be dependent upon the child/young person's inner resilience, personal and family coping strategies and the stage of the child/young person's development. It may also be dependent upon whether they were born with this condition, whether they developed it in early childhood or whether it is something that has recently occurred. These factors may dictate how the child or young person might cope and can be associated with an adjustment disorder (Goodman & Scott, 2005).

There are those who experience significant difficulties and require intensive mental health nursing care within tier 3 and 4 services. For many children/young people and their families, this can be a frightening experience and can carry a certain element of stigma with it. Where possible, it is better to avoid the mental health 'label' when working with children and young people as this can have a negative effect upon their future lives. However, it is sometimes unavoidable that children are sectioned under the Mental Health Act (1983), and although these cases are rare, we should instead encourage the use of the Children's Act (1989) where possible, only using the Mental Health Act when absolutely necessary. For a mental health diagnosis to be made, under the World Health Organization's International Classification of Diseases 10, the criteria state that these 'difficulties' must have a strict impairment on the child or young person's day-to-day life.

The majority of children and young people with cardiac conditions are nursed on children's wards by children's nurses. These areas are not traditionally thought to be a part of child and adolescent mental health services but do in fact sit on the filter line between tier 1 and tier 2 services as defined by the Health Advisory Service (1995). As such, these areas see more children and young people with emotional, psychological and mental health disorders than any other single discipline. Although the care given on these wards is predominantly physically based, it has long been recognised that we care for the whole child, which also encompasses their mental health. It is therefore vital that children's nurses have the knowledge and skills to recognise when a child or young person is showing signs and symptoms of mental health disorder and can act appropriately. Standard 9 of the *National Service Framework for Children, Young People and Maternity Services* (Department of Health [DH], 2004) considers their psychological wellbeing and highlights the importance of recognition and early intervention. The mental health of our children and young people is high on the health agenda, and it should be noted that child and adolescent mental health is every nurse's business and not exclusively that of the mental health nurse (Royal College of Nursing [RCN], 2004).

With improving care and technology, more children and young people with cardiac conditions are living longer now than was previously expected. It could be argued that their QoL is much better from the point of view of physical health. However, there can be a negative impact on their mental health, especially in adolescence (McDougall, 2006). Adolescence is the period in life when young people experiment and tend to engage in risk-taking behaviours such as drugs, alcohol and sexual activity. It is also an important time in the formation of identity and, according to Erikson (1974), is the time when we decide what we want to be and where we are going in life. These are going to be difficult decisions for the young person who is likely to face his or her own death within the foreseeable future.

What we might consider to be normal adolescent behaviour may impact significantly on a young person with a heart problem. The negative risk factors associated with smoking and drinking alcohol are well documented and pose an even greater risk to this client group. Likewise, the effects of recreational drugs will be amplified. Amphetamines (commonly known as speed) are a widely used range of drugs; the side-effects of these are a raised heart rate and palpitations. Using crack cocaine is linked to heart disease, as is ecstasy. Although not all young people use drugs, there is evidence to suggest that 10% will have experimented between the ages of 11 and 15 years of age (Health Advisory Service, 2001). Risky sexual activity is an issue for all young people and has resulted in an increased rate of sexually transmitted infections and unwanted pregnancies (DH, 2003). Again, this risk has implications for the young person with a life-limiting cardiac condition.

One of the biggest risks associated with young people currently is self-harm, with the rates thought to be 1 in 10 (Camelot Foundation and Mental Health Foundation, 2006). There are many factors associated with self-harming behaviours, including chronic physical illness, disturbed education and relationship difficulties. It is inevitable that young people who have a chronic illness will miss time at school through repeated hospital admissions and general illness related to their condition, which can

Box 4.1 Case study: Charlotte's healthcare episode

Charlotte is a 15-year-old girl who was born with congenital heart disease. She has always been compliant with her medication and care routine. She has never been allowed to partici-pate in any physical activities due to her condition. Her parents describe her as their 'special' child and have, by their own admission, wrapped her in cotton wool. Charlotte is a quiet girl and doesn't have many friends. She has lost a lot of time from school and rarely goes out. Her life expectancy is late teens to early twenties but lately her condition has deteriorated, which has resulted in longer periods of hospitalisation. Charlotte has spent a lot of her childhood on the ward and knows it well.

During her last admission, Charlotte became very quiet, tearful and isolated; she hardly mixed with the other young people on the ward, which is unlike her. She had a reduced appetite and an altered sleeping pattern. No one appeared to have noticed this change in her despite the fact that she had lost some weight. One of the other young people noticed cuts on Charlotte's arms and told a nurse.

The ward was very busy and Charlotte's care was time-consuming, but when she was having some treatment she told one of the nurses that she felt very down, much more than usual. The nurse said that this was to be expected in the circumstances and not to worry about it, she was 'bound to be down'.

Charlotte was discharged home the next day.

also result in a school phobia. It has also been identified that these young people find it difficult to make long-term relationships and are poorly supported by their class-mates (Cooper et al, 2005). Additionally, this is linked to low self-esteem, poor body image and depression. There are strong links between depression and self-harming behaviour (National Institute for Health and Clinical Excellence, 2004) and high rates of depression amongst children with life-limiting disorders (Goodman & Scott, 2005).

In relation to chronic illness, emotional distress and coping strategies vary and may present in a variety of ways. Whilst many of these young people may engage in risk-taking behaviour, it is important to note that others internalise the problem and exhibit alternative behaviours. Box 4.1 shows one particular example of how a young person may react.

We can see from Charlotte's case study that she has been described as a quiet girl who doesn't socialise well, but it should be evident to nursing staff that she is even quieter than normal. She has been a regular patient on this unit, and by now the nurses should have a good insight into Charlotte's 'normal' behaviour. She has told the nurse that she feels even more down than usual, and it has been noted that she has lost some weight and has not been sleeping well. It is hoped that the nurse would also have noticed the marks on Charlotte's arms. These are the signs and symptoms of depression that the nurse needs to be aware of (Cooper et al, 2005). It would appear that the nurse sees this as normal behaviour 'in the circumstances' and has not con-sidered that Charlotte has actually tried to tell someone how she is feeling.

The nurse spent 25 minutes giving intravenous drugs – a missed opportunity to talk to Charlotte about how she was coping and any worries or concerns that she might have. Whilst the children's nurse may not be an expert in mental health, she should be able to recognise that there is a problem. She should be able to make some form of psychological assessment and refer to the CAMHS if needed. The first marker of good practice within Standard 9 of the National Service Framework (DH, 2004) highlights that all staff working directly with children and young people should have sufficient knowledge and training to identify early indicators of psychological difficulty and mental ill health.

Charlotte may be facing her own death within the next few years, and it is perhaps understandable that she 'feels down', as the nurse describes it. However, feeling down is very different from suffering with a depressive illness, and we need to have the knowledge and skills to be able to differentiate. Even though children's wards can be busy and there are time constraints, there are opportunities when nurses can talk and listen to children and young people. This may be when undertaking treatments or procedures, and we should see this as an opportunity to provide emotional care. As children's nurses, we have a responsibility to care for the mental health of children and young people as well as their physical health. After all, child and adolescent mental health is every nurse's business (RCN, 2004).

The adult with CHD – long-term physical and social issues

To address the long-term physical and social issues, it is appropriate to consider initially some of the relevant medical problems that adults with CHD may encounter and the impact of these on their lives. It is also recognised that increasing numbers of young people with CHD are now presenting with complex lesions and many unique problems that require specialist management at a recognised adult CHD (ACHD) centre. The vast majority of adults with CHD require lifelong follow-up for moderate or complex disease and the potential to develop late complications. Some will need further surgery. Despite the recent organisation and expansion of services, there are still only a limited number of specialist clinics; consequently three levels of care have been recommended (European Society of Cardiology [ESC], 2003):

- level 1: exclusive follow-up in the specialist congenital heart unit;
- level 2: shared care with appropriate general adult cardiac services;
- level 3: patients who can be managed in non-specialist clinics.

Approximately 25–50% of the ACHD population require level 1 and 2 follow-up (ESC, 2003). Less than 10% of adults with CHD need to be admitted as inpatients to a specialist ACHD centre (British Cardiac Society, 2002). However, lifelong outpatient follow-up is necessary.

Whilst the vast majority of CHD is diagnosed in the antenatal period or early in life, it is important to be aware that a number of patients with CHD are diagnosed in adult life with structural and/or valvar abnormalities such as atrial septal defect (ASD) or pulmonary stenosis. This may be due to a complication of an asymptomatic lesion such as infective endocarditis in a bicuspid aortic valve, or to the development of an arrhythmia such as atrial fibrillation, paradoxical embolus and stroke associated with an ASD.

A multiprofessional team approach is essential to provide holistic care to adults with CHD. The specialist team should include a CHD specialist, adult cardiologist, congenital cardiac surgeon and anaesthetist, electrophysiologist, nurses, obstetrician, haematologist, geneticist, psychologist, general practitioner and social worker. Good communication between the specialist centre, district general hospital and primary healthcare team is essential. The ACHD specialist has a responsibility to keep the primary healthcare physician informed of the patient's diagnosis, any residual problems and possible changes. This is important because, for the patients, their general practitioner is the first port of call. If admission is necessary, the district hospital requires a cardiologist with an interest in CHD who has good contacts with the specialist unit and can identify when to refer the patient.

Relevant medical issues

The long-term outlook for patients with moderate or significant CHD varies considerably, depending on the outcome of previous surgical interventions and the haemodynamic status (Kovacs et al, 2005), and is similar for those who have not had surgery. Many face the prospect of further operations, arrhythmias, complications and, if managed inappropriately, an increased risk of heart failure and premature death (Somerville, 1997; Gatzoulis et al, 2003). Patients may be at risk of developing specific medical problems later in life related to their underlying cardiac anatomy. Those with complex cyanotic CHD can develop problems related to the effects of chronic cyanosis such as polycythaemia, iron deficiency anaemia, abnormal clotting and bleeding tendencies. Patients with a haemoglobin level of over 20 g/dL and a haematocrit of over 65% may experience symptoms of hyperviscosity such as headache, blurred vision and poor concentration. There is risk of cerebral abscess and cerebrovascular accident. Patients who are persistently cyanosed and those with Eisenmenger syndrome, irrespective of the underlying cardiac anatomy, may develop joint problems, scoliosis, abnormal renal function, gallstones, acne and gout.

Heart failure is not an uncommon presenting feature in some patients with unrepaired lesions, in patients who have had a previous palliation such as the Fontan procedure or in those who were considered to have had a 'successful' repair in the past such as the Mustard operation. Patients may develop side-effects from long-term medications such as amiodarone, beta-blockers, angiotensin-converting enzyme inhibitors and diuretics. They need to be carefully monitored and, because of ventricular dysfunction, may develop resultant pulmonary vascular changes.

Many adults with CHD may have elevated pulmonary vascular resistance and distortion of the pulmonary vessels due to previous surgery. Eisenmenger syndrome occurs when pulmonary vascular disease becomes irreversible due to a persistent communication between the systemic and pulmonary circulations. Careful evaluation of the pulmonary vascular bed is necessary before any surgical or catheter intervention is undertaken.

Arrhythmia and pacing

The improved survival of patients with CHD has led to an increase in the number of adult patients presenting with arrhythmias. These are one of the most common causes of hospitalisation in this age group and can lead to significant morbidity and mortality. The electrophysiological evaluation and treatment of CHD patients with catheter ablation is becoming an increasingly important focus of management. The aetiology of arrhythmias is most commonly related to previous surgery and scar tissue resulting from incisions and patches in the atria or ventricles, ischaemia, hypertrophied tissue and fibrosis. In some cases, the arrhythmic potential is further compounded by chronic volume and/or pressure overload leading to conduction delay.

In those patients who have undergone operative intervention, four cardiac lesions are associated with a high incidence of atrial arrhythmias. Patients with an ASD are at risk both before and after repair, particularly if repair is undertaken late in adulthood. Those who have undergone surgical correction of tetralogy of Fallot, atrial switch for simple TGA (Mustard/Senning operation) or have single-ventricle physiology treated with the Fontan procedure are also at risk. Ventricular arrhythmias are less common in those with CHD, although ventricular tachycardia associated with previous surgical right ventricular outflow tract intervention in patients with tetralogy of Fallot is well known. Radiofrequency ablation in the catheter laboratory may offer treatment if arrhythmic pathways can be demonstrated, or it may be that antiarrhythmic surgery is required to improve the haemodynamic status.

The availability of dual-chamber sensing and pacing to maintain atrioventricular synchrony and sensor-driven rate-response pacing has been a significant advance for patients with heart block and sinoatrial (sinus) node disease (Gregoratos et al, 2002). The advent of biventricular pacing for the treatment of congestive cardiac failure by resynchronization of the left ventricular wall motion is now possible. Antitachycardic pacing may also be a possible treatment.

Cardiological interventions

The impact of percutaneous interventions on the adult with CHD is gaining important recognition. This is in areas such as ASD device closure (Berger et al, 1999), muscular ventricular septal defect (VSD) device closure, balloon dilatation and stenting of pulmonary artery stenosis. The use of a percutaneous pulmonary valve in conduit stenosis has also been undertaken (Bonhoeffer et al, 2000). As an adjunct to the surgical procedure, concurrent interventional approaches to a complex lesion, such as coil embolisation of important collaterals and systemic-to-pulmonary-artery shunts have been performed.

Cardiac surgical management

Due to the complex nature of the surgery and the lack of long-term outcome data, the risk of late mortality and morbidity is not fully understood yet. Success is not guaranteed, and patients and families/carers need a great deal of support and patience when decisions are being made about whether or not surgery should be performed. Patients find attendance at a preadmission clinic helpful and particularly value the opportunity to address questions to the surgeon personally. They require considerable information, written as well as verbal, and should the patient die, this support for the family will often be needed for some time afterwards. However, it is important to emphasise that risk is minimised in units where there is a multidisciplinary team approach to the management and ongoing care of these patients.

Non-cardiac surgical procedures

Many adults with CHD have health problems in addition to their heart conditions, requiring support from other medical services. Non-cardiac surgery may be complicated by haemodynamic deterioration related to anaesthesia, hypovolaemia or the injudicious manipulation of vascular tone. All inhalational anaesthetic agents affect vascular resistance, and most are negatively inotropic. This may be dangerous if there is pulmonary hypertension or the potential for intracardiac shunting. Shunting refers to the movement of blood through a congenitally abnormal or surgically created connection between two circuits, at the level of the atria, ventricles or great vessels (Gatzoulis et al, 2005). This means that blood may move from the right side of the heart to the left without being oxygenated via the lungs, inducing cyanosis. Cyanotic patients are at risk of haemorrhage, dehydration and paradoxical emboli. For this reason, adults with CHD who require general surgery under general anaesthesia may require preoperative assessment by a CHD specialist and anaesthesia supervised by a cardiac anaesthetist.

Physical activity and exercise

The beneficial effects of physical exercise on fitness, psychological wellbeing, confidence and social integration are widely known. The ability to exercise is one measure of QoL and is used to assess the effect of disease. Exercise capacity in young people with CHD is determined by the underlying defect and has been shown to be diminished in patients with both unrepaired and repaired CHD.

There have been a number of studies of exercise tolerance in children and adolescents with CHD but very few in adults. Trojnarska (2007) commented on the lack of uniform functional classifications for adults with CHD. The NYHA classification of heart failure is the conventional measure of HRQoL in both ACHD and left ventricular failure in the general population. However, subjective functional evaluation of the NYHA classification does not reflect the actual level of the heart's exercise tolerance in patients with CHD. The Ability Index (Warnes & Somerville, 1986) was designed specifically for the adult population with CHD; despite limited exercise capacity and left ventricular ejection fraction, many patients lead nearly normal lives as judged by the Ability Index, but it has not been widely used.

The benefits of an objective spiroergometric exercise test have been documented; patients with various types of CHD differed in their level of exercise capacity. Those with simple non-cyanotic CHD demonstrated better exercise tolerance than those with complex cyanotic CHD, particularly those with a functional single ventricle and pulmonary hypertension. Similarly, patients with sinus rhythm had a higher value of peak oxygen consumption compared with patients with atrial fibrillation or atrial flutter. Trojnarska (2007) also reviewed the possible correlation between the spiroergometric exercise test and NYHA class; however, the subjective evaluation tends to be somewhat more optimistic. Even asymptomatic patients showed significantly decreased oxygen consumption compared with the healthy population.

This lack of perception of progressive exercise intolerance may result from lifelong adaptation of many patients with CHD to exercise limitation. However, interventions to improve physical functioning should be promoted for all patients with CHD. Restrictions apply to those with pulmonary hypertension and obstructive lesions of the left heart, who should not participate in competitive sports because of the risk of syncope and sudden death. Patients who have aortic anomalies, those on oral anticoagulants and those with pacemakers should avoid contact sports. Cardiac rehabilitation programmes have been developed primarily for people with coronary artery disease, and adults with CHD, including those with cyanotic CHD, may benefit from directed exercise therapy.

Psychosocial issues

In addition to their physical problems, some patients face lifelong social, emotional and psychological difficulties caused by chronic illness and hospitalisation, disrupted education and distorted body image. This is an area that has been relatively neglected, and the long-term implications of living with CHD are uncertain.

Many patients have a high level of anxiety about their underlying heart condition and prognosis. Brandhagen et al (1991) reported high levels of psychological problems amongst patients with CHD that were unrelated to the clinical severity of the original cardiac defect. Some experience difficulties with social interaction and express loneliness and feelings of being different from their peers. The desire to be normal is strong, which may result in a reluctance to admit limitations and/or symptoms, as well as to discuss problems (ESC, 2003). Some patients indulge in risk-taking behaviour whilst others remain dependent on parents and physicians, are less well informed about their illness and are overanxious about relatively trivial residual problems.

Some factors may contribute to emotional and behavioural problems in adults with operated CHD, for example patients' perceptions of the scar, their physical condition and restrictions imposed by physicians (Van Rijen et al, 2004). Anxiety and depressive symptoms have been found amongst patients who had been thought to be 'well adjusted' (Bromberg et al, 2003). Lip et al (2005) performed a Cochrane systematic review of the literature to identify interventions for depression in adolescents and adults with CHD. Depression is common in patients with CHD and can exacerbate the physical consequences of the illness. Effective treatments exist, such as psychotherapy, cognitive-behavioural therapies and talking therapies in addition to pharmacological treatments; however, no trials could be identified showing the effectiveness of non-pharmacological treatments for depression. In contrast, Utens et al (1998) investigated long-term psychological outcome in 166 young adults aged 19–25 who underwent surgery for CHD in infancy and childhood using the Young Adult Self-Report form. Overall satisfactory psychosocial functioning was reported.

The extent of psychological dysfunction in adults with CHD appears conflicting. Kovacs et al (2005) revealed that interview data may suggest more psychological disturbance than self-report data. The use of self-denial and high achievement motivation among adults with CHD might artificially inflate ratings of emotional states on self-report measures (van Rijen et al, 2003). It may be premature to generalise international differences in the emotional functioning of adults with CHD because of cultural differences in healthcare provision and service arrangements for the long-term management of adults with CHD. The role of disease severity remains unclear (Kovacs et al, 2005) and in one study was only marginally associated with QoL (Moons et al, 2005).

A sensitive and supportive approach is necessary to enable patients to deal with difficulties as they arise. It is important to pay attention to patients' personal experiences concerning issues related to their CHD. Some patients may need counselling or formal psychological assessment and intervention.

Careers/employment

Prolonged hospitalisation in childhood may lead to interrupted education that results in poor educational achievement. This, combined with lack of self-confidence, may limit job opportunities in adult life. In the Netherlands, Van Rijen et al (2003) examined the emotional and social functioning of 362 patients aged 20–46 years belonging to five diagnostic groups – ASD, VSD, tetralogy of Fallot, TGA and pulmonary stenosis – 20–33 years after their initial open heart surgery. All the patients were seen by the same psychologist, who examined their psychosocial functioning using a structured interview and questionnaires. Lower educational and occupational levels were reported in all groups. The proportion of patients with a history of special education was high (27%), due in part to the impact of the CHD on their schooling and also due to the presence of some sort of learning disability.

A more recent but smaller Dutch study (van der Rijken et al, 2007) examined the long-term physical, educational, behavioural and emotional outcome of 101 patients who underwent surgical correction of CHD at school age (6–16 years). The patients and their parents completed the Outcome of Congenital Heart Disease and Surgery Questionnaire, the RAND 36-Item Health Survey, and the Child Behaviour Checklist/Youth Self-Report/Young Adult Self-Report. While the patients reported a good subjective state of health and did not report any behavioural or emotional problems, they did experience academic difficulties. They had received special education more frequently than their healthy peers, and many had needed to repeat a grade or had received remedial teaching. Consequently, the educational level of patients was lower than that of their healthy peers. However, some reports are contradictory. Brandhagen et al (1991) investigated the long-term psychological implications of CHD and found an even higher educational level in adults with CHD compared with reference groups.

Nevertheless, early careers advice is necessary, and important decisions about the general certificate of education (GCSE) exams may need to be made that may impact on choice of career in later life. Careers advice needs to be realistic and based on physical and intellectual capacity, as well as on specific issues such as the presence of arrhythmias, which may preclude certain types of work, perhaps lorry-driving or joining the armed forces. Restrictions for employment exist when the safety of others is the direct responsibility of the individual with CHD. This includes possession of a heavy goods vehicle licence, becoming a commercial airline pilot and joining the police force or fire service. The armed forces exclude most applicants with a previous history of CHD.

Studies have shown discrimination against job applicants with CHD based on speculative concerns about performance, absenteeism, premature retirement and medical insurance (ESC, 2003). The ability to obtain and maintain employment depends not only on intellect, motivation and communication skills, but also on physical capacity and stamina, which can be problematic for some adults with CHD. Kamphuis et al (2002) investigated employment and career-related problems among 76 patients with complex CHD, 80 individuals with mild CHD and reference groups between 17 and 32 years of age. Patients older than 25 years with complex CHD had lower job participation (64%) than the general population (83%). Among this group, 55% reported having at least one problem in their career related to CHD, 51% felt restricted in their choice of jobs, 9% were excluded after a medical examination and 3% were not promoted. The main reasons patients stopped working were physical disability, tiredness and emotional problems.

Unemployment has major adverse effects that lower self-esteem and social contact, and it is associated with depression in cyanotic patients with CHD (Popelova et al, 2001). Many people with CHD feel different from their peers and report feelings of loneliness and isolation. Disclosing a chronic health condition to colleagues is something that most adults with CHD will avoid, either because they do not want to share such personal information or because they are worried that it will influence colleagues' perception of their ability to do the job. Whilst how much they want to reveal is ultimately the patient's decision, it can make the situation easier if they decide on a strategy for disclosing at least some information. Healthcare professionals can greatly increase patients' employment opportunities by providing appropriate support and interacting directly with the prospective employer if necessary, as objective data for many conditions are still not available.

Under the Disability Discrimination Act (1995), the employers of people suffering from many forms of illness, chronic conditions or disabilities have a duty to make reasonable changes to the working environment to enable the individuals in question to do their job. However, Crossland et al (2005), in a British study using a questionnaire with 299 adults with CHD and 177 of their friends without heart defects as controls, still elicited that employment difficulties were of concern. Whatever the severity of their disease, adults with congenitally malformed hearts were more likely to be unemployed than matched controls. They were less likely to receive useful advice regarding potential careers, and found the advice given less useful than did controls. Receiving suitable advice was, however, associated with being employed in the population with congenital cardiac disease (Crossland et al, 2005).

Many patients with CHD are not physically capable of undertaking a job involving manual labour. Their education may have been interrupted, lessening their chances in the job market, although Gersony et al (1993) in the USA reported that those patients who had survived after surgery for aortic stenosis, pulmonary stenosis or VSD had a QoL similar to that of the general population. The websites of the Department for Work and Pensions, the Equality and Human Rights Commission and ACAS are good sources of information for patients and good employers. Help and information can also be obtained from the Grown Up Congenital Heart (GUCH) Patients Association or the Citizens' Advice Bureau.

Insurance

Health and life insurance can be difficult or impossible to obtain, particularly if there is complex disease. Life insurance may be denied, be offered at normal rates or carry a heavily loaded additional premium. The actual risks quoted by insurance companies usually bear little relation to long-term outcome (Celermajer & Deanfield, 1993). Nowadays, companies providing free health insurance and running their own pension schemes may be reluctant to insure someone who may require more than the usual medical care. There appears to be little consistency between the various policies available, which may be due to a lack of appropriate guidelines, so the best advice to give patients with CHD is to shop around. Crossland et al (2004), in a study of 299 adults with CHD, noted that they were significantly more likely to have difficulty obtaining life insurance or a mortgage than were controls. Refusal rates appeared to be independent of the severity of CHD. The GUCH Patients Association is a good source of useful advice and assistance.

Travel

Most adults with CHD, even those with cyanosis and Eisenmenger syndrome, can travel by air (Harinck et al, 1996). The reduced oxygen content in the cabins of commercial aircraft is well tolerated even by those with cyanotic CHD, and in-flight oxygen is rarely required for chronically hypoxaemic people. Venous thrombosis is a risk during prolonged flights (>12 hours) and in people with known risk factors (Gatzoulis et al, 2005). General in-flight advice is to maintain hydration because of the low humidity of commercial aircraft, avoid alcohol and move around as much as possible. Those with pulmonary hypertension should be cautious when travelling to areas of high altitude and should seek medical advice beforehand. In general, all patients with complex CHD should discuss their travel plans with their specialist.

Contraception

Young people with CHD need appropriate advice about contraception from an early age so that pregnancy can be planned appropriately. Many women with CHD do not know the most appropriate method of contraception for them or have received incorrect advice. It is often those with less severe defects who receive the most inappropriate advice (Leonard et al, 1996).

The combined oral contraceptive pill is suitable for the majority of women with CHD but it is contraindicated in women with cyanotic CHD and Eisenmenger syndrome because of the risk of thromboembolism. Progesterone-only methods are safe in all types of CHD and are available in a number of different preparations: the oral progesterone-only pill Cerazette; the subdermal implant Implanon, which only needs replacing every 3 years; and the injectable Depo-Provera, which is given by deep intramuscular injection every 12 weeks. Barrier methods of contraception are suitable for all women with CHD but, as a sole method, failure rates are often not acceptable. The Mirena intrauterine system does not have the risks of increased vaginal bleeding and pain that are associated with the older copper intrauterine devices. Sterilization may be considered, but the slight risks of surgery and anaesthesia mean that it should be performed in a hospital where specialist anaesthetic and cardiac care is available. Emergency contraception is safe for women with heart disease as it contains no oestrogen.

Pregnancy

The majority of women with CHD can cope well with pregnancy. However, heart disease remains the second leading cause of maternal morbidity and mortality in the UK (Lewis, 2007). The risk to the mother and baby is dependent on the specific congenital heart defect and the individual patient. In cases of Eisenmenger syndrome, maternal mortality in pregnancy is as high as 30–50% (Gleicher et al, 1979; Daliento et al, 1998). The greatest risk of death is in the peripartum period. Early termination is often recommended because it is less risky than continuing with the pregnancy (Gatzoulis et al, 2005).

In general, pregnancy for women with CHD can be stratified into high-, medium- and low-risk groups. Women who have Marfan syndrome with a dilated aortic root, severe aortic or mitral valve stenosis, poor systemic ventricular function or cyanotic heart disease are considered to be at high risk. These women should be managed in a specialised unit that includes an obstetrician, specialist cardiologist, anaesthetist and paediatrician. Risky pregnancies should be closely monitored, the mode and place of delivery planned well in advance, and the post-delivery care of both mother and infant clarified and recorded in a delivery plan. Patients in this group may need admission to the specialist cardiac unit for bed rest and cardiac monitoring as the pregnancy advances and for eventual delivery. Joint care between the ACHD specialist and the obstetric team with regular clinical assessment is the ideal for medium-risk patients. The specialist team should provide a consultation service for obstetricians and physicians managing 'lower'-risk women in other centres. For the majority of women, vaginal delivery is preferable to caesarean section unless there are obstetric indications.

All women with CHD should receive preconception counselling with a specialist in an adult congenital heart clinic in order to discuss the risks and genetic implications of pregnancy. In addition, an assessment of functional status should be made prior to conception. The haemodynamic changes of pregnancy have a significant impact on the circulation: plasma volume increases by 40–50% and sets the stage for a rise in cardiac output of 30–50% that peaks at 20–24 weeks' gestation and continues throughout gestation in response to increased heart rate and stroke volume. It is therefore important that a woman and her partner understand the haemodynamic effect of pregnancy on the physiology of the underlying defect. The need to discuss long-term prognosis is also of importance as many women with CHD worry they will not live to see their children grow up. Advice is needed about the risk of occurrence of CHD in the offspring. This ranges from 2% to 50% (ESC, 2003) and the risk is higher when the mother rather than the father has CHD (Nora & Nora, 1987). All pregnant women should be offered fetal echocardiography at 16–18 weeks' gestation. Genetic counselling should be available; the highest recurrence risks occur in single-gene disorders and/or chromosomal abnormalities such as Marfan syndrome, Noonan syndrome and Holt–Oram syndrome (ESC, 2003).

The risks of maternal and fetal complications such as low birth weight, prematurity and fetal death are greater when resting oxygen saturation levels in air are less than 85%. Hypertension, diabetes and heavy smoking are additional risk factors. The safety of anticoagulation in pregnancy is a serious concern. Heparin may not prevent mechanical valve thrombosis, and warfarin may cause fetal embryopathy. The use of anticoagulation in pregnancy requires careful management. It is preferable to discontinue warfarin prior to conception and for the first trimester because of the harmful effect on the fetus, and to use intravenous heparin as an alternative. Optimising and changing medication is therefore important prior to conception.

Sexual health

Published data on sexual health among males with CHD are scarce; many patients are concerned about the risk of death as a result of having sex. Erectile dysfunction can create relationship and mental health problems. There is a strong link between erectile dysfunction and heart failure, diabetes, hypertension and coronary artery disease. The medication, particularly beta-blockers, used to treat these conditions can contribute to sexual problems. It is important to educate patients about the potential side-effects of medication so that any problems can be dealt with promptly. This is an area where further research is necessary (Horner, 2009).

Driving

In principle, no one should drive if their performance is compromised by drugs and/or a medical condition. The overriding concern is that a medical problem may increase the individual's risk to drive due to a sudden loss of consciousness or significant alteration of mental state. The Driver and Vehicle Licensing Agency (DVLA) issues medical standards applicable to people who have cardiovascular disorders that include CHD; these are reviewed every 6 months. The recommendations cover issues most likely to be seen in the adult with CHD. Restrictions exist for people who have arrhythmia and those who require an implantable cardioverter–defibrillator; further disqualification will occur for 6 months after any shock therapy and/or symptomatic antitachycardia pacing. It is the physician's responsibility to advise the patient that he or she should not drive, and it is the patient's duty to contact the DVLA. People with minor CHD and those who have been successfully corrected may be (re-)licensed subject to specialist evaluation.

Quality of life of adults with CHD

Few studies of QoL using validated measures have been undertaken in large populations of adolescent or adults with CHD (ESC, 2003). The findings from studies that have been performed appear ambiguous and somewhat contradictory.

One of the first studies to examine QoL, among 276 adult patients aged 16–85 years with all types of CHD registered at the ACHD clinic in Birmingham, UK, was undertaken by Lane et al (2002) using the 36-item Short-Form Health Survey (SF-36). Patients with inoperable or cyanotic conditions and, paradoxically, those deemed surgically cured had the poorest QoL among adults with CHD. However, all patients had significantly poorer levels of physical functioning and overall general health perception than similarly aged people in the general population.

In the Netherlands, van den Bosch et al (2004) examined mortality, morbidity and QoL in 36 patients who had had a Fontan procedure using an electrocardiogram, exercise testing and an echocardiogram. QoL was assessed using the SF-36 Health Survey. Physical functioning, mental health and general health perception were found to be significantly lower for individuals who had undergone a Fontan procedure than for controls from the normal Dutch population. Reoperations, arrhythmias and thromboembolic events all compromised QoL. McCrindle et al (2006) investigated the relationship between health status, socio-demographic and medical characteristics in children and adolescents after the Fontan procedure. A parent unable to work because of the patient's health and lower family income had a negative impact on both physical and psychological functioning.

Saliba et al (2001) evaluated QoL in 89 adult patients aged 17–49 years with a uni-ventricular heart using the Duke Health Profile. Despite repeated hospital admissions, surgical interventions and other disease-related everyday stresses, a satisfying QoL for this group of adults was reported. These patients probably developed adaptive coping mechanisms that eased the psychological stress and resulted in better scores on the Duke Profile. This is not dissimilar to the difficulty of correlating the symptoms/subjective QoL assessment and the actual burden of illness and objective cardiopulmonary testing amongst this group of heterogenous patients with very different backgrounds.

Many adults with CHD have concerns about the future and worry about a shortened life expectancy and disability. However, most patients will say they are asymptomatic when questioned. Whilst some may have adjusted to and learnt to cope with their health problems and limitations, others may be reluctant to admit to them and to discuss problems. Horner et al (2000) examined the psychosocial profile of 29 patients with complex CHD aged 26–56 years using interview and questionnaires to perform a psychiatric evaluation. Many patients met symptomatic criteria for psychiatric diagnoses, but most were functional in day-to-day life and used denial in adapting to their CHD.

In a qualitative study, Claessens et al (2005) described how patients feel their lives are different from those of people without CHD because of physical limitations imposed by the condition and the visible signs of the heart defect. They struggle constantly with themselves and with their environment to be accepted as normal. Adults with CHD have to strike a balance between being different and not being different, being sick and being healthy, revealing their CHD or hiding it and living with a hidden handicap. Consequently, they might hide their symptoms from healthcare professionals and sometimes even from themselves (Berghammer et al, 2006), hence the importance of sensitive handling and education and the advocacy role of the ACHD team (ESC, 2003).

A further aspect is the financial burden of living with CHD, which may be considerable. The costs of regular trips to the specialist centre for outpatient follow-up and assessment soon accumulate, and prescription charges are not insignificant. Loss of income may be incurred for the self-employed. The cost escalates for those who require intermittent admission to hospital, lose income and may have to stop working because of progressive disability. Adults with CHD may be eligible for financial support in the form of incapacity benefit, which is awarded to those unable to work because of illness or disability. Disability Living Allowance is paid to people who are so severely disabled, either physically or mentally, that they have personal care needs, mobility needs or both. Entitlement is based on how much help with personal care and/or mobility is needed. This is used as a broad indicator of the extra costs arising from disability. Healthcare teams should recognise the difficulties some people face and provide the appropriate support when necessary.

Independent living

The ability to live independently is important for people with long-term conditions, but the reality is that many of them are living at home with one or both parents. People with learning disabilities in particular need to be prepared for independent living whenever possible. Not surprisingly, young adults with CHD have been found to live a more dependent lifestyle, living with their parents more frequently than healthy peers (Kokkonen & Paavilainen, 1992). Parental overprotection increases the dependency of young people and might explain why younger adults are not able to organise their lives independently of their parents and tend to live longer with them (Tong et al, 1998). Other factors that have been found to affect independence in adults with CHD are the severity of the condition, continuing medication, a lower level of education, lower self-esteem and the unknown outcome of CHD (Niwa et al, 2002). More importantly, those with intellectual disabilities face some barriers to establishing independent social lives, such as lack of access to a peer group or adult supervision; they are also less likely to gain paid employment.

The impact on the family

Caring for a child with a chronic illness has been identified as one of the most stressful experiences for any family (Bouma & Schweitzer, 1990). For the family of the child with CHD, the emotional and psychological significance associated with the heart can result in adjustment difficulties out of proportion to the severity of the lesion (Wray & Sensky, 1998), with the families of children with CHD experiencing more difficulties and stress than families of children with other congenital anomalies (Emery, 1989). The birth and subsequent care of a child with CHD has an impact on the functioning of the family as a unit (Mussatto, 2006), as well as on the individual family members, irrespective of the severity of the lesion (Wray & Maynard, 2005). Whilst some adverse affects have been reported, other studies have identified a resiliency in families, with positive outcomes in terms of family adjustment and coping. It is therefore important for health professionals to have an open mind, rather than preconceived ideas, about how a particular family may cope, and to identify constructive ways of helping and supporting families through difficult times that are tailored to the needs of the individual family.

Parents and the diagnosis

The diagnosis of CHD in a child may create a crisis for the parents (Higgins & Kashani, 1986) and may elicit a whole range of emotions, such as grief, anxiety, fear, denial, depression, shock, anger and guilt, as they experience and mourn the loss of the imagined healthy child and cope with a lack of knowledge of the disease, as well as the difficulties of providing care for their infant (Cohn, 1996; Rona et al, 1998; Upham & Medoff-Cooper, 2005). The diagnosis of CHD in the neonatal period, necessitating urgent transfer of the baby to a specialist centre, can disrupt the usual pattern of parent–infant bonding (Shor, 1978; Bentovim, 1983). The impact of the diagnosis at this time may be heightened by other stressors (such as the birth itself) and may be exacerbated by the need to make difficult treatment decisions urgently (Fisk, 1986).

In more recent years fetal echocardiography has become widely established and advances in technology have allowed for a more accurate and earlier detection of congenital heart defects prenatally. In addition to improving the outcome for some infants born with severe forms of CHD, a prenatal diagnosis allows for improved management of the remainder of a pregnancy and greater planning regarding the birth and subsequent treatment of the child. The increased use of fetal echocardiography to identify patients who are suitable for in utero intervention is also likely to be part of the next era of treatment of CHD.

Psychologically, fetal echocardiography allows for the counselling of parents whose child has a cardiac diagnosis, as well as reassurance for parents who have a normal scan. In a study of women who gave birth to a child with CHD, those who had undergone fetal echocardiography felt less responsible for their infant's defects and had a better relationship with the father of their baby than did those whose children were diagnosed postnatally (Sklansky et al, 2002). Fathers whose children were diagnosed antenatally were also found to be less distressed and were more optimistic than those who received a diagnosis after birth (Hoehn et al, 2004). Fetal echocardiography is also important for families who already have a child with CHD and has been shown to reduce maternal anxiety when scans are normal (Bjorkhem et al, 1997). Whilst the antenatal diagnosis of CHD has many positive facets, it is important for professionals to elicit the perspective of the individual parent and to support such families from the time of diagnosis (Rempel et al, 2004), particularly through the decision-making processes that follow.

Parenting an infant with CHD

Parents of infants with CHD have reported higher levels of stress, more problems with depression and a lowered sense of competence than parents of healthy infants or parents of children with other chronic illnesses, with mothers reporting higher levels of stress than fathers (Goldberg et al, 1990a; Darke & Goldberg, 1994). It has also been suggested that significantly fewer infants with CHD, compared with healthy babies, have secure relationships with their mothers (Goldberg et al, 1991). In this latter study, the quality of the relationship was not found to be influenced by parental stress levels or the severity of the diagnosis but it did have a bearing on later social and physical development. In a comparative study of the parents of infants with CHD or cystic fibrosis and the parents of healthy infants, the most securely attached infants in the healthy group had the most positive mother–child interaction at 2 years of age, but this was not the case in either the CHD or cystic fibrosis groups (Goldberg et al, 1990b). The authors suggest that the influence of the early parent–child relationship may be altered by a child's health status and that parent–child attachments are less consistent in the presence of chronic illness.

In a longitudinal study of mothers' attachment style and mental health, maternal avoidant attachment at diagnosis was the best predictor of deterioration in the mother's mental health and marital satisfaction at 7 years, particularly in the group whose children had severe CHD. Furthermore, mothers' attachment insecurities (both anxiety and avoidance) at diagnosis were associated with their children's emotional problems and poor self-image 7 years later (Berant et al, 2008).

A number of babies with CHD are born prematurely and, due to this and their heart lesion, require more prolonged hospitalisation. Preterm infants hospitalised for longer than a month at birth have been found to have a significantly different pattern of attachment (more anxious-resistant) compared with healthy preterm infants (Plunkett et al, 1986). A further important and frequently mentioned factor for the parents of infants with CHD is feeding difficulties and the impact of this on the parents. Whilst it seems likely that feeding difficulties are related to organic difficulties in the child rather than to problems with the child–mother interaction (Clemente et al, 2001), it has been suggested that feeding problems in their infants can result in parental anxiety and feelings of inadequacy such that some parents withdraw emotional support from their child (Gudermuth, 1975; D'Antonio, 1976). It is clear, therefore, that the parents of children with CHD may require additional support to deal with the practical and emotional impact of feeding difficulties.

Parenting and the older child with CHD

Whilst significant levels of stress have been reported in the families of younger children with CHD (Goldberg et al, 1990b; Pelchat et al, 1999), for the majority of families of older children there is no detrimental impact on family activities or on family relationships (Wray & Maynard, 2005). In the latter study, 43% of mothers reported that family relationships had become closer as a result of their child's heart condition, and in only 8% had they been 'pulled apart'. These findings support earlier studies that did not find higher divorce rates among the parents of children with CHD when compared with the parents of healthy children, although these studies did not assess parental satisfaction and happiness with the marital relationship.

Within other chronic illness groups elevated levels of marital distress have been found, but this was not the case in a recent study of parents of children undergoing cardiac surgery (Wray & Sensky, 2004). Furthermore, there were some positive changes in levels of marital happiness from before to 1 year after surgery, suggesting that largely corrective surgery had a positive impact on parents' relationships, supporting other research which has shown that coping with disease can have a positive effect on parents' relationships (Vance et al, 1980; Taanila et al, 1996).

Assessment of parental adjustment has largely focused on mothers, and as has been found in other chronic illness groups, psychological adjustment is associated with coping strategies and daily stressors rather than the severity of the disease (Davis et al, 1998; DeMaso et al, 1991; Thompson et al, 1992, 1994). In a study of 52 mothers of children with CHD, just over one-third met the criteria for poor adjustment, and the increased use of palliative coping strategies and high levels of daily stress were negatively related to maternal adjustment (Davis et al, 1998).

Elevated levels of psychological distress have also been reported for the parents of children awaiting elective cardiac surgery, with mothers demonstrating higher distress levels and greater problems with coping than fathers (Utens et al, 2000). A longitudinal evaluation of both mothers and fathers before and 1 year after surgery found a significant reduction in distress levels over time, from 63% to 25% in mothers and 48% to 17% in fathers (Wray & Sensky, 2004).

The results of longer-term follow-up studies, however, are less clear. In one follow-up of mothers 5 years after their child's corrective surgery, 25% continued to experience high levels of stress, particularly if their child had behaviour problems (Majnemer et al, 2006b), whereas distress levels were found to be lower than those of reference groups in an evaluation of parents of children aged 7–15 years old with CHD (Spijkerboer et al, 2007). One factor that may be underestimated is the impact of corrective surgery in terms of parenting. It has been suggested that some parents go through another grieving stage where they mourn the ill child that they had and come to terms with the well child that they now have. Whilst parents are relieved, happy and grateful that their child is able to participate more normally in everyday life, mothers in particular can feel redundant in terms of their caring role and feel that one of their defining characteristics as a parent has been taken away.

For some parents, adjusting to such changes can be challenging. In a large study involving the parents of 1092 children with CHD, rates of distress and hopelessness were higher than those seen in the parents of children with other illnesses or the parents of healthy children (Lawoko & Soares, 2002). Corroborating previous findings, it was the presence of CHD rather than its severity that was the determinant of psychological distress, and caregiving burden, socio-economic difficulties and social support were important contributory factors to distress levels.

A number of children with CHD also have other co-morbidities and it would seem that, irrespective of the cardiac diagnosis, the addition of other health problems has a significant impact on the perceived ability to carry out normal activities, highlighting the importance of assessing all aspects of health rather than focusing exclusively on the cardiac condition (Wray & Maynard, 2005).

Parental coping and parenting attitudes

Little information has been published about the coping strategies used by the parents of children with CHD, but in studies of other groups of chronically ill children, parental coping strategies have been found to influence adjustment in the children (Sanger et al, 1991; Sloper et al, 1994) and to vary according to the specific disease involved

(Eiser & Havermans, 1992). A number of studies of CHD have found that mothers use social support more than fathers (Utens et al, 2000; Wray & Sensky 2004; Spijkerboer, et al, 2007) and that higher levels of perceived social support are associated with more positive outcomes in terms of the physical and psychological functioning of children and their families (Tak & McCubbin, 2002). However, parents have also reported finding trust in medical care and the use of autonomy more helpful than social or family support (Eiser & Havermans, 1992). Overall, however, there is no clear-cut picture about the use of other specific coping strategies in the parents of children with CHD.

Studies of parental personality characteristics and their relationship to parenting attitudes have found similar findings for the parents of children with CHD and the parents of healthy children. A study of school absenteeism found that children from families with a high external locus of control beliefs tended to have increased school absence compared with children from families with an internal health locus of control beliefs. This finding was applicable to both children with CHD and healthy children (Fowler et al, 1987). A comparison of the parenting attitudes of mothers of children with acyanotic heart disease with the mothers of healthy children found no overall differences between the two groups. However, parental personality style was significantly correlated with parenting attitude, irrespective of the child's health status (Boll et al, 1978). Other research addressing parenting style has identified elevated levels of parental vigilance regarding their sick child (Carey et al, 2002) and difficulty with setting limits and disciplining the child with CHD (Uzark & Jones, 2003; Brosig et al, 2007).

In contrast to the literature on structural congenital heart defects, there is very little information about the impact on parents of having a child with conditions such as hypertrophic cardiomyopathy or congenital long QT syndrome, both of which cover the spectrum of being asymptomatic to sudden death as the presenting event. In a qualitative study of 31 parents of children with long QT syndrome, fear of their child dying was a prevalent theme, with the impact on family life being more significant when the child was diagnosed in adolescence rather than early childhood (Farnsworth et al, 2006). Issues such as management of the children and the impact on family life have not been well studied, but what is evident is the need for health professionals to understand the lifestyle implications of such a diagnosis and for psychosocial input to be provided for these families.

Information, communication and support

A review of the needs of parents of chronically sick children identified three main themes – the need for normality and certainty, the need for information and the need for partnership (Fisher, 2001). Almost half of parents of children with CHD recently surveyed reported that they wanted more information, which mainly referred to the surgical and treatment aspects of their child's condition, as well as information about services available to help them cope with different aspects of the heart condition and its impact on everyday life (Wray & Maynard, 2006). A number of studies assessing parental knowledge about their child's heart condition have identified a significant proportion of parents who are unaware of important aspects of their child's previous or ongoing treatment (Cheuk et al, 2004; van Deyk et al 2004; Wray et al, 2004; Chessa et al, 2005), indicating the requirement to address the information needs of families. It has been suggested that the overall improvements in the status of children with

CHD may lead health professionals to underestimate the levels of concern and distress experienced by families (Van Horn et al, 2001). Parents may find it difficult to communicate anxieties or concerns or ask questions during busy outpatient visits, and the recall and understanding of new information at stressful times may be less than optimal. Concerns about communication with professionals have been voiced by parents (Kendall et al, 2003) and the importance of optimising communication and ensuring that there is sufficient time to talk to families cannot be overemphasised.

The vast majority of families receive support from family and friends, but community support appears to be more patchy. An area that has not been well investigated is that of respite care provision for children with more complex CHD. As the surgical and medical management of such children improves, the number now living with significant morbidity is increasing, with ever-increasing demands on their families. The recent shift in emphasis from hospital to home care has resulted in families managing much of their child's care at home, but accessing appropriate respite care provision can be difficult, if not impossible, for some families.

Providing adequate practical and emotional support for these families therefore needs to be seen as a priority. One important area of support that is becoming more accessible is that of support groups, although it is evident that they are still not perceived by all families as being available to them. Whilst not all families choose to access them, the majority of those that do report finding them extremely helpful. However, a small minority have found them unhelpful, so it is important that, as they become more prominent, the involvement that support groups have with potentially vulnerable families continues to be constructive.

Siblings

The presence of a sick child in a family can be a particularly difficult experience for a healthy child (Coddington, 1972). Chronic illness threatens the integrity of the sibling relationship both directly and indirectly (Eiser, 1993), and healthy siblings lose their equal relationship with their sick brother or sister (Trahd, 1986). Relationships between parents and their well children are also affected (Gallo, 1988), and healthy siblings can feel 'displaced and unimportant' (Martinson et al, 1990). Chronic illness alters the quality and quantity of intra- and extrafamilial communication (McKeever, 1983), often with significant consequences for the healthy siblings. It is therefore perhaps not surprising that some researchers have concluded that, within the family, healthy siblings bear the greatest burden of stress (Spinetta, 1981).

Two meta-analyses have indicated that healthy siblings in families where there is a child with a chronic illness are at a significantly increased risk of adjustment difficulties (Lavigne & Faier-Routman, 1992; Sharpe & Rossiter, 2002). Parents tend to report a greater impact on the healthy siblings than is reported by the siblings themselves, and in those situations where the chronic illness necessitates daily caretaking regimens, siblings are more affected. Compared with controls, the siblings of a child with a chronic illness were found to have poorer psychological functioning and lower cognitive development scores, and there was also a negative impact on peer activities.

Despite CHD being the most common congenital defect, studies on the healthy siblings of such children are few in number. In the most recent meta-analysis by Sharpe & Rossiter (2002), only two of the 51 studies included siblings of children with CHD. Early studies reported behaviour problems and/or psychosomatic disorders in the siblings of cardiac patients (Maxwell & Gane, 1962; Apley et al, 1967; Boon, 1972). However, in more recent studies, the siblings of cardiac children compare favourably with the siblings of children with other chronic illnesses (Lavigne & Ryan, 1979; Faux, 1991) and have not been found to have a higher prevalence of behaviour problems than a normative sample (Janus & Goldberg, 1997).

In a study addressing, amongst other things, the impact of CHD on family life, less time was given to the healthy siblings in one-quarter of families, and in those families where a child had undergone transplantation this rose to half of healthy siblings having reduced time with their parents (Wray & Maynard, 2005). Parents reported that the main difficulties for healthy siblings were feeling left out, fear of getting too close to their sick sibling, being prevented from doing things as a family because of their sibling's condition, resentment of the extra time given to the sick child and their perceptions of differences in parenting (e.g. with regard to discipline). A small number of parents also identified that they wanted more help for their healthy children in the form of emotional support for them, practical assistance when the ill child was hospitalised and help to allow them (the parents) to spend more time with their healthy children (Wray & Maynard, 2006).

Whilst healthy siblings may not demonstrate clinically significant behavioural problems, it is evident that for some there will be a detrimental impact of their sick sibling's condition. What is also clear is that many siblings show a resiliency and adapt positively, but this should not be confused with not caring or being unaffected. In providing care for children with CHD and their family, it is therefore imperative to consider the (often unexpressed) needs of the healthy siblings.

Diversity and culture

It has been estimated that up to 15 million children die or are crippled annually by potentially treatable or preventable cardiac disease (Yacoub, 2007). Children with CHD in the developing world are recognised to be at risk of delayed care, and a number of factors have been identified which contribute to this, such as living in a rural area or far from a surgical centre and a lack of social security or equivalent membership (Kowalsky et al, 2006). Increasingly, there is recognition of the need to help countries in the developing world set up specialist cardiac centres and provide them with the necessary infrastructure, training, equipment and other resources, and there are now a growing number of organisations involved in facilitating this worldwide.

Within the industrialised world, the prevalence of CHD within different ethnic and culturally diverse groups is, in the main, stable across populations, although specific groups have been identified as being at increased risk of poorer outcome. For example, black and Hispanic individuals have been found to be at a higher risk of death following cardiac surgery for CHD in the USA (Benavidez et al, 2006), with disparities being only partially explained by gender and region within the USA. In an evaluation of patients who had undergone the Fontan procedure, ethnic differences in coagulation factor abnormalities were identified, with Chinese patients having a different coagulation profile from Caucasian patients (Cheung et al, 2006); this had important consequences for their postoperative management. In contrast, whilst a number of studies have addressed the physical and medical outcomes associated with diversity and culture, far fewer studies have looked at the psychological factors for patients and families from different ethnic and cultural backgrounds being treated in large cosmopolitan cardiac centres within industrialised nations.

Understanding the significance of diversity is vital for optimising the delivery of care to children and families within a multicultural setting. An appreciation and understanding of different cultures and their association with healthcare practice will facilitate the development of culturally sensitive interventions, thereby optimising outcomes for children with CHD and their families.

Conclusion

The impact of CHD on young people and their families covers a broad spectrum, from those who are seemingly unaffected by the condition to young people and families for whom the impact is severe and multidimensional. Assessment of factors other than the purely physical needs to be an integral part of the ongoing management of children with heart disease and their families, and included in this should be an evaluation of aspects such as HRQoL, development and cognitive abilities, behaviour, physical activity, adherence and family functioning. Given the significant population of children and young people with heart disease this is clearly a tall order, and one of the first requirements is to develop effective screening tools to identify children and young people who are at risk of poor psychosocial outcome.

Similarly, there is much to be learned from the majority of children and families who adjust well to the impact of living with heart disease, and identifying factors and characteristics that are associated with good outcomes is also important. With the paradigm shift from mortality to morbidity, the onus is on health professionals to broaden the scope of their care to reduce psychosocial morbidity in this population and help young people to maximise their QoL and achieve their potential in all aspects of their lives as they move into and through adulthood.

References

Alden, B., Gilljam, T. & Gillberg, C. (1998). Long-term psychological outcome of children after surgery for transposition of the great arteries. *Acta Paediatrica, 87,* 405–410.

Angold, A., Weissman, M.M., John, K., Merikangas, K.R., Prusoff, B.A., Wickramaratne, P. et al (1987). Parent and child reports of depressive symptoms in children at low and high risk of depression. *Journal of Child Psychology and Psychiatry, 28,* 901–915.

Apley, J., Barbour, R.F. & Westmacott, I. (1967). Impact of congenital heart disease on the family: preliminary report. *British Medical Journal, 1,* 103–105.

Baum, M., Chinnock, R., Ashwal, S., Peverini, R., Trimm, F. & Bailey, L. (1993). Growth and neurodevelopmental outcome of infants undergoing heart transplantation. *Journal of Heart and Lung Transplantation, 12,* S211–S217.

Baum, M., Freier, M.C., Freeman, K., Babikian, T., Ashwal, S., Chinnock, R. & Bailey, L. (2004). Neuropsychological outcome of infant heart transplant recipients. *Journal of Pediatrics, 145,* 365–372.

Behrman, R.E., Kliegman, R.M., Nelson, W.E. & Vaughan, V.C. (1992). *Nelson textbook of pediatrics.* 14th edn. Philadelphia: W.B. Saunders.

Bellinger, D.C., Jonas, R.A., Rappaport, L.A., Wypij, D., Wernovsky, G., Kuban, K.C.K. et al (1995). Developmental and neurologic status of children after heart surgery with hypothermic circulatory arrest or low-flow cardiopulmonary bypass. *New England Journal of Medicine, 332,* 549–555.

Bellinger, D.C., Rappaport, L.A., Wypij, D., Wernovsky, G. & Newburger, J.W. (1997). Patterns of developmental dysfunction after surgery during infancy to correct transposition of the great arteries. *Journal of Developmental and Behavioral Pediatrics, 18,* 75–83.

Bellinger, D.C., Wypij, D., Kuban, K.C.K., Rappaport, L.A., Hickey, P.R., Wernovsky, G. et al (1999). Developmental and neurological status of children at 4 years of age after heart surgery with hypothermic circulatory arrest or low-flow cardiopulmonary bypass. *Circulation*, *100*, 526–532.

Bellinger, D.C., Wypij, D., duPlessis, A.J., Rappaport, L.A., Jonas, R.A., Wernovsky, G. & Newburger, J.W. (2003a). Neurodevelopmental status at eight years in children with dextro-transposition of the great arteries: the Boston Circulatory Arrest Trial. *Journal of Thoracic and Cardiovascular Surgery*, *126*, 1385–1396.

Bellinger, D.C., Bernstein, J.H., Kirkwood, M.W., Rappaport, L.A. & Newburger, J.W. (2003b). Visual-spatial skills in children after open-heart surgery. *Journal of Developmental and Behavioral Pediatrics*, *24*,169–179.

Benavidez, O.J., Gauvreau, K. & Jenkins, K.J. (2006). Racial and ethnic disparities in mortality following congenital heart surgery. *Pediatric Cardiology*, *27*, 321–328.

Bentovim, A. (1983). Psychiatric and intellectual assessment. *Paediatric Cardiology*, *5*, 309–316.

Berant, E., Mikulincer, M. & Shaver, P.R. (2008). Mothers' attachment style, their mental health, and their children's emotional vulnerabilities: a 7-year study of children with congenital heart disease. *Journal of Personality*, *76*, 31–65.

Berger, F., Vogel, M., Alexi-Meskishvili, V. & Lange, P.E. (1999). Comparison of results and complications of surgical and Amplatzer device closure of atrial septal defects. *Journal of Thoracic and Cardiovascular Surgery*, *118*, 674–678.

Berghammer, M., Dellborg, M. & Ekman, I. (2006). Young adults' experiences of living with congenital heart disease. *International Journal of Cardiology*, *110*, 340–347.

Birks, Y., Sloper, P., Lewin, R. & Parsons, J. (2007). Exploring health-related experiences of children and young people with congenital heart disease. *Health Expectations*, *10*, 16–29.

Bjorkhem, G., Jorgensen, C. & Hanseus, K. (1997). Parental reactions to fetal echocardiography. *Journal of Maternal-Fetal Medicine*, *6*, 87–92.

Bloom, A.A., Wright, J.A., Morris, R.D., Campbell, R.M. & Krawiecki, N.S. (1997). Additive impact of in-hospital cardiac arrest on the functioning of children with heart disease. *Pediatrics*, *99*, 390–398.

Boll, T.J., Dimino, E.& Mattsson, A.E. (1978). Parenting attitudes: the role of personality style and childhood long term illness. *Journal of Psychosomatic Research*, *22*, 209–213.

Bonhoeffer, P., Boudjemline, Y., Saliba, Z. et al (2000). Percutaneous replacement of pulmonary valve in a right-ventricle to pulmonary-artery prosthetic conduit with valve dysfunction. *Lancet*, *356*, 1403–1405.

Boon, A.R. (1972). Tetralogy of Fallot – effect on the family. *British Journal of Preventative and Social Medicine*, *26*, 263–268.

Bouma, R. & Schweitzer, R. (1990). The impact of chronic childhood illness on family stress: a comparison between autism and cystic fibrosis. *Journal of Clinical Psychology*, *46*, 722–730.

Brandhagen, D.J., Feldt, R.H. & Williams, D.E. (1991) Long-term psychologic implications of congenital heart disease: a 25-year follow-up. *Mayo Clinic Proceedings*, *66*, 474–479.

British Cardiac Society (2002). Grown-up congenital heart (GUCH) disease: current needs and provision of service for adolescents and adults with congenital heart disease in the UK. *Heart*, *88*, i1–i14.

Bromberg, J.I., Beasley, P.J., D'Angelo, E.J., Landzberg, M. & DeMaso, D.R. (2003). Depression and anxiety in adults with congenital heart disease: a pilot study. *Heart Lung*, *32*, 105–110.

Brosig, C.L., Mussatto, K.A., Kuhn, E.M. & Tweddell, J.S. (2007). Psychosocial outcomes for preschool children and families after surgery for complex congenital heart disease. *Pediatric Cardiology*, *28*, 255–262.

Camelot Foundation and Mental Health Foundation (2006). *Truth hurts*. London: MHF.

Carey, L.K., Nicholson, B.C. & Fox, R.A. (2002). Maternal factors related to parenting young children with congenital heart disease. *Journal of Pediatric Nursing*, *17*, 174–183.

Casey, F.A., Craig, B.G. & Mulholland, H.C. (1994). Quality of life in surgically palliated complex congenital heart disease. *Archives of Disease in Childhood, 70*, 382–386.

Celermajer, D.S. & Deanfield, J.E. (1993). Employment and insurance for young adults with congenital heart disease. *British Heart Journal, 69*, 539–543.

Cetta, F., Bell, T.J., Podlecki, D.D. & Ros, S.P. (1993). Parental knowledge of bacterial endocarditis prophylaxis. *Pediatric Cardiology, 14*, 220–222.

Chervin, R.D., Dillon, J.E., Bassetti, C., Ganoczy, D.A. & Pituch, K.J. (1997). Symptoms of sleep disorders, inattention, and hyperactivity in children. *Sleep, 20*, 1185–1192.

Chervin, R.D., Archbold, K.H., Dillon, J.E., Panahi, P., Pituch, K.J., Dahl, R.E. & Guilleminault, C. (2002). Inattention, hyperactivity, and symptoms of sleep-disordered breathing. *Pediatrics, 109*, 449–56.

Chessa, M., De Rosa, G., Pardeo, M., Negura, D.G., Butera, G., Giamberti, A. et al (2005). What do parents know about the malformations afflicting the hearts of their children? *Cardiology in the Young, 15*, 125–129.

Cheuk, D.K.L., Wong, S.M.Y., Choi, Y.P., Chau, A.K.T. & Cheung, Y.F. (2004). Parents' understanding of their child's congenital heart disease. *Heart, 90*, 435–439.

Cheung, Y.F., Chay, G.W. & Ma, E.S. (2006). Ethnic differences in coagulation factor abnormalities after the Fontan procedure. *Pediatric Cardiology, 27*, 96–101.

Claessens, P., Moons, P., de Casterle, B.D. et al (2005). What does it mean to live with a congenital heart disease? A qualitative study on the lived experiences of adult patients. *European Journal of Cardiovascular Nursing, 4*, 3–10.

Clemente, C., Barnes, J., Shinebourne, E. & Stein, A. (2001). Are infant behavioural feeding difficulties associated with congenital heart disease? *Child: Care Health and Development, 27*, 46–59.

Coddington, R.D. (1972). The significance of life events as etiologic factors in the diseases of children – II: a study of a normal population. *Journal of Psychosomatic Research, 16*, 205–213.

Cohen, M., Mansoor, D., Langut, H. & Lorber, A. (2007). Quality of life, depressed mood and self-esteem in adolescents with heart disease. *Psychosomatic Medicine, 69*, 313–318.

Cohn, J.K. (1996). An empirical study of parents' reaction to the diagnosis of congenital heart disease in infants. *Social Work in Health Care, 23*, 67–79.

Cooper, M., Hooper, C. & Thompson, M. (2005). *Child and adolescent mental health theory and practice.* Oxford: Edward Arnold.

Crossland, D.S., Jackson, S.P., Lyall, R. et al. (2004). Life insurance and mortgage application in adults with congenital heart disease. *European Journal of Cardio-thoracic Surgery, 25*, 931–934.

Crossland, D.S., Jackson, S.P., Lyall, R. et al. (2005). Employment and advice regarding careers for adults with congenital heart disease. *Cardiology in the Young, 15*, 391–395.

Culbert, E.L., Ashburn, D.A., Cullen-Dean, G., Joseph, J.A., Williams, W.G., Blackstone, E.H., McCrindle, B.W. & the Congenital Heart Surgeons Society (2003). Quality of life of children after repair of transposition of the great arteries. *Circulation, 108*, 857–862.

Daliento, L., Somerville, J., Presbitero, P. et al (1998). Eisenmenger syndrome. Factors relating to deterioration and death. *European Heart Journal, 19*, 1845–1855.

D'Antonio, I.J. (1976). Mothers' responses to the functioning and behavior of cardiac children in child-rearing situations. *Maternal-Child Nursing Journal, 5*, 206–259.

Darke, P.R. & Goldberg, S. (1994). Father–infant interaction and parent stress with healthy and medically compromised infants. *Infant Behavior and Development, 17*, 3–14.

Davis, C.C., Brown, R.T., Bakeman, R. & Campbell, R. (1998). Psychological adaptation and adjustment of mothers of children with congenital heart disease: stress, coping, and family functioning. *Journal of Pediatric Psychology, 23*, 219–228.

Davis, I.D., Chang, P. & Nevins, T.E. (1990). Successful renal transplantation accelerates development in young uremic children. *Pediatrics, 86*, 594–600.

Department of Health (1983). *The Mental Health Act*. London: HMSO.

Department of Health (1989). *The Children Act*. London: HMSO.

Department of Health (1995). *Disability Discrimination Act* 1995. London: HMSO.

Department of Health (2003). *Effective sexual health promotion: A toolkit for primary care trusts and others working in the field of promoting good sexual and HIV prevention*. London: HMSO.

Department of Health (2004). *The National Service Framework for children, young people and maternity services*. London: HMSO.

DeMaso, D.R., Campis, L.K., Wypij, D., Bertram, S., Lipshitz, M. & Freed, M. (1991). The impact of maternal perceptions and medical severity on the adjustment of children with congenital heart disease. *Journal of Pediatric Psychology, 16*, 137–149.

DeMaso, D.R., Lauretti, A., Spieth, L., van der Feen, J.R., Jay, K.S., Gauvreau, K. et al (2004). Psychosocial factors and quality of life in children and adolescents with implantable cardioverter-defibrillators. *American Journal of Cardiology, 93*, 582–587.

Dua, J.S., Cooper, A.R., Fox, K.R. & Stuart, A.G. (2007). Physical activity levels in adults with congenital heart disease. *European Journal of Cardiovascular Prevention and Rehabilitation, 14*, 287–293.

Dunbar-Masterson, C., Wypij, D., Bellinger, D.C., Rappaport, L.A., Baker, A.L., Jonas, R.A. & Newburger, J.W. (2001). General health status of children with d-transposition of the great arteries after the arterial switch operation. *Circulation, 104*, 138–142.

Du Plessis, A.J. (1997). Cardiac surgery in the young infant: an in vivo model for the study of hypoxic–ischemic brain injury? *Mental Retardation and Developmental Disabilities Research Reviews, 3*, 49–58.

Eiser, C. (1981). Psychological sequelae of brain tumours in childhood: a retrospective study. *British Journal of Clinical Psychology, 20*, 35–38.

Eiser, C. (1993). *Growing up with a chronic disease: the impact on children and their families*. London: Jessica Kingsley.

Eiser, C. & Havermans, T. (1992). Mothers' and fathers' coping with chronic childhood disease. *Psychology and Health, 7*, 249–257.

Eiser, C. & Morse, R. (2001). Can parents rate their child's health-related quality of life? Results of a systematic review. *Quality of Life Research, 10*, 347–357.

Eke, C.C., Gundry, S.R., Baum, M.F., Chinnock, R.E., Razzouk, A.J. & Bailey, L.L. (1996). Neurologic sequelae of deep hypothermic circulatory arrest in cardiac transplant infants. *Annals of Thoracic Surgery, 61*, 783–788.

Emery, J.L. (1989). Families with congenital heart disease. *Archives of Disease in Childhood, 64*, 150–154.

Erikson, E. (1974). *Dimensions of a new identity: The 1973 Jefferson Lectures on the Humanities*. New York: Norton.

European Society of Cardiology (2003). Management of grown up congenital heart disease: the Task Force on the Management of Grown Up Congenital Heart Disease of the European Society of Cardiology. *European Heart Journal, 24*, 1035–1084.

Farnsworth, M.M., Fosyth, D., Haglund, C. & Ackerman, M.J. (2006). When I go in to wake them … I wonder: parental perceptions about congenital long QT syndrome. *Journal of the American Academy of Nurse Practitioners, 18*, 284–290.

Faux, S.A. (1991). Sibling relationships in families with congenitally impaired children. *Journal of Pediatric Nursing, 6*, 175–184.

Fekkes, M., Kamphuis, R.P., Ottenkamp, J., Verrips, E., Vogels, T., Kamphuis, M. & Verloove-Vanhorick, S.P. (2001). Health-related quality of life in young adults with minor congenital heart disease. *Psychology and Health, 16*, 239–250.

Ferry, P.C. (1987a). Neurologic sequelae of cardiac surgery in children. *American Journal of Diseases in Childhood, 141*, 309–312.

Ferry, P.C. (1987b). Neurologic sequelae of open-heart surgery in children: an 'irritating question'. *American Journal of Diseases in Childhood*, *144*, 369–373.

Fisher, H.R. (2001). The needs of parents with chronically sick children: a literature review. *Journal of Advanced Nursing*, *36*, 600–607.

Fisk, R. (1986). Management of the pediatric cardiovascular patient after surgery. *Critical Care Quarterly*, *9*, 75–82.

Fixler, D.E., Pastor, P., Sigman, E. & Eifler, C.W. (1993). Ethnicity and socio-economic status: impact on the diagnosis of congenital heart disease. *Journal of American Colloquium of Cardiology*, *21*, 1722–1726.

Fletcher, G.F., Balady, G., Blair, S.N., Blumenthal, J., Caspersen, C., Chaitman, B. et al (1996). Statement on exercise: benefits and recommendations for physical activity programs for all Americans: a statement for health professionals by the committee on exercise and cardiac rehabilitation of the council on clinical cardiology, American Heart Association. *Circulation*, *94*, 857–862.

Forbess, J.M., Visconti, K.J., Hancock-Friesen, C., Howe, R.C., Bellinger, D.C. & Jonas, R.A. (2002). Neurodevelopmental outcome after congenital heart surgery: results from an institutional registry. *Circulation*, *106*(12 Suppl. 1), 195–202.

Fowler, M.G., Johnson, M.P., Welshimer, K.J., Atkinson, S.S. & Loda, F.A. (1987). Factors related to school absence among children with cardiac conditions. *American Journal of Diseases in Childhood*, *141*, 1317–20.

Fredriksen, P.M., Kahrs, N., Blaasvaer, S., Sigurdsen, E., Gundersen, O., Roeksund, O. et al (2000). Effect of physical training in children and adolescents with congenital heart disease. *Cardiology in the Young*, *10*, 107–114.

Fredriksen, P.M., Veldtman, G., Hechter, S., Therrien, J., Chen, A., Warsi, M.A. et al (2001). Aerobic capacity in adults with various congenital heart diseases. *American Journal of Cardiology*, *87*, 310–314.

Freier, M.C., Babikian, T., Pivonka, J., Burley Aaen, T., Gardner, J.M., Baum, M. et al (2004). A longitudinal perspective on neurodevelopmental outcome after infant cardiac transplantation. *Journal of Heart and Lung Transplantation*, *23*, 857–864.

Gallo, A.M. (1988). The special sibling relationship in chronic illness and disability: parental communication with well siblings. *Holistic Nursing Practice*, *2*, 28–37.

Gatzoulis, M.A., Webb, G.D. & Daubeney, P.E.F. (2003). *Diagnosis and management of adult congenital heart disease*. Edinburgh: Churchill Livingstone.

Gatzoulis, M.A., Swan, L., Thierrien, J. & Pantely, G.A. (2005). *Adult congenital heart disease: A practical guide*. Oxford/London: Blackwell Publishing/BMJ Books.

Gersony, W.M., Hayes, C.J., Driscoll, D.J., Keane, J.F., Kidd, L., O'Fallon, W.M. et al (1993). Second natural history study of congenital heart defects. Quality of life of patients with aortic stenosis, pulmonary stenosis, or ventricular septal defect. *Circulation*, *87*, 152–165.

Gleicher, N., Midwall, J., Hochberger, D. & Jaffin, H. (1979). Eisenmenger's syndrome and pregnancy. *Obstetrical and Gynaecological Survey*, *34*, 721–741.

Goldberg, S., Morris, P., Simmons, R.J., Fowler, R.S. & Levison, H. (1990a). Chronic illness in infancy and parenting stress: a comparison of three groups of parents. *Journal of Pediatric Psychology*, *15*, 347–358.

Goldberg, S., Washington, J., Morris, P., Fischer-Fay, A. & Simmons, R.J. (1990b). Early diagnosed chronic illness and mother–child relationships in the first two years. *Canadian Journal of Psychiatry*, *35*, 726–733.

Goldberg, S., Simmons, R.J., Newman, J., Campbell, K. & Fowler, R.S. (1991). Congenital heart disease, parental stress and infant–mother relationships. *Journal of Pediatrics*, *119*, 661–666.

Goodman, R. & Scott, S. (2005). *Child psychiatry*. 2nd edn. Oxford: Blackwell Publishing.

Goslin, E.R. (1978). Hospitalisation as a life crisis for the preschool child: a critical review. *Journal of Community Health*, *3*, 321–346.

Green, M. & Levitt, E.E. (1962). Constriction of body image in children with congenital heart disease. *Pediatrics, 29*, 438–441.

Gregoratos, G., Abrams, J., Epstein, A.E. et al. (2002). ACC/AHA/NASPE Guideline update for implantation of cardiac pacemakers and antiarrhythmia devices. *Circulation, 106*, 2145–2161.

Gudermuth, S. (1975). Mothers' reports of early experiences of infants with congenital heart disease. *Maternal-Child Nursing Journal, 4*, 155–164.

Hagemo, P.S., Rasmussen, M., Bryhn, G. & Vandvik, I.H. (1997). Hypoplastic left heart syndrome: multi-professional follow-up in the mid-term following palliative procedures. *Cardiology in the Young, 7*, 248–253.

Harinck, E., Hutter, P.A., Hoorntje, T.M. et al (1996). Air travel and adults with cyanotic congenital heart disease. *Circulation, 93*, 272–276.

Health Advisory Service (1995). *Child and adolescent mental health services thematic review: Together we stand*. London: Health Advisory Service HMSO.

Health Advisory Service (2001). *Tackling drugs: Arrest referral statistical update*. London: HMSO.

Higgins, S.S. & Kashani, I.A. (1986). The cyanotic child: heart defects and parental learning needs. *American Journal of Maternal Child Nursing, 11*, 259–262.

Hoehn, K.S., Wernovsky, G., Rychik, J., Tian, Z.Y., Donaghue, D., Alderfer, M.A. et al (2004). Parental decision-making in congenital heart disease. *Cardiology in the Young, 14*, 309–314.

Holm, I., Fredriksen, P.M., Fosdahl, M.A., Ostad, M. & Vollestad, N. (2007). Impaired motor competence in school-aged children with complex congenital heart disease. *Archives of Pediatrics and Adolescent Medicine, 161*, 945–950.

Horner, A. (2009). *Male health issues* [online]. Available at: http://www.guch.org.uk/experiences/mhealth [Accessed 25 March 2009].

Horner, T., Liberthson, R. & Jellinek, M.S. (2000). Psychosocial profile of adults with complex congenital heart disease. *Mayo Clinic Proceedings, 75*, 31–36.

Hovels-Gurich, H.H., Seghaye, M.-C., Dabritz, S., Messmer, B. & von Bernuth, G. (1997). Cognitive and motor development in preschool and school-aged children after neonatal arterial switch operation. *Journal of Thoracic and Cardiovascular Surgery, 114*, 578–585.

Hovels-Gurich, H.H., Seghaye, M.-C., Sigler, M., Kotlarek, F., Bartl, A., Neuser, J. et al (2001). Neurodevelopmental outcome related to cerebral risk factors in children after neonatal arterial switch operation. *Annals of Thoracic Surgery, 71*, 881–888.

Hovels-Gurich, H.H., Konrad, K., Wiesner, M., Minkenberg, R., Herpertz-Dahlmann, B., Messmer, B. & von Bernuth, G. (2002a). Long term behavioural outcome after neonatal arterial switch operation for transposition of the great arteries. *Archives of Disease in Childhood, 87*, 506–510.

Hovels-Gurich, H.H., Seghaye, M.-C., Schnitker, R., Wiesner, M., Huber, W., Minkenberg, R. et al (2002b). Long-term neurodevelopmental outcomes in school-aged children after neonatal arterial switch operation. *Journal of Thoracic and Cardiovascular Surgery, 124*, 448–458.

Hovels-Gurich, H.H., Kunz, D., Seghaye, M., Miskova, M., Messmer, B.J. & von Bernuth, G. (2003). Results of exercise testing at a mean age of 10 years after neonatal arterial switch operation. *Acta Paediatrica, 92*, 190–196.

Hovels-Gurich, H.H., Konrad, K., Skorzenski, D., Nacken, C., Minkenberg, R., Messmer, B.J. & Seghaye, M.C. (2006). Long-term neurodevelopmental outcome and exercise capacity after corrective surgery for tetralogy of Fallot or ventricular septal defect in infancy. *Annals of Thoracic Surgery, 81*, 958–966.

Hovels-Gurich, H.H., Konrad, K., Skorzenski, D., Herpertz-Dahlmann, B., Messmer, B.J. & Seghaye, M.C. (2007). Attentional dysfunction in children after corrective cardiac surgery in infancy. *Annals of Thoracic Surgery, 83*, 1425–1430.

Hovels-Gurich, H.H., Bauer, S.B., Schnitker, R., Willmes-von Hinckeldey, K., Messmer, B.J., Seghaye, M.C. & Huber, W. (2008). Long-term outcome of speech and language in children after corrective surgery for cyanotic or acyanotic cardiac defects in infancy. *European Journal of Paediatric Neurology, 12*, 378–386.

Janus, M. & Goldberg, S. (1997). Treatment characteristics of congenital heart disease and behaviour problems of patients and healthy siblings. *Journal of Paediatrics and Child Health, 33*, 219–225.

Kamphuis, M., Vogels, T., Ottenkamp, J., van der Wall, E.E., Verloove-Vanhorick, S.P. & Vliegen, H.W. (2002). Employment in adults with congenital heart disease. *Archives of Pediatric and Adolescent Medicine, 165*, 1143–1148.

Karsdorp, P.A., Everaerd, W., Kindt, M. & Mulder, B.J.M. (2007). Psychological and cognitive functioning in children and adolescents with congenital heart disease: a meta-analysis. *Journal of Pediatric Psychology, 32*, 527–541.

Kendall, L., Sloper, P., Lewin, R.J.P. & Parsons, J.M. (2003). The views of parents concerning the planning of services for rehabilitation of families of children with congenital cardiac disease. *Cardiology in the Young, 13*, 20–27.

Kendall, L., Parsons, J.M., Sloper, P. & Lewin, R.J.P. (2007). A simple screening method for determining knowledge of the appropriate levels of activity and risk behaviour in young people with congenital cardiac conditions. *Cardiology in the Young, 17*, 151–157.

Kern, J.H., Hinton, V.J., Nereo, N.E., Hayes, C.J. & Gersony, W.M. (1998). Early developmental outcome after the Norwood procedure for hypoplastic left heart syndrome. *Pediatrics, 102*, 1148–1152.

Kirshbom, P.M., Flynn, T.B., Clancy, R.R., Ittenbach, R.F., Hartman, D.M., Paridon, S.M. et al (2005). Late neurodevelopmental outcome after repair of total anomalous pulmonary venous connection. *Journal of Thoracic and Cardiovascular Surgery, 129*, 1091–1097.

Knirsch, W., Hassberg, D., Beyer, A., Teufel, T., Pees, C., Uhlemann, F. & Lange, P.E. (2003). Knowledge, compliance and practice of antibiotic endocarditis prophylaxis of patients with congenital heart disease. *Pediatric Cardiology, 24*, 344–349.

Kochilas, L., Shores, J.C., Novello, R.T., Wernovsky, G., Clancy, R.R., Gaynor, J.W. et al (2001). Aortic morphometry and microcephaly in the hypoplastic left heart syndrome. *Journal of the American College of Cardiology, 37*, 470.

Kokkonen, J. & Paavilainen, T. (1992). Social adaptation of young adults with congenital heart disease. *International Journal of Cardiology, 36*, 23–29.

Kovacs, A.H., Sears, S.F. & Saidi, A.S. (2005). Biopsychosocial experiences of adults with congenital heart disease: review of the literature. *American Heart Journal, 150*, 193–201.

Kowalsky, R.H., Newburger, J.W., Rand, W.M. & Castaneda, A.R. (2006). Factors determining access to surgery for children with congenital cardiac disease in Guatemala, Central America. *Cardiology in the Young, 16*, 385–391.

Kramer, H.H., Awiszus, D., Sterzel, U., van Halteren, A. & Classen, R. (1989). Development of personality and intelligence in children with congenital heart disease. *Journal of Child Psychology and Psychiatry, 30*, 299–308.

Krol, Y., Grootenhuis, M.A., DestreeVonk, A., Lubbers, LJ., Koopman, H.M. & Last, B.F. (2003). Health related quality of life in children with congenital heart disease. *Psychology and Health, 18*, 251–260.

La Greca, A.M. & Schuman, W.B. (1995). Adherence to prescribed medical regimens. In Roberts, M.C., ed. *Handbook of pediatric psychology*. 2nd edn. New York: Guilford. pp. 55–83.

Landolt, M.A., Valsangiacomo Buechel, E.R. & Latal, B. (2008). Health-related quality of life in children and adolescents after open-heart surgery. *Journal of Pediatrics, 152*, 349–355.

Lane, D.A., Lip, G.Y.H. & Millane, T.A. (2002). Quality of life in adults with congenital heart disease. *Heart, 88*, 71–75.

Lavigne, J.V. & Faier-Routman, J. (1992). Psychological adjustment to pediatric physical disorders: a meta-analytic review. *Journal of Pediatric Psychology, 13*, 363–378.

Lavigne, J.V. & Ryan, M. (1979). Psychologic adjustment of siblings of children with chronic illness. *Pediatrics, 63*, 616–627.

Lawoko, S.& Soares, J.J.F. (2002). Distress and hopelessness among parents of children with congenital heart disease, parents of children with other diseases, and parents of healthy children. *Journal of Psychosomatic Research, 52*, 193–208.

Leonard, H., O'Sullivan, J.J. & Hunter, S. (1996). Family planning requirements in the adult congenital heart disease clinic. *Heart, 76*, 60–62.

Lewis, G., ed. (2007). *Why mothers die 2000–2002. The sixth report of Confidential Enquiries into Maternal Death in the United Kingdom.* London: RCOG Press.

Limperopoulos, C., Majnemer, A., Shevell, M.I., Rosenblatt, B., Rohlicek, C. & Tchervenkov, C. (1999). Neurologic status of newborns with congenital heart defects before open heart surgery. *Pediatrics, 103*, 402–408.

Limperopoulos, C., Majnemer, A., Shevell, M.I., Rohlicek, C., Rosenblatt, B., Tchervenkov, C. & Darwish, H.Z. (2002). Predictors of developmental disabilities after open heart surgery in young children with congenital heart defects. *Journal of Pediatrics, 141*, 51–58.

Lip, G.Y.H., Lane, D.A. & Millane, T.A. (2005). Psychological interventions for depression in adolescent and adult congenital heart disease. *Cochrane Database of Systematic Reviews*, Issue 2: CD004372.

Mahle, W.T., Clancy, R.R., Moss, E.M., Gerdes, M., Jobes, D.R. & Wernovsky, G. (2000). Neurodevelopmental outcome and lifestyle assessment in school-aged and adolescent children with hypoplastic left heart syndrome. *Pediatrics, 105*, 1082–1089.

Majnemer, A., Limperopoulos, C., Shevell, M., Rosenblatt, B., Rohlicek, C. & Tchervenkov, C. (2006a). Long-term neuromotor outcome at school entry of infants with congenital heart defects requiring open-heart surgery. *Journal of Pediatrics, 148*, 72–77.

Majnemer, A., Limperopoulos, C., Shevell, M., Rohlicek, C., Rosenblatt, B. & Tchervenkov, C. (2006b). Health and well-being of children with congenital cardiac malformations, and their families, following open-heart surgery. *Cardiology in the Young, 16*, 157–164.

Marcus, B.H., Williams, D.M., Dubbert, P.M., Sallis, J.F., King, A.C., Yancey, A.K. et al; American Heart Association Council on Nutrition, Physical Activity and Metabolism (Subcommittee on Physical Activity); American Heart Association Council on Cardiovascular Disease in the Young & Interdisciplinary Working Group on Quality of Care and Outcomes Research (2006). Physical activity intervention studies: what we know and what we need to know. A scientific statement from the American Heart Association council on nutrition, physical activity, and metabolism (subcommittee on physical activity); council on cardiovascular disease in the young; and the interdisciplinary working group on quality of care and outcomes research. *Circulation, 114*, 2739–2752.

Marino, B.S., Pasquali, S.K., Wernovsky, G. Bockoven, J.R., McBride, M., Cho, C.J., et al (2006). Exercise performance in children and adolescents after the Ross Procedure. *Cardiology in the Young, 16*, 40–47.

Martinson, I.M., Gilliss, C., Colaizzo, D.C., Freeman, M. & Bossert, E. (1990). Impact of childhood cancer on healthy school-age siblings. *Cancer Nursing, 13*, 183–190.

Maxwell, G.M. & Gane, S. (1962). The impact of congenital heart disease upon the family. *American Heart Journal, 64*, 449–454.

McBride, M.G., Kirshbom, P.M., Gayanor, J.W., Ittenbach, R.F., Wernovsky, G., Clancy, R.R. et al (2007). Late cardiopulmonary and musculoskeletal exercise performance after repair for total anomalous pulmonary venous connection during infancy. *Journal of Thoracic and Cardiovascular Surgery, 133*, 1533–1539.

McCrindle, B.W., Williams, R.V., Mitchell, P.D., Hsu, D.T., Paridon, S.M., Atz, A.M. et al. (2006). Relationship of patient and medical characteristics to health status in children and adolescents after the Fontan procedure. *Circulation, 113*, 1123–1129.

McCrindle, B.W., Williams, R.V., Mital, S., Clark, B.J., Russell, J.L., Klein, G. & Eisenmann, J.C. (2007). Physical activity levels in children and adolescents are reduced after the Fontan procedure, independent of exercise capacity, and are associated with lower perceived general health. *Archives of Disease in Childhood, 92*, 509–514.

McCusker, C.G., Doherty, N.N., Molloy, B., Casey, F., Rooney, N., Mulholland, C. et al (2007). Determinants of neuropsychological and behavioural outcomes in early childhood survivors of congenital heart disease. *Archives of Disease in Childhood*, *92*, 137–141.

McDougall, T. (2006). *Child and adolescent mental health nursing*. Oxford: Blackwell Publishing.

McKeever, P. (1983). Siblings of chronically ill children: a literature review with implications for research and practice. *American Journal of Orthopsychiatry*, *53*, 209–218.

Miatton, M., De Wolf, D., Francois, K., Thiery, E. & Vingerhoets, G. (2007a). Intellectual, neuropsychological, and behavioral functioning in children with tetralogy of Fallot. *Journal of Thoracic and Cardiovascular Surgery*, *133*, 449–455.

Meltzer, H., Green, H., McGinnity, A., Ford, T. Goodman, R. *The mental health of children and adolescents in Great Britain 2004*. London: Stationery Office.

Miatton, M., De Wolf, D., Francois, K., Thiery, E. & Vingerhoets, G. (2007b). Neuropsychological performance in school-aged children with surgically corrected congenital heart disease. *Journal of Pediatrics*, *151*, 73–78.

Miatton, M., De Wolf, D., Francois, K., Thiery, E. & Vingerhoets, G. (2007c). Behavior and self-perception in children with a surgically corrected congenital heart disease. *Journal of Developmental and Behavioral Pediatrics*, *28*, 294–301.

Moons, P., Van Deyk, K., Budts, W. & De Geest, S. (2004). Caliber of quality of life assessments in congenital heart disease: a plea for more conceptual and methodological rigor. *Archives of Pediatrics and Adolescent Medicine*, *158*, 1062–1069.

Moons, P., Van Deyk, K., De Geest, S., Gewillig, M. & Budts, W. (2005). Is the severity of congenital heart disease associated with the quality of life and perceived health of adult patients? *Heart*, *91*, 1193–1198.

Moons, P., Barrea, C., De Wolf, D., Gewillig, M., Massin, M., Mertens, L. et al (2006a). Changes in perceived health of children with congenital heart disease after attending a special sports camp. *Pediatric Cardiology*, *27*, 67–72.

Moons, P., Barrea, C., Suys, B., Ovaert, C., Boshoff, D., Eyskens, B. et al (2006b). Improved perceived health status persists three months after a special sports camp for children with congenital heart disease. *European Journal of Pediatrics*, *165*, 767–772.

Morris, R.D., Krawiecki, N.S., Wright, J.A. & Walter, L.W. (1993). Neuropsychological, academic and adaptive functioning in children who survive in-hospital cardiac arrest and resuscitation. *Journal of Learning Disabilities*, *26*, 46–51.

Moyen Laane, K., Meberg, A., Otterstad, J.E., Froland, G., Sorland, S., Lindstrom, B. & Eriksson, B. (1997). Quality of life in children with congenital heart defects. *Acta Paediatrica*, *86*, 975–980.

Mulhern, R.K., Fairclough, D.L., Smith, B. & Douglas, S.M. (1992). Maternal depression, assessment methods and physical symptoms affect estimates of depressive symptomatology among children with cancer. *Journal of Pediatric Psychology*, *17*, 313–326.

Mussatto, K. (2006). Adaptation of the child and family to life with a chronic illness. *Cardiology in the Young*, *16*(Suppl. 3), 110–116.

Mussatto, K. & Tweddell, J. (2005). Quality of life following surgery for congenital cardiac malformations in neonates and infants. *Cardiology in the Young*, *15*(Suppl. 1), 174–178.

National Institute for Health and Clinical Excellence (2004). *Self-harm. The short-term physical and psychological management and secondary prevention of self-harm in primary and secondary care*. London: NICE.

Newburger, J.W., Silbert, A.R., Buckley, L.P. & Fyler, D.C. (1984). Cognitive function and age at repair of transposition of the great arteries in children. *New England Journal of Medicine*, *310*, 1495–1499.

Newburger, J.W., Jonas, R.A., Wernovsky, G., Wypij, D., Hickey, P.R., Kuban, K. et al (1993). A comparison of the perioperative neurologic effects of hypothermic circulatory arrest versus low-flow cardiopulmonary bypass in infant heart surgery. *New England Journal of Medicine*, *329*, 1057–1064.

Newburger, J.W., Wypij, D., Bellinger, D.C., du Plessis, A.J., Kuban, K.C., Rappaport, L.A. et al (2003). Length of stay after infant heart surgery is related to cognitive outcome at age 8 years. *Journal of Pediatrics*, 143, 67–73.

Niwa, K., Tateno, S., Tatebe, S. et al (2002). Social concern and independence in adults with congenital heart disease. *Journal of Cardiology*, 39, 259–266.

Nora, J.J. & Nora, A.H. (1987). Maternal transmission of congenital heart diseases: new recurrence risk figures and the questions of cytoplasmic inheritance and vulnerability to teratogens. *American Journal of Cardiology*, 59, 459–463.

Norozi, K., Gravenhorst, V., Hobbiebrunken, E. & Wessel, A. (2005). Normality of cardiopulmonary capacity in children operated on to correct congenital heart defects. *Archives of Pediatrics and Adolescent Medicine*, 159, 1063–1068.

Oates, R.K., Turnbull, J.A., Simpson, J.M. & Cartmill, T.B. (1994). Parent and teacher perceptions of child behaviour following cardiac surgery. *Acta Paediatrica*, 83, 1303–1307.

Oates, R.K., Simpson, J.M., Cartmill, T.B. & Turnbull, J.A.B. (1995). Intellectual function and age of repair in cyanotic congenital heart disease. *Archives of Disease in Childhood*, 72, 298–301.

O'Brien, L.M., Holbrook, C.R., Mervis, C.B., Klaus, C.J., Bruner, J.L., Raffield, T.J. et al (2003). Sleep and neurobehavioral characteristics of 5- to 7-year-old children with parentally reported symptoms of attention-deficit/hyperactivity disorder. *Pediatrics*, 111, 554–563.

O'Dougherty, M., Wright, F.S., Loewenson, R.B. & Torres, F. (1985). Cerebral dysfunction after chronic hypoxia in children. *Neurology*, 35, 42–46.

Parsons, S.K., Barlow, S.E., Levy, S.L., Supran, S.E. & Kaplan, S.H. (1999). Health-related quality of life in pediatric bone marrow transplant survivors: according to whom? *International Journal of Cancer Supplement*, 12, 46–51.

Pelchat, D., Ricard, N., Bouchard, J.-M., Perreault, M., Saucier, J.F., Berthiaume, M. & Bisson, J. (1999). Adaptation of parents in relation to their 6-month-old infant's type of disability. *Child: Care, Health and Development*, 25, 377–397.

Plunkett, J.W., Meisels, S.J., Stiefel, G.S., Pasick, P.L. & Roloff, D.W. (1986). Patterns of attachment among preterm infants of varying biological risk. *Journal of the American Academy of Child Psychiatry*, 25, 794–800.

Polinsky, M.S., Kaiser, B.A., Stover, J.B., Frankenfield, M. & Baluarte, H.J. (1987). Neurologic development of children with severe chronic renal failure from infancy. *Pediatric Nephrology*, 1, 157–165.

Ponton, L.E. (1997). *The romance of risk*. New York: Basic Books.

Popelova, J., Slavik Z. & Skovranek, J. (2001). Are cyanosed adults with congenital cardiac malformations depressed? *Cardiology in the Young*, 11, 379–384.

Rempel, G.R., Cender, L.M., Lynam, M.J., Sandor, G.G. & Farquharson, D. (2004). Parents' perspectives on decision making after antenatal diagnosis of congenital heart disease. *Journal of Obstetric, Gynecologic, and Neonatal Nursing*, 33, 64–70.

Reybrouck, T. & Mertens, L. (2005). Physical performance and physical activity in grown-up congenital heart disease. *European Journal of Cardiovascular Prevention & Rehabilitation*, 12, 498–502.

Rhodes, J., Curran, T.J., Camil, L., Rabideau, N., Fulton, D.R., Gauthier, N.S. et al (2005). Impact of cardiac rehabilitation on the exercise function of children with serious congenital heart disease. *Pediatrics*, 116, 1339–1345.

Rogers, B.T., Msall, M.E., Buck, G.M., Lyon, N.R., Norris, M.K., Roland, J.-M.A. et al (1995). Neurodevelopmental outcome of infants with hypoplastic left heart syndrome. *Journal of Pediatrics*, 26, 496–498.

Rogers, R., Reybrouck, T., Weymans, M., Dumoulin, M., Van Der, H.L. & Gewillig, M. (1994). Reliability of subjective estimates of exercise capacity after total repair of Tetralogy of Fallot. *Acta Paediatrica*, 83, 866–869.

Rona, R.J., Smeeton, N.C., Beech, R., Barnett, A. & Sharland, G. (1998). Anxiety and depression in mothers related to severe malformation of the heart of the child and foetus. *Acta Paediatrica, 87*, 201–205.

Royal College of Nursing (2004). *Children and young people's mental health – every nurse's business.* London: RCN.

Saliba, Z., Butera, G., Bonnet D., Bonhoeffer, P., Villain, E., Kachaner, J. et al (2001). Quality of life and perceived health status in surviving adults with univentricular heart. *Heart, 86*, 69–73.

Salzer-Muhar, U., Herle, M., Floquet, P., Freilinger, M., Greber-Platzer, S., Haller, A. et al (2002). Self-concept in male and female adolescents with congenital heart disease. *Clinical Pediatrics, 41*, 17–24.

Sanger, M.S., Copeland, D.R. & Davidson, E.R. (1991). Psychosocial adjustment among pediatric cancer patients: a multidimensional assessment. *Journal of Pediatric Psychology, 16*, 463–74.

Sharpe, D. & Rossiter, L. (2002). Siblings of children with a chronic illness: a meta-analysis. *Journal of Pediatric Psychology, 27*, 699–710.

Shaw, R.J. (2001). Treatment adherence in adolescents: development and psychopathology. *Clinical Child Psychology and Psychiatry, 6*, 137–150.

Shor, V.S. (1978). Long term implications of cardiovascular disease. *Issues in Comprehensive Pediatric Nursing, 2*, 36–50.

Silbert, A., Wolff, P.H., Mayer, B., Rosenthal, A. & Nadas, A.S. (1969). Cyanotic heart disease and psychological development. *Pediatrics, 43*, 192–200.

Sklansky, M., Tang, A., Levy, D., Grossfeld, P., Kashani, I., Shaughnessy, R. & Rothman, A. (2002). Maternal psychological impact of fetal echocardiography. *Journal of the American Society of Echocardiography, 15*, 159–166.

Sloper, T., Larcombe, I.J. & Charlton, A. (1994). Psychosocial adjustment of five-year survivors of childhood cancer. *Journal of Cancer Education, 9*, 163–169.

So, S.K.S., Chang, P.N., Najarian, J.S., Mauer, S.M., Simmons, R.L. & Nevins, T.E. (1987). Growth and development in infants after renal transplantation. *Journal of Pediatrics, 110*, 343–50.

Somerville, J. (1997). Near misses and disasters in the treatment of grown-up congenital heart patients. *Journal of the Royal Society of Medicine, 90*, 124–127.

Spijkerboer, A.W., Helbing, W.A., Bogers, A.J.J.C., Van Domburg, R.T., Verhulst, F.C. & Utens, E.M.W.J. (2007). Long-term psychological distress, and styles of coping, in parents of children and adolescents who underwent invasive treatment for congenital cardiac disease. *Cardiology in the Young, 17*, 638–645.

Spinetta, J.J. (1981). The sibling of the child with cancer. In Spinetta, J.J. & Deasy-Spinetta, P., eds. *Living with childhood cancer.* St Louis: C.V. Mosby. pp. 133–142.

Stewart, S.M., Uauy, R., Waller, D.A., Kennard, B.D. & Andrews, W.S. (1987). Mental and motor development correlates in patients with end-stage biliary atresia awaiting liver transplantation. *Pediatrics, 79*, 882–888.

Suddaby, E.C., Samango-Sprouse, C., Vaught, D.R. & Custer, D.A. (1996). Neurodevelopmental outcome of infant cardiac recipients. *Journal of Transplant Coordination, 6*, 9–13.

Swan, L. & Hillis, W.S. (2000). Exercise prescription in adults with congenital heart disease: a long way to go. *Heart, 83*, 685–687.

Taanila, A., Kokkonen, J. & Jarvelin, M.R. (1996). The long-term effects of children's early-onset disability on marital relationships. *Developmental Medicine and Child Neurology, 38*, 567–577.

Tabbutt, S., Nord, A.S., Jarvik, G.P., Bernbaum, J., Wernovsky, G., Gerdes, M. et al (2008). Neurodevelopmental outcomes after staged palliation for hypoplastic left heart syndrome. *Pediatrics, 121*, 476–483.

Tak, Y.R. & McCubbin, M. (2002). Family stress, perceived social support and coping following the diagnosis of a child's congenital heart disease. *Journal of Advanced Nursing, 39*, 190–8.

Takken, T., Tacken, M.H., Blacnk, A.C., Hulzebos, E.H., Strengers, J.L. & Helders, P.J. (2007). Exercise limitation in patients with Fontan circulation: a review. *Journal of Cardiovascular Medicine, 8,* 775–781.

Therrien, J., Fredriksen, P.M., Walker, M., Granton, J., Reid, G.J. & Webb, G. (2003). A pilot study of exercise training in adult patients with repaired tetralogy of Fallot. *Canadian Journal of Cardiology, 19,* 685–689.

Thompson, P.D., Buchner, D., Piña, I.L., Balady, G.J., Williams, M.A., Marcus, B.H. & Berra, K. (2003). Exercise and physical activity in the prevention and treatment of atherosclerotic cardiovascular disease: a statement from the Council on Clinical Cardiology (subcommittee on exercise, rehabilitation, and prevention) and the Council on Nutrition, Physical Activity, and Metabolism (subcommittee on physical activity). *Circulation, 107,* 3109–3116.

Thompson, R.J., Gustafson, K.E., Hamlett, K.W. & Spock, A. (1992). Stress, coping and family functioning in the psychological adjustment of mothers of children and adolescents with cystic fibrosis. *Journal of Pediatric Psychology, 17,* 573–585.

Thompson, R.J., Gil, K.M., Gustafson, K.E., George, L.K., Keith, B.R., Spock, A. & Kinney, T.R. (1994). Stability and change in the psychological adjustment of mothers of children and adolescents with cystic fibrosis and sickle cell disease. *Journal of Pediatric Psychology, 19,* 171–188.

Tong, E., Sparacino, P., Messias, D., Foote, D., Chesla, C. & Gilliss, C. (1998). Growing up with congenital heart disease: the dilemmas of adolescents and young adults. *Cardiology in the Young, 8,* 303–309.

Trahd, G.E. (1986). Siblings of chronically ill children: helping them cope. *Pediatric Nursing, 12,* 191–193.

Trojnarska, O. (2007). Heart failure in the adult patient with congenital heart disease. *Cardiology Journal, 14,* 127–136.

Upham, M. & Medoff-Cooper, B. (2005). What are the responses and needs of mothers of infants diagnosed with congenital heart disease? *MCN American Journal of Maternal Child Nursing, 30,* 24–29.

Utens, E.M., Versluis-Den Bieman, H.J., Verhulst, F.C., Meijboom, F.J., Erdman, R.A. & Hess, J. (1998). Psychopathology in young adults with congenital heart disease follow-up results. *European Heart Journal, 19,* 647–651.

Utens, E.M., Versluis-Den Bieman, H.J., Verhulst, F.C. & Witsenburg, A.J.J.C. (2000). Psychological distress and styles of coping in parents of children awaiting elective cardiac surgery. *Cardiology in the Young, 10,* 239–244.

Utens, E.M.W.J., Versluis-Den Bieman, H.J., Witsenburg, M., Bogers A.J.J.C., Verhulst, F.C. & Hess, J. (2001). Cognitive and behavioural and emotional functioning of young children awaiting elective cardiac surgery or catheter intervention. *Cardiology in the Young, 11,* 153–160.

Uzark, K. & Jones, K. (2003). Parenting stress and children with heart disease. *Journal of Pediatric Health Care, 17,* 163–168.

Uzark, K., VonBargen-Mazza, P., & Messiter, E. (1989). Health education needs of adolescents with congenital heart disease. *Journal of Pediatric Health Care, 3,* 137–143.

Uzark, K.C., Sauer, S.N., Lawrence, K.S., Miller, J., Addonizio, L. & Crowley, D.C. (1992). The psychosocial impact of pediatric heart transplantation. *Journal of Heart and Lung Transplantation, 11,* 1160–1167.

Uzark, K., Lincoln, A., Lamberti, J.J., Mainwaring, R.D., Spicer, R.L. & Moore, J.W. (1998). Neurodevelopmental outcomes in children with Fontan repair of functional single ventricle. *Pediatrics, 101,* 630–633.

Uzark, K., Jones, K., Burwinkle, T.M. & Varni, J.W. (2003). The Pediatric Quality of Life Inventory in children with heart disease. *Progress in Pediatric Cardiology, 18,* 141–148.

Vance, J.C., Fazan, L.E., Satterwhite, B. & Pless, I.B. (1980). Effects of nephrotic syndrome on the family: a controlled study. *Pediatrics, 65,* 948–955.

van den Bosch, A.E., Roos-Hesselink, J.W., van Domburg, R., Bogers, A.J., Simoons, M.L. & Meijboom, F.J. (2004). Long-term outcome and quality of life in adult patients after the Fontan operation. *American Journal of Cardiology, 93,* 1141–1145.

van der Rijken, R.E., Maassen, B.A., Walk, T.L., Daniels, O. & Hulstijn-Dirkmaat, G.M. (2007). Outcome after surgical repair of congenital cardiac malformations at school age. *Cardiology in the Young, 17*, 64–71.

Van Deyk, K., Moons, P., Gewillig, M. & Budts, W. (2004). Educational and behavioral issues in transitioning from pediatric cardiology to adult-centered health care. *Nursing Clinics of North America, 39*, 755–768.

Van Horn, M., DeMaso, D.R., Gonzalez-Heydrich, J. & Erickson, J.D. (2001). Illness-related concerns of mothers of children with congenital heart disease. *Journal of the American Academy of Child and Adolescent Psychiatry, 40*, 847–854.

van Houten, J.P., Rothman, A. & Bejar, R. (1996). High incidence of cranial ultrasound abnormalities in full-term infants with congenital heart disease. *American Journal of Perinatology, 13*, 47–53.

van Rijen, E.H.M., Utens, E.M.W.J., Roos-Hesselink, J.W., Meijboom, F.J., van Domburg, R.T., Roelandt, J.R.T.C. et al (2003). Psychosocial functioning of the adult with congenital heart disease, a 20–33 years follow-up. *European Heart Journal, 24*, 673–683.

van Rijen, E.H.M., Utens, E.M.W.J., Roos-Hesselink, J.W., Meijboom, F.J., van Domburg, R.T., Roelandt, J.R.T.C. et al (2004). Medical predictors for psychopathology in adults with operated congenital heart disease. *European Heart Journal, 25*, 1605–1613.

Vargas, S. & Camill, G. (1999). A meta-analysis of research on sensory integration treatment. *American Journal of Occupational Therapy, 53*, 189–198.

Vernon, D.T.A., Schulman, J.L. & Foley, J.M. (1966). Changes in children's behavior after hospitalisation. *American Journal of Diseases in Childhood, III*, 581–593.

Walker, R.E., Gauvreau, K. & Jenkins, K.J. (2004). Health-related quality of life in children attending a cardiology clinic. *Pediatric Cardiology, 25*, 40–48.

Warnes, C.A. & Somerville, J. (1986). Tricuspid atresia in adolescents and adults: current state and late complications. *Heart, 56*; 535–543.

Wayman, K.I., Cox, K.L. & Esquivel, C.O. (1997). Neurodevelopmental outcome of young children with extrahepatic biliary atresia 1 year after liver transplantation. *Journal of Pediatrics, 131*, 894–898.

Webster-Stratton, C. (1990). Stress: a potential description of parent perceptions and family interactions. *Journal of Clinical Child Psychology, 19*, 302–312.

Wernovsky, G., Stiles, K.M., Gauvreau, K., Gentles, T.L., duPlessis, A.J., Bellinger, D.C. et al (2000). Cognitive development after the Fontan operation. *Circulation, 102*, 883–889.

White-Koning, M., Arnaud, C., Dickinson, H.O., Thyen, U., Beckung, E., Fauconnier, J. et al (2007). Determinants of child–parent agreement in quality-of-life reports: a European study of children with cerebral palsy. *Pediatrics, 120*, e804–e814.

WHOQOL Group (1993). Study protocol for the World Health Organisation project to develop a quality of life assessment instrument (WHOQOL). *Quality of Life Research, 2*, 153–159.

Wray, J. & Maynard, L. (2005). Living with congenital or acquired heart disease in childhood: what is the impact on the child and family? *Cardiology in the Young, 15*, 133–140.

Wray, J. & Maynard, L. (2006). The needs of families of children with congenital or acquired heart disease. *Journal of Developmental and Behavioral Pediatrics, 27*, 11–17.

Wray, J. & Radley-Smith, R. (2004). Developmental and behavioural status of infants and young children awaiting heart or heart–lung transplantation. *Pediatrics, 113*, 488–495.

Wray, J. & Radley-Smith, R. (2005). Beyond the first year after pediatric heart or heart–lung transplantation: changes in cognitive function and behaviour. *Pediatric Transplantation, 9*, 170–177.

Wray, J. & Radley-Smith, R. (2006). Anxiety, depression and social competence in children and adolescents undergoing transplantation. *Journal of Heart and Lung Transplantation, 25*(2S), S153.

Wray, J. & Sensky, T. (1998). How does the intervention of cardiac surgery affect the self perception of children with congenital heart disease? *Child: Care, Health and Development, 24*, 57–72.

Wray, J. & Sensky, T. (1999). Controlled study of preschool development after surgery for congenital heart disease. *Archives of Disease in Childhood*, *80*, 511–516.

Wray, J. & Sensky, T. (2001). Congenital heart disease and cardiac surgery in childhood: effects on cognitive function and academic ability. *Heart*, *85*, 687–691.

Wray, J. & Sensky, T. (2004). Psychological functioning in parents of children undergoing elective cardiac surgery. *Cardiology in the Young*, *14*, 131–139.

Wray, J., Radley-Smith, R. & Yacoub, M. (1992). Effect of cardiac or heart–lung transplantation on the quality of life of the paediatric patient. *Quality of Life Research*, *1*, 41–46.

Wray, J., Pot-Mees, C., Zeitlin, H., Radley-Smith, R. & Yacoub, M. (1994). Cognitive function and behavioural status in paediatric heart and heart–lung transplant recipients: the Harefield Experience. *British Medical Journal*, *309*, 837–841.

Wray, J., Long, T., Radley-Smith, R. & Yacoub, M. (2001). Returning to school after heart or heart-lung transplantation: how well do children adjust? *Transplantation*, *72*, 100–106.

Wray, J., Small, G., Freedman, B. & Franklin, R.C.G. (2004). Carer knowledge of children's medical problems in a paediatric cardiology outpatient setting. *Heart*, *90*, 213–214.

Wray, J., Waters, S., Radley-Smith, R. & Sensky, T. (2006). Adherence in adolescents and young adults following heart or heart–lung transplantation. *Pediatric Transplantation*, *10*, 694–700.

Wright, M. & Nolan, T. (1994). Impact of cyanotic heart disease on school performance. *Archives of Disease in Childhood*, *71*, 64–70.

Yacoub, M.H. (2007). Establishing pediatric cardiovascular services in the developing world: a wake-up call. *Circulation*, *116*, 1876–1878.

Website

Grown Up Congenital Heart Disease Patients Association: www.guch.org.uk

5 What are 'communication skills'?

Jean Simons

The term 'communication skills', in relation to healthcare, is likely to elicit in the reader a variety of opinion ranging from didactic certainty to puzzled incomprehension about what, exactly, such skills are, in what situations they are best employed, and by whom.

Despite years of research studies and teaching of healthcare professionals (the majority of such work, until very recent years, focusing on doctor–patient communication), the tendency has been in practice for healthcare professionals to conflate the concept of 'communication' with situation-specific giving of information (breaking bad news, imparting a diagnosis). Patients and families, however, have placed at least equal value on a reciprocal exchange that enables them to express the emotional and social impact upon themselves of their condition and its problems, and to feel that they are able to adopt a 'negotiating and partnership' style with the healthcare professional (Maguire & Pitceathly, 2002).

Such a view was widely expressed at the Children's Heart Federation Conference in September 2001, at a crowded Support for Families workshop. Participants said they often felt 'bombarded' with information (not all of it useful or relevant to their particular child), but consistent appreciation was expressed for the cardiac liaison nurses who could 'get to know them as a family' as well as impart specialist knowledge and advice.

The changing climate

Perceived failings in some aspects of paediatric care in the NHS and social care services in the last decade, leading to major public enquiries, accelerated an appreciation of the need for cultural change in the health service, and emphasised the crucial importance of open, family-centred communication throughout the whole of the 'patient journey', as an 'integral part of all activity in the care and treatment of the child and family' (Department of Health [DH], 2002a). The findings of the Bristol Royal Infirmary (BRI) Inquiry (DH, 2002a) further highlighted a catalogue of poor communication, not only in the necessary engagement between healthcare professionals and the family, but also between clinicians and teams in the care setting, in the community and between professional groups.

The first recommendation of the BRI Inquiry report is:

In a patient-centred healthcare service patients must be involved, wherever possible, in decisions about their treatment and care.

This encapsulates the changed thinking that provoked a raft of legislation and guidelines, under the 'umbrella' of Patient and Public Involvement, emphasising the key concepts of 'engagement', 'reciprocity' and 'partnership' as central to effective communication between all parties in healthcare. Phrases such as 'patient-centred care' and 'shared decision-making' entered the national vocabulary.

In the National Health Service (NHS), the Knowledge and Skills Framework was designed to improve staff communication competence, and the Royal College of Paediatrics and Child Health published its framework for competences for basic specialist training in paediatrics (DH, 2004). Both of these latter initiatives continued the practice of providing guidelines for communication but not a detailed template for personal interaction or a consistent vocabulary by which those engaged in the communication might recognise, appraise and improve their skills.

There is evidence that healthcare professionals assume that they do communicate in a patient-centred way, if only they follow written guidelines. However, guidelines may be inadequate to achieve real engagement without training in the skills and behaviours that should accompany their use. The issue of 'consent', particularly contentious following the Redfern Report (DH, 1999), exemplifies some common misunderstandings about the concept of 'patient-centredness'.

Consent

Patient Advice and Liaison Service officers, and others, have reported anecdotally that many patients/parents continue to be dissatisfied with the 'consent' process (Box 5.1), despite a thorough overhaul of the guidelines governing the process, changes in the law and the devising of careful and detailed new consent forms. Laudable attempts to ensure that patients and parents are fully and comprehensively informed about post mortem or anticipated surgery (a stated wish of individual parents and groups representing their interests following the BRI Inquiry and the Redfern Report [DH, 1999]) can still backfire if the focus is all on facts and figures, with no attempt to explore the patient's own feelings and expectations.

Expressions of dissatisfaction from patients and families may be met with incomprehension on the part of the challenged healthcare professional, who will insist that

---

Box 5.1 An example of a discussion regarding consent

After a consent discussion with a locum junior doctor whom she had not previously known, a mother said, 'I felt as if I was about to sign his life away, and with the signature, I was agreeing that I would not blame anyone if it all went wrong. I wouldn't have wanted to blame anyone; the staff have always been brilliant and done their utmost for him and us. All I wanted was to hear what the surgeon thought were the risks for [my son] given all the knowledge we all have, and what the surgeon could try if things didn't go well. Quoting figures about risk or survival percentages in an impersonal way meant nothing to me. I felt more frightened after the 'consent discussion'. I felt a bit let down by the people we have always trusted; as if it wasn't about my son or our family, and what a huge thing this all is for us, but as if the hospital were 'covering their backs'.

he or she 'went through the form' meticulously. It seems not to be well understood that 'to make consent properly patient-centred, clinicians need to ask patients what they want from treatment before they discuss treatment strategies' (Bridson et al, 2004, p. 1159) and that patients' 'objectives may differ from the assumptions made by clinicians' (p. 1159).

It is anecdotally reported that the rather mechanistic signing of forms, as the aim or culmination of the 'consent discussion', leads some patients to a cynical assumption that the process is designed for healthcare professionals' security rather than to engage and inform the patient and family. This impression is strengthened when the process is referred to by staff as 'getting the patient consented', still a commonly heard expression despite the criticism of its use, at the BRI Inquiry, for its implied assumption of patient passivity.

> Many patients are uncomfortable questioning clinicians and may not declare their objectives unless asked. The onus, therefore, is on clinicians to explore patients' aims rather than merely discussing risks and benefits associated with procedures. (Bridson et al, 2003, p. 1161)

The 'explanatory' or 'exploratory' communication style

A qualitative analysis of verbal interactions in all circumstances between healthcare professionals of all grades, and patients and families, consistently confirms that healthcare professionals are often overly reliant on professional- or organisation-centred 'explanatory' rather than patient-centred 'exploratory' forms of communication (Maguire & Pitceathly, 2002).

'Explanatory' communication, as the term suggests, tends to mean that the healthcare professional does most of the speaking in the interaction, which can make for a rather one-sided 'engagement'. Even if the patient has asked for the explanation, as will most often be the case when discussing clinical issues, equal emphasis must be given to exploring the patient's understanding, feelings and wishes. Explanatory styles of communication may also sound, and be, essentially defensive, militating against the desired reciprocity of interaction.

The more desirable patient-centred, exploratory, approach, shown by Nurse A in Box 5.2, involves skills that 'promote patient disclosure' and involve an interviewing style that:

> shows genuine interest in patients as individuals, their reasons for seeking help, their perceptions of what might be wrong, their feelings about this and the impact of any problems on their daily lives, mood and personal relationships ... [this approach] leads to greater patient compliance with advice and treatment, as well as greater patient satisfaction. (Maguire & Pitceathly, 2002, p. 697)

Ford and Hall describe as crucial the ability to 'respond to verbal cues suggestive of emotional distress' and ask 'more questions about patients' feelings', which is outlined in Boxes 5.3 and 5.4.

Recommendation 59 of the report of the BRI Inquiry (DH, 2002a) recognises and confirms the necessity of reciprocity and attention to emotional as well as practical considerations:

Box 5.2 An example of breaking bad news

Nurse A is familiar with the situation of 'breaking the bad news' to families that their child's operation has had to be cancelled at the last minute for reasons relating to the hospital's organisation rather than the child's condition. She has observed that the tendency of many healthcare professionals is to explain at length that there is a shortage of intensive care nurses, that the intensive care facilities have had to be allocated overnight to an even sicker child, etc., and to apologise fulsomely, but to avoid engagement with the feelings and reactions of the parent, especially if they are angry, as is often the case.

In one such instance, Nurse A acknowledged the feelings of an angry and weeping mother by asking what effect the cancellation had had on her and her family, and listened to her story of near family breakdown because of the emotional stress of the child's condition and the uncertainties of the anticipated operation. Having been heard, the mother acknowledged that she was thankful that it was not her child who had been so critically ill as to need the intensive care facilities, and arranged a further admission, with no more mention of her earlier threat to 'sue the hospital'.

Box 5.3 Recognising cues

A cue indicates the most important issue for the person at any particular time, and is usually about an emotion, feeling or concern:

- ■ 'I'm worried about …'
- ■ 'It's puzzling …'
- ■ 'I don't know what to think/do/feel …'

If a person offers a cue, they want you to ask about it. Explore what is said. Don't guess what may be felt. Respond to the cue with an **open question** or invitation:

- ■ 'Why (are you worried)?'
- ■ 'What (have you thought of doing)?'
- ■ 'How (do you feel)?'
- ■ 'Can you tell me about that?'

Education in communication skills must be an essential part of the education of all healthcare professionals. Communication skills include the ability to engage patients on an emotional level, to listen, to assess how much information a patient wants to know, and to convey information with clarity and sympathy. (DH, 2002a, p. 445)

This recommendation, like any other guideline, does not set out to include any detail about the 'how to' of 'engaging patients on an emotional level' or assessing the desired level of information. Staff often have to find their own way of interpreting these kinds of guideline, and few have the confidence, without specific training and supervision, to explore the emotional and psychological issues inherent in real engagement.

Box 5.4   Asking open questions

Follow up a cue with an **open question**. Relate the question to the cue, for example:

■ 'I feel so upset.'
■ 'What (are you upset) about?'
■ 'Why (are you upset)?'

This confirms that you are ready to listen, and the approach invites the person to tell you what they want to say.

– It enables a disclosure of emotional and psychological issues.
– It leaves the person in control of how much – and what – they tell you.
– It implies confidence in the person's capacity to think things through with you.

Remember, it is not rude, nosy or inappropriate to *explore* an offered cue.

Box 5.5   Premature reassurance

This is also known as 'meaningless reassurance' – with good reason. It is offered instead of an **open, exploratory question**, in response to a cue:

■ 'I feel so UPSET.'
■ 'Oh, there's no need to be. It'll all be OK.'

This prevents an exploration of concerns. It closes down communication, or keeps it very superficial.
   This approach is often driven by an assumption about the person which may be inaccurate:

■ 'I'm worried about the operation.'
■ 'Oh, it's nothing to worry about; it's a very common procedure.'
■ 'I'm full of anxiety.'
■ 'But you're so strong. You'll cope.'

You can't reassure without first exploring the concern.

Unfortunately, the organisation-focused, explanatory approach remains prevalent; it often involves:

■ ignoring cues;
■ an overreliance on information-giving;
■ the use of assumption and premature (meaningless and ineffective) reassurance, which is further explored in Box 5.5.

Premature reassurance is a potential and actual hindrance in virtually all interactions in healthcare. It is often employed in (to staff) seemingly trivial encounters, where

> **Box 5.6** A mother's example of her short-term and subsequently long-term feelings about her daughter's heart transplant
>
> A mother said, 'She wouldn't be alive if it wasn't for the transplant, and we are eternally grateful to the donor and the team, but after the initial euphoria of coming through the operation we are living a nightmare. Of course she isn't 'better'; it's a very long haul, and she is very depressed about her appearance. She shouts at me,
> 'Why did you let them? I wish I HAD died', which is devastating for us to hear, and it's a struggle to get her to take all the medication; sometimes I have to give up.
> 'They did talk to us about potential side-effects, of course, but you can't have any real idea, and I seem to remember that most conversations with my daughter focused on encouraging her by the idea that 'when you get your new heart, you'll be *normal* again'.
> 'I'm not saying we would have made a different decision, nor would I expect the surgeon to dwell on things like steroid effects, which to him probably seem a minor matter, but we would have been more prepared, and perhaps not have expected so much, too soon.'

patients' cues are ignored, probably without great ill effect, but missing the opportunity for effective engagement:

■ 'I'm having a bad day today; I'm quite worried.'
■ 'I'm sure you'll feel better tomorrow; you'll be able to get up.'
■ 'I don't think I'm ever going to feel better.'
■ 'Oh, come on, you just have to give it time.'

Premature reassurance is an especially difficult issue to overcome when serious medical or surgical procedures with an uncertain outcome are under discussion.

Families with a member undergoing transplantation report an emphasis on the short-term success of the operation itself (as can be seen in Box 5.6), sometimes at the expense of focus on the longer-term, quality of life issues. This is a very understandable attitude from the healthcare professional's point of view; teenage patients, however, have reported depression, even thoughts of suicide, because of the effects upon their appearance of steroids and other necessary long-term medication.

An organisational research project

The more recent acceptance throughout the NHS that high-quality care was and is always dependent upon good communication is a theme reiterated and explored in several government initiatives. In 2003, the DH published *Building on the Best: Choice, Responsiveness and Equity* and highlighted the fact that:

> Most people express a stronger desire for responsiveness to them as individuals alongside a desire for a more human approach where people feel listened to, valued and respected as individuals. (p. 18)

In this context, the cardiorespiratory and critical care (CRACC) division at a large paediatric hospital received an evaluation of their service following the Paediatric and Congenital Cardiac Services Review (DH, 2002b). As anticipated, the Review praised the clinical service as exemplary, but suggested that 'communication' was an area where improvement could be made.

The current author with colleagues undertook to design and deliver an organisational research study, in partnership with Constructive Dialogue for Clinical Accountability (CDCA), a group of parents and professionals committed to addressing key communication issues arising from the events examined by the BRI Inquiry (DH, 2002a). The study aimed to assess whether a programme designed to improve the competence and confidence in interactive communication of multiprofessional team members was effective and could lead to better patient care through appropriate and enhanced interactive skills.

Between October 2002 and May 2003, 40 multiprofessional staff from the CRACC division at the hospital were exposed to a planned programme of skills training and assessment. In order to avoid the misconceptions associated with the term 'communication skills', the study referred to 'interactive skills', and the transferability of these skills to any situation in the clinical or non-clinical environment (or in telephone interaction) was emphasised throughout.

The teaching methods involved were:

■ exposition through patient simulators and professional role players;
■ experiential practice;
■ self-assessment through reflective practice and diary recordings;
■ recorded audiotapes of interactive skills in simulated clinical situations.

The three main 'exploratory' skills, deemed 'tools' for all effective interaction and dialogue, were assessed, taught and practised intensively throughout the training; these being:

■ cue recognition;
■ the ability to ask open questions;
■ the ability to avoid premature reassurance.

Participants were provided by the CDCA with a diary for recording 'self-reflective practice'. The diary contained a summary, with examples (shown in Box 5.7), of the skills to be acquired and practised during the training.

The participants undertook three sessions of 3 hours' duration, and worked with parent/patient simulators and professional role players to practise and discuss the use of the skills in realistic scenarios commonly met in their workplace(s). The simulators and professionals 'played' the patient on all occasions; no participant was ever required to assume a role other than their own during skills practice.

Some didactic teaching and group exercises at the beginning of each session enabled the establishment of a consistent understanding of the terms used; even very senior staff acknowledged that, at the outset, they did not necessarily share a common understanding of the term 'open question', for example. The acquisition of these simple concepts, via a common vocabulary, had an effect that surprised even the trainers. Peer review, self-assessment, reflective practice and debriefing became far more focused and effective.

Participants were able to suggest, having watched a scenario between a member of their team and a parent simulator, that their colleague had succeeded in establishing a rapport with the mother because he had recognised the mother's cues and, using

Box 5.7 Examples of skills to be acquired and practised during communication training

A very simple example of a **cue** from a patient or parent was illustrated by the words:

■ 'I'm worried about the operation.'

A reply from the healthcare professional that constituted **premature reassurance**, was illustrated by the words:

■ 'Oh, he'll be fine. We do a lot of these procedures here, and we've got an excellent team.'

An example of the desirable **open question** was:

■ 'What are you worried about?'

open questions, had enabled the mother to express and describe her real worry. Before the vocabulary to pinpoint the above skills had been learnt, participants were much more likely to say that their colleague was a 'good communicator' because he 'made eye contact', 'sounded kind', 'gave the mother time' or some such vague praise that did not really further the participants' skills or enable them to build on a solid conceptual base and use the required skills in other situations.

Similarly, participants' difficulties or uncertainties in interacting with patients and families before the acquisition of the basic skills and vocabulary were often explained away as some fault on the *patient's* part. For example, a participant mentioned an interview in which he had not succeeded in engaging with a worried father despite having 'tried everything' to 'draw him out'. He explained his lack of success, and consequent frustration, as being due to the father 'obviously not being ready to talk'.

A more effective analysis, when the participant described in detail what had been said, and using the newly acquired vocabulary to analyse the interaction, proved to be that the participant had ignored the father's cues in favour of his own overreliance on giving information, and had offered premature reassurance instead of an exploratory open question to the one concern that the father had managed to raise, thus effectively closing down the potential conversation.

Having acquired the ability to recognise these concepts, and to describe and analyse a conversation consistently, participants were quick to spot the potential value of these skills and the attendant vocabulary for appraisal sessions, ward round teaching or videoed consultation debriefings. During the study, participants were required to record three audiotaped, simulated interviews over the period of the project, and the tapes were rated and reported on by an independent professional trainer and experienced rater.

The results

As a group, the participants' skills improved significantly after training, and the improvement appeared to be sustained in those who undertook a further audiotaped

> **Box 5.8** A surgeon giving premature reassurance to a 15-year-old about his
> proposed operation
>
> A surgeon was talking to a 15-year-old patient about a proposed operation. The young man
> gave several cues about his concerns. He said he was 'worried about coming into hospital' and
> that he 'didn't want to be in hospital for ages, if anything went wrong'. Without exploring any
> of these particular worries, the surgeon reiterated that the youngster 'needed' the operation,
> that there was no reason to think anything would go wrong, and that he would 'feel better'
> and 'have a lot more energy' afterwards.
>
>   All of these remarks were designed to reassure the patient, and may have done so to some
> extent, but to the team's concern, the patient was still hesitant about agreeing to the opera-
> tion. A social worker visited him later that day and asked him, in a simple open question, *why*
> he was worried. It emerged that his mother was depressed and was not coping at home with
> a rebellious, truanting younger sister. His father had left the family some years before and
> the patient felt 'responsible' for the family's difficulties; he was also reluctant to expect his
> mother to be with him and support him through another period of hospitalisation and
> convalescence.
>
>   Having explored the concern, timely reassurance was able to be given, in the form of
> planned, practical support for his admission and surgery.

interview 3 months after training. The most noticeable domain of improvement was
in questioning strategies (highly correlated with ability to engage in patient-centred
interaction).

All participants, however, continued, although improved, to show a tendency for
premature reassurance, as shown in Box 5.8. This is an issue that is known to bedevil
effective staff–patient interaction and should be constantly exposed by trainers in
their teaching and appraisal of junior staff. Unfortunately, many senior staff of all
disciplines do not themselves have the ability to recognise their own tendency to
exhibit this problematic behaviour, or to detect and help eradicate it in those they are
training, leaving junior staff unconfident and lacking understanding in potentially
ineffective interactions.

The templates and the competency in interactive communication

Following the insights gained from this organisational research study, and the clear
confirmation gained about 'what worked', the current authors developed some simple
templates for use in any interactive situation (Boxes 5.3–5.5, 5.9, 5.11 and 5.12), the
whole designed to form an 'infrastructure' for a competency in interactive communication (Box 5.9) that can be taught and measured during workplace learning and
teaching:

- Acknowledge **cues** from the patient/family about their thoughts, feelings and
  concerns.
- Ask **open questions** to explore and clarify the patient and family agenda.
- Acknowledge the expressed emotion.
- (Re)negotiate the focus and agenda as necessary.

> **Box 5.9**   Core competency for interactive communication skills
>
> **Competency statement**
> Engage verbally with the child/family and the healthcare team at all stages of the patient journey, to facilitate shared decision-making and a respectful partnership of care.
>
> **Outcome criteria**
> The healthcare professional will be able to initiate engagement with the patient/family, using the four key steps below:
>
> ■ Introduce self and establish the identity of all other participants.
> ■ 'Set out the stall' regarding the reason for the interview.
> ■ Negotiate and establish expectations, including the time available.
> ■ Gain permission to proceed.

■ Check understanding and employ screening questions to ensure that the patient/family agenda has been fully explored.
■ Give **appropriate reassurance**, but only if requested.
■ Come to a shared decision.
■ Establish an action plan.

As evidence of achievement, the healthcare professional will have demonstrated, from live, audio or video observation or written recording:

■ consistent practice in the four key tasks of initial engagement (see Box 5.9);
■ the ability to recognise and explore the patient's verbal cues;
■ the ability to employ open, screening and checking questions, and to avoid inappropriate closed or leading questions;
■ the ability to offer appropriate reassurance and avoid premature reassurance;
■ the ability to record an action plan.

Several enquiries were received from within and outside the trust as to whether the skills would be applicable to other settings. The current authors realised how entrenched was the assumption that 'communication' was almost always linked to a particular topic during healthcare professionals' training, and usually focused primarily on information delivery rather than the acquisition of core, transferable skills.

Seminars or training sessions in 'Breaking bad news' or 'Taking consent' are typically promoted in professional journals as designed to improve 'communication skills'. Participants, however, mentioned that although these types of training or study day were often interesting and informative, they rarely conferred specific and lasting skills, usually offering only guidelines for communication, for example emphasising the need to be 'sensitive' (as seen in the example in Box 5.10) to the needs of shocked or distressed parents or to 'elicit the patient's own views', without specific teaching on how to apply both these suggestions.

Certainly, parents were unanimous at the Children's Heart Federation Workshop that they could cope with healthcare professionals being much franker in their discussion of risk and their proactive raising of issues such as post mortem examination and organ donation. One parent, in acknowledging that such discussion was 'hard'

> **Box 5.10** An example of healthcare professionals' being 'sensitive'
>
> One of the participants, referring to the then recent Bristol Royal Infirmary Inquiry, remarked that perhaps the healthcare professionals at the centre of the Inquiry had thought they **were** being 'sensitive' (interpreted as 'kind' or 'sparing feelings') in allegedly not including parents in full and truthful discussions about their child's situation and treatment recommendations, the lack of such inclusion eventually being a key reason for the parents' demand for the Inquiry to take place.

> **Box 5.11** Pre-interaction strategy
>
> Before the anticipated interactions, take a few moments to think and decide:
>
> ■ What is the purpose of the proposed interaction?
> ■ Who should be present?
> ■ Who should say what and to whom (in broad terms, not a detailed 'script')?
> ■ What must be agreed before the end of the interaction?
> ■ How should the result of the interaction be recorded and where?

> **Box 5.12** Organising the interaction
>
> ■ Introduce yourself and anyone else present.
> ■ Explain any unfamiliar titles or terms.
> ■ Check the identities and relationships of others present.
> ■ 'Set out your stall' and confirm the time available.
> ■ Check expectations and (re)negotiate the purpose of the interaction if necessary.
> ■ Gain permission to proceed.

for doctors, remarked that it was 'even harder' for parents, and that it was part of a paediatrician's 'job' to 'partner parents, not patronise them'.

In response to requests for guidance about the context in which these interactive skills could be best delivered, two further templates were devised (Boxes 5.11 and 5.12), for the 'Pre-interaction strategy' and for 'Organising the interaction'. The whole 'package' of transferable templates forms the basis of a very simple and easily delivered training, which is itself interactive, adaptable to the needs of any group and compliant with evidenced best practice in continuing medical education, in terms of course content and training methods.

Using the templates

The two templates, in Boxes 5.11 and 5.12, were found to be helpful to the confidence of the staff, some of whom quite frequently went into potentially difficult interactive situations without much idea of what or whom they would find, or what should be the agreed outcome of the interaction, let alone how they could achieve it. This can be seen in Box 5.13 in the example of a junior doctor's discussion with a distressed mother.

Box 5.13 A junior doctor's discussion with an upset mother

A junior doctor was asked by the charge nurse to, 'have another talk with [a particular mother]; she's been crying all morning', making the assumption that the recently delivered diagnosis was causing the upset, probably because of a misunderstanding. The doctor began on a reiteration of the diagnostic findings and treatment protocol, until the mother was able to indicate that her earlier cry to the charge nurse of 'I can't understand it' was a general comment on her feeling that the child's illness must have been caused by some unsuspected problem in her pregnancy, and did not relate to the information she had been given.

The junior doctor did not have a confident strategy for exploring the mother's feelings of guilt other than to offer her the premature reassurance that she 'shouldn't blame herself'. A staff discussion proved helpful, when the ward team took a few minutes to think about who should talk to the mother and what should be the focus of the conversation (see also Box 5.11). Allowing her to disclose and explore her feelings, using open questions, was appropriate, rather than merely repeating clinical information.

Box 5.14 A misunderstanding to avoid

Having been told that 'the doctor will come and explain everything this afternoon', a mother called several family members together, involving time off work and travelling a distance for some of them. The doctor paused briefly on the ward round to confirm the diagnosis and the outline plan for future surgery, but had clearly made no arrangement for a longer discussion.

With regard to Box 5.12, and despite the frequently heard protest from healthcare professionals that they 'don't have time' to communicate appropriately, the current author and colleagues have tried the template with numerous groups of staff and confirmed that, with practice, it takes about 2 or 3 minutes to apply, often saving a great deal *more* time in misdirected communication, misunderstanding or simply unconfident or muddled information.

'Gaining permission to proceed' involves only a simple 'OK then?' or 'I'll begin, shall I?' or something similar, but it pays dividends in terms of family and patient engagement, compared with the still commonly reported situation whereby the healthcare professional simply comes into the room and immediately starts talking. This latter practice, without attention paid to the suggestions in Box 5.12, is more likely to lead to the need for repeated explanations from different staff, and less confident understanding and compliance on the part of the patient and family.

Participants in the research study also confessed that, to their own and the patient's detriment, they had often failed to introduce themselves properly, or to check who any other people were who were in the room. Anecdotes were shared about giving test results to the wrong child, taking the wrong set of notes into a discussion with a family, introducing the consultant to the wrong family on the ward, assuming that the child's grandmother was the mother throughout a diagnostic discussion, and discovering after a diagnostic discussion that the male who had dominated the conversation and cowed the child's mother was currently subject to a court order to prevent him having any contact with his child. Checking expectations, within the team as well as with the patient, can also save much misunderstanding and wasted time, as seen in the example in Box 5.14.

Time available

Families are also frequently unclear about how much time the staff can spare for discussion, and are reluctant to say or ask all the things they may want to when a staff member gives the impression of being rushed. It is respectful and patient centred to say how much time can be given to the discussion, so that the patient/parent can prioritise their concerns.

If families have no idea if and when they can talk to an appropriate staff member, they may resort to the tactic of 'catching' someone in the corridor or asking their questions of an inappropriate person (pressing the radiographer to say what the X-ray shows), resulting in frustration and irritation all round.

Transferability of the templates

Training using these templates has been successfully delivered to senior doctors to assist with appraisal skills, a paediatric intensive care unit to assist with making the handover and ward round process more efficient, an emergency paediatric admissions team to simplify the telephone referral system, a group of GP trainers and trainees to support their learning through videoed consultations, a Patient Advice and Liaison Service team, and the staff of a telephone helpline supporting parents who have a child in a neonatal, paediatric or cardiac intensive care unit, as well as many groups of healthcare professionals in non-paediatric settings.

Competency-based training promotes consistency of practice, and the transferability of the competency as a tool for interactive engagement in any situation, irrespective of the specific topic under discussion, has been evidenced in all of the above settings.

Child protection

A very important issue was revealed by cardiac unit staff in a large paediatric hospital when invited to undertake child protection update training. All staff are aware of the guidelines to follow when suspecting that they may be faced with a child protection issue. It was apparent across the particular trust, however, that there were several instances of guidelines being ignored or inefficiently operated, to the potential detriment of the child patient. It seems reasonable to extrapolate that similar units will experience similar issues.

The initial response from the trust was to emphasise the training opportunities for understanding the guidelines, on the assumption that staff were not fully familiar with them. Anecdotal reports and subsequent discussion with several staff revealed, however, that the problem was not one of lack of knowledge but of lack of confidence. In cases where a child protection issue may be suspected, staff – and not only nurses – often hesitate to engage with families, as they assume that 'partnering parents' is a concept incompatible with what they may see as confrontation.

A senior nurse, writing to the child protection coordinator of the trust in a personal communication, said:

> Recent experience of training with a group of nurses elicited honest opinion from
> many of them that they know what they should be doing and they can recognise

> **Box 5.15** An example of a nurse's anxiety in raising an issue with a parent
>
> A nurse noticed marks on a child's chest which she thought might be cigarette burns but said nothing as the child was about to be discharged from the ward. In addition, she felt very reluctant and unconfident to raise this with the mother. At handover, after the child had left the ward, she mentioned her observation, thus obliging other staff, at this later stage, to take more time-consuming investigative action in the community.
>
> Luckily, the health visitor knew that the child was recovering from an acute skin reaction. The mother, hearing of the staff's concern, expressed surprise that no one had asked her about the marks while in the ward; she had assumed that her child's notes had contained information about the recent skin problem. She was upset that staff had 'gone behind her back' with their concern, as she felt she had hitherto had a 'good relationship' with ward staff.

> **Box 5.16** An example of a nurse immediately questioning a mother
>
> On another occasion, a nurse, noticing what she thought were bruises, immediately asked the mother if she had noticed the 'marks' and what she thought about them. The mother was non-committal, giving an implausible story, and the nurse said (as she would where there was concern over any symptom) that she would ask the doctor to 'come and have a look'.
>
> Thus, the nurse established right away that the bruises had been noticed and that they would be investigated, and the mother had been given an opportunity to explain or express an opinion. The nurse did not need to make assumptions, jump to conclusions, interrogate or accuse the mother, but simply ask openly about her initial observation. The nurse took a few minutes with her senior colleague to consider the issues in Box 5.12, and the social worker was informed and took over the coordination of investigation according to the trust's child protection policy.

signs indicative of potential abuse, but they are anxious about engaging with the family in case they have 'got it wrong' or may 'make things worse' [such as the situation explained in Box 5.15] and there is confusion about the paramountcy of the child's best interests against maintaining a good relationship with the parents. There is an overeagerness to "get someone else to deal with it" (e.g. social worker or health visitor) without having engaged with the family or child within the remit of their own professional role.

Work in conjunction with the child protection training coordinator, based on the competency and using the 'tool' templates, helped staff to recognise how they could use interactive skills to explore a patient's situation without being judgemental or accusatory. This can be seen in the example in Box 5.16 of where a nurse immediately questioned a mother about some marks on her child.

Ethical or communication issues?

The clinical ethics committee of a specialist paediatric hospital noticed that many of the situations referred to them were about consent issues and were not strictly ethical problems but more usually difficult interactions that staff felt unconfident to handle.

Box 5.17 A teenager refusing to consent to treatment

A teenage girl was refusing to consent to a potentially life-saving course of treatment after years of hospital admissions and increasing disability. She had become withdrawn from her distraught parents who were trying to persuade her to take the treatment; as she was aged 16, they could still have overridden her wishes. Ward staff had begun to discuss the possibility of legal action, insisting that although it had been clearly stated to the girl that she would die without the treatment, she was 'obviously not able fully to appreciate the implications of this'.

A member of the ethics committee who had not met the girl before sat with her and asked why she felt the way she did. It emerged that, far from not understanding the implications of her refusal of further treatment, she regarded her decision as the last act of control she could take over her own life. She said she was not frightened of death itself (which she had 'accepted' some years previously as eventually inevitable) but worried a lot about how her parents would cope with her decision. She said it would 'hurt them too much' to discuss her feelings, but she was very disappointed that staff whom she had tried to cue about her thoughts and feelings had not responded by engaging with her in discussion; they had all seemed to assume that she could not really be capable of such a mature and difficult decision. They had instead resorted to the premature reassurance of repeating how strong and brave she had always been and how she would 'come through' the proposed treatment.

She talked with a member of the palliative care team, who enabled her, through open questioning, to express her thoughts and doubts, and answered all her questions straightforwardly. She wanted to consider visiting a hospice, and this was arranged. Having regained control, as she saw it, the girl agreed to the proposed treatment, on the understanding that she could refuse to continue at any point, and move to a palliative care regime.

Box 5.17 outlines an example of a teenager refusing to consent to a course of treatment.

Adolescents

Communicating with adolescents is often considered to be a separate skill, requiring special training: certainly the emotional and practical needs of this age group are likely to be more varied and challenging than those of younger paediatric patients or older, fully adult individuals. However, communicating at an individual, interactive level does not require a different approach, as the above example illustrates. The types of cue given and the response to open questioning may be unexpectedly frank, or even shocking, if staff are not used to engaging with adolescent patients, but the templates are still transferable and applicable.

Summary

The examples above may help to illustrate that the need of every patient and family member, no matter what their condition, situation or age, whether or not the interview has to be conducted via an interpreter or in less than ideal physical circumstances, is for truly patient-centred engagement, allowing the expression of difficult thoughts and feelings, as well as the acquisition of factual information, in order to achieve properly shared decision-making. The templates offer a practical guide to the necessary skills, which, when mastered, will enable healthcare professionals to gain confidence in their ability to engage effectively with patients and parents in any circumstances.

Research has consistently confirmed that the skills outlined and discussed above are valued by patients and families as enabling their proper engagement in their own and their children's care. It has also been shown that healthcare staff do not necessarily acquire these skills in their initial professional training, nor are they more likely to be acquired automatically as a professional becomes more senior. The skills are no more likely to be exhibited by any particular profession, but all professionals and volunteer staff can acquire them with a specific training, and there is evidence that, once learnt, the skills are not lost as long as they are subject to regular practice and revalidation.

Within the field of paediatric cardiac care, the skills are appropriate for the many professional and volunteer staff who engage with the child and family, often over many years. The importance of consistency and continuity in support personnel, and the need for long-term engagement between the caring team and the family, often over many years, makes it vital that the members of the professional team can engage flexibly and openly with the family at all stages.

The templates do not offer a rigid script of 'what to say' but suggest a framework for engagement that emphasises the qualities of real reciprocity and partnership between professionals, patients and their families.

References

Bridson, J., Hammond, C., Leach, A. & Chester, M.R. (2004). Making consent patient centred. *British Medical Journal*, *327*, 1159–1161.

Department of Health (1999). *Report of the Royal Liverpool Children's Inquiry* [The Redfern Report]. London: HMSO.

Department of Health (2002a). *Learning from Bristol: the Department of Health's response to the Report of the Public Inquiry into children's heart surgery at the Bristol Royal Infirmary 1984–1995*. London: DH.

Department of Health (2002b). *Paediatric and congenital cardiac services review report*. London: DH.

Department of Health (2003). *Building on the best: Choice, responsiveness and equity in the NHS: A summary*. London: DH.

Department of Health (2004). *A framework of competencies for basic specialist training in paediatrics*. London: Royal College of Paediatrics and Child Health.

Maguire, P. & Pitceathly, C. (2002). Key communication skills and how to acquire them [review]. *British Medical Journal*, *325*, 697–700.

6 Transition to adult services

Lorraine Priestley-Barnham, Fiona Kennedy, Jo Wray

Each week in the United Kingdom (UK), an average of 90 babies are born with some form of congenital heart disease (CHD) (Department of Health, 2003). Forty years ago, 70% of such children would have died before reaching their 10th birthday. However, scientific and technological advances in cardiothoracic care have improved the prognoses for these children (British Heart Foundation, 2003) resulting in a tremendous increase in survival, whereby there are now an overwhelming 135,000 young people and adults currently living with CHD in the UK (Department of Health, 2003; British Cardiac Society, 2002). Consequently, there are a number of adolescents and young adults undergoing medical follow-up at adult services with diseases previously unseen or managed by adult teams, but where life long management and review is crucial to long term survival. A study by Somerville (1997), reported disasters resulting from the treatment of grown-up congenital heart (GUCH) patients by adult cardiologists with little knowledge of the anatomy of CHDH, hence the evolution of GUCH clinics around the UK. Current international guidelines recommend that just over half of adult patients with CHD should be seen every 12 to 24 months by an adult cardiologist with specific expertise in CHD (Warnes et al, 2001; Therrien et al, 2001). It is therefore essential to long-term survival and to minimise the incidence of loss to follow up that health care providers prepare and support all those young people making the move from paediatric to adult care, a process now widely defined and universally known as 'Transition'.

The Society for Adolescent Medicine has now standardised a definition for transition which describes the concept as 'a purposeful, planned process that addresses the medical, psychosocial and educational needs of adolescents and young adults with chronic physical and medical conditions as they move from child-centred to adult orientated health care systems' (Rosen et al, 2003).

Transitional care is a key element of adolescent care irrespective of the presence or absence of chronic illness. All young people will eventually move from childhood to adulthood, school to university or living at home to living independently. Many young people will make this transition successfully; however some will find this process difficult for various reasons, particularly those with a chronic illness. Further explanations, which contribute to either a triumphant or failed transition, will be unfolded and the reasons for this thrashed out throughout this chapter. In healthcare, transition should incur a gradual process of change allowing sufficient time to ensure that young people and their families are not just prepared but feel ready to make the move into adult health care system. A summary of the diverse models of care and logistics of transition will be explored shortly.

The primary objective of the transition cycle is for specialist teams to understand, accept and acknowledge that transitioning adolescents to adult care is not the same as transferring care. The term 'transfer' has been widely used by many when referring to transition of care from the paediatric to adult health services. However, this 'transfer' is not recommended by DH guidelines, which state that transfer is not an appropriate term for this process as it indicates that transition may be seen as a one-off event. For transition to be successful, it must be perceived as an ongoing process (DH, 2006). Failure to meet the needs of adolescents and their families during the transition process will result in disastrous consequences, an area to be discussed later in this chapter.

Preparation

CHD is a lifelong condition that affects quality of life. Lifetime management for patients with CHD is now the model for care delivery due to moderate or complex disease and the potential to develop late complications. Mortality from CHD, once greatest in infancy, now occurs in adult life (Somerville, 1997). Few congenital heart conditions can be regarded as completely corrected, perhaps with the exception of an early successfully surgically ligated and divided ductus arteriosus. All other repaired defects have the potential to develop late complications long after primary interventions have been completed.

The onset of cardiac-related problems in this group of patients can be subtle and subclinical. Early recognition of changes enables appropriate intervention to reduce progressive myocardial and circulatory deterioration. Young people who have lived with a chronic cardiac problem may not notice or may ignore slight changes in exercise capacity until they become significant. By the time the individual becomes aware of dyspnoea and exercise limitation, underlying valvular and ventricular dysfunction is often severe and potentially irreversible. Consequently, people who have CHD need to receive regular specialist assessment.

Many children reach adolescence with a limited knowledge of their diagnosis and little understanding of the implications of their cardiac condition. Several studies have assessed the level of knowledge that young people with CHD have of their condition and reveal a poor level of knowledge about their heart defect, their symptoms of deterioration and the reasons for long-term follow-up (Veldtman et al, 2000; Moons et al, 2001; Dore et al, 2002). There may be a number of reasons for this, for example that parents need to understand their child's heart condition in order to enable their child to understand. However, it appears that parental understanding is related to parental education: the children of parents who were less educated tended to lack knowledge themselves (Beeri et al, 2001).

Many parents want to protect their child from the reality of an uncertain future and more operations by limiting the amount of information they provide about the heart condition and avoiding direct discussion. However, this means that the young people then have to adjust to and accept their limitations later in life and may require considerable support in making this adjustment. The most common reason for the lack of parental knowledge may be because detailed information was provided at the time of diagnosis or surgery, when high levels of anxiety affected their ability to retain the information. This lack of knowledge may have potentially harmful consequences for some patients and result in a number dropping out of the system during their teen and early adult years as they make the transition from paediatric to adult care.

Many patients view themselves as 'cured' because they have not been told anything different by their parents or doctors (Greenaway, 2008). A Canadian study (Reid et al, 2006) examined perceptions of life expectancy among adolescents and young adults with moderate-to-complex CHD and found that patients expect to live almost as long as their healthy peers. Young people need accurate information about their condition delivered in a sensitive manner to make informed life choices about education, careers and family.

Although medical care for these young people has improved a great deal, the complexity of the anatomy and physiology and symptoms that these patients present in adulthood often exceeds the expertise of many healthcare professionals in primary and secondary healthcare, who require support from a specialist adult congenital heart (ACH) unit (Gatzoulis, 2006). This point is further illustrated by a survey undertaken in North America revealing that patients with CHD are more likely than the general population to seek urgent medical care in the emergency department setting. Over half of the doctors working in this field felt they had received insufficient training in adult CHD (ACHD; Cross & Santucci, 2006).

This is of concern for patients who require emergency care and admission to hospital, highlighting the importance for people with CHD to be knowledgeable about their cardiac condition in order to inform other medical teams. Improving care for young people with CHD involves educating them about their heart condition, providing them with key information about treatment in childhood and extending this education to include all health professionals involved in their care. Transitional programmes are an important way of providing structured education (Dore et al, 2002).

Aims of the transition service

The purpose of a transition service for patients with CHD is to ensure continuous and coordinated management between paediatric and adult care, to develop skills in self-care, to promote independence and to support parents (DH Vascular Programme Team, 2006). The process ideally starts in early adolescence, before the teen years, and continues until the young person is participating fully in adult healthcare (Jordan & McDonagh, 2006). In order to achieve this, healthcare professionals need to enable young people to develop the necessary skills to manage their own heart condition and learn how to negotiate adult healthcare services independently. Adolescence is a time when adult behaviours become established, and it offers a window of opportunity to promote healthy behaviour (McDonagh & Viner, 2006). Learning new behaviour takes time, with a lot of shifting back and forth before attitudes and behaviours become consistent. It is important to understand and accept that acute episodes of illness or the need for hospital admission can cause temporary regression to previous behaviours and coping strategies for both the patient and their parent (Kools et al, 2002).

Cognitive development in adolescence

An understanding of cognitive development in the adolescent is necessary for communication to be effective. Adolescence can be divided into three stages: early (11–14 years), middle (15–18 years) and late (19 years+). In early adolescence, young people begin to develop abstract thinking, which enables them to think hypothetically about the future and assess multiple outcomes. This capacity is essential if young people are to give informed consent to treatment and manage their own conditions. Health professionals also need to remember that adolescents characteristically do not share an adult's understanding of society or possess adult cognitive abilities to decide between treatment alternatives in the light of future risks to health. Teenagers do not see medical issues in the same way as adults, as Bull (1998) indicated in her paper about the Fontan procedure and the past lessons learned. They see themselves as invincible, which can lead to risk-taking behaviour, and many are struggling to maintain their self- esteem despite their medical history and do not want to stand out from the crowd. Middle-aged people tend to value long life; however the inclination of adolescents is to attach more value to the quality of the next year of their lives than to long-term survival (Bart, 1983). Assessment of the adolescent's stage of development should be the first step in the transition process. Development is an individual process and adolescents progress through developmental stages at different rates (Tong & Kools, 2004). Therefore, it is important to introduce new information in a manner appropriate to the individual's development. Christie & Viner (2005) suggest using only here-and-now concrete examples for adolescents, avoiding abstract concepts discussions (if ..., then ...) for communication to be meaningful. Information should be reinforced and expanded as the patient develops cognitive maturity. Health care professionals need to be supportive but firm in helping young people to understand the consequences of their behaviour.

Transitional issues

For anyone who has had a chronic disease since birth, the transitional move from paediatric to adolescent and subsequently adult care brings a number of additional considerations for both the young person and their parents. Many patients and their families have been looked after by the same team since birth, during which time a trusting relationship has developed. They now have to establish a new bond with the adult team, and it is desirable that the paediatric cardiologist is involved in the transition service together with the adult specialist, as this allows for greater continuity and helps to reduce anxiety. Many patients and their parents are apprehensive about moving to adult care and find the change stressful. Good communication is essential in order to facilitate continuity of care and is considered by young people to be the most important issue (DH Vascular Programme Team, 2006).

It is vital that patients and their families/carers are given time to prepare for the move to adult care. The transition period should be a gradual, structured process for both the patient and the medical team, during which the focus of communication shifts from the parent to the young person. It is particularly effective for key healthcare professionals from both the adult and paediatric centres to run the transition clinic together. A number of models for transition have recently been proposed that can provide a useful framework for developing services (European Society of Cardiology, 2003; RCN, 2004). These will be discussed in greater detail later.

The transition from childhood to adulthood is a challenging period for youngsters with learning disabilities. These patients need education and preparation appropriate to their level of understanding and may have complex support needs, which will be covered later. During their school years, young people with learning disability need to be prepared for the world of work and encouraged to become as independent as possible. Development of healthy self-esteem is important and involvement in various recreational activities (Pueschel, 1996).

Room for improvement

The first study to quantify the number of young adults with CHD to transfer to adult care at the appropriate time reported that approximately 50% of the study group (360 patients) transferred successfully. However, more than a quarter of patients revealed no cardiac medical care from the age of 18 years. Those engaging in multiple risky health behaviours involving substance use such as binge drinking, illegal drug use, drinking and driving, and risky sexual behaviour were less likely to attend medical appointments. These young people require a continuing programme of education, counselling and treatment to make substantial changes in their behaviour, which in turn will hopefully lead to effective transfer. Successful transition is associated with developmentally appropriate staged discussions involving the patient, both with and without the parents, throughout adolescence in the paediatric setting (Reid et al, 2004).

An understanding of the relationship between physical and psychological needs and an awareness of individual and family processes in chronic illness are important components of transitional care. Adult teams need to recognise and value the understanding of the illness that patients and their families have acquired over the years (Kools et al, 2002). It is important to young people with CHD that their anxiety and past experiences are recognised by the adult team if a trusting relationship is to develop. A sensitive and understanding approach is crucial as this is a particularly stressful time for many patients and their families/carers.

Education

It is essential not to overwhelm the young person with large volumes of information provided on a single occasion; this is likely to induce denial and lack of attendance. Transition of care should be a gradual process for the patient and medical team. Adolescents and young adults need education about their condition, healthcare needs and prognosis. Such education forms an important part of the transition process intended to encourage young people to take more responsibility for their own health. An individual patient education programme regarding the heart condition and need for follow-up, how to recognise changes, how to seek help and where to find support, information and advice is designed to enable the young person to operate within the adult healthcare system. Patients need to understand their condition and should be able to describe the heart defect. Each patient should be given a diagram to help them visualise the structure of their heart. A personal health record containing details of medical and surgical treatment and contact information about the specialist unit is particularly useful for young people who are studying or working away from home. Patients also need to understand the reasons for medication, side effects and relevant interactions with other drugs and foods.

In addition, patients require information and advice about lifestyle issues such as the prevention of infective endocarditis, cardiovascular risk factor management, physical exercise, including extreme sports, healthy eating and avoiding obesity and the use and effects of tobacco, alcohol, stimulant drinks, and recreational drugs on the circulation. Sensitive issues such as contraception, the prevention of sexually transmitted diseases, family planning, and pregnancy and recurrence risk need to be addressed at an early stage and reinforced subsequently (Kennedy, 2007). Information should also be provided about employability and insurance.

Recently recommendations for infective endocarditis prophylaxis in England and Wales have changed practice. Antibiotic prophylaxis is no longer offered routinely for interventional procedures. There is little evidence to support the routine use of antibiotics as a preventative measure for people at risk of infective endocarditis undergoing interventional procedures. (National Institute for Health and Clinical Excellence Clinical Guideline 64, 2008). Nevertheless people with CHD at risk of infective endocarditis require clear and consistent information about prevention which should include the importance of maintaining good oral health, symptoms that may indicate infective endocarditis and when to seek expert advice. The risks of undergoing invasive procedures, including non-medical procedures such as body piercing or tattooing need to be discussed. Further information can be found at: www.nice.org.uk/CG064. Oral explanations should be reinforced with written material whenever possible.

Young people need to be prepared for the way in which adult services work, particularly the outpatient clinics. Each patient must receive written information about the adult unit, information about the adult clinics and most importantly, a named contact person and telephone number. Many young people and their parents are fearful that the people who attend the adult clinic are old, this is actually not the case and it is important to identify any areas of concern and to clarify any misconceptions.

Tension exists between the philosophies underpinning the care of children and the care of adults in hospital. Paediatric care promotes family-centred care and focuses on the child as part of a family. Parents are supported to continue caring for their child to the extent they feel comfortable doing so while in hospital. Adult care, on the other hand, promotes self-care with the focus of care on the patient as an individual. The transition process offers an opportunity to prepare young people and their families for this change by promoting and gradually introducing the concept of self-management. Many young people embrace this change and are more than ready to move to adult services; however, there are others who require more support. The CHD nurse specialist has a pivotal role in assessing the needs of each young person and providing an individual patient education programme.

In summary, transition of care from paediatric to adult services is a process of change that requires careful planning and management. Young people with CHD have unique needs that do not fit into the existing paediatric and adult models of care. The development of specialist health care services for young people has been slow and the need not widely recognised. It is crucial that we listen to what younger people say about our services and how they would like their needs to be addressed in the future. Services must be designed around the needs of young people rather than the needs of the service. Poorly planned transition is associated with increased risk of non-adherence to treatment and loss to follow-up (Watson, 2000). Successful transition will engage young people in a lifelong relationship with their medical team.

Logistics

Models of transition

The specific health needs of adolescents have been recognised for many years in the UK (Platt (1959), Court Report (1976), British Paediatric Association (1985), House of Commons Health Committee (1997), NSF (2004), Department of Health (2006)). Not only has there been this recognition of adolescents from government bodies but many professional bodies in the UK particularly the Royal Colleges have now also recently developed major policies and guidance notes on how to provide appropriate services for adolescents undergoing transition within the paediatric and adult settings (RCPCH, 2003; RCN, 2004; BMA, 2003).

Various research projects from individual specialties such as rheumatology and cystic fibrosis have provided clues to the type of support and service configurations that should be in place in order to ensure positive transition. From this research, several models have emerged and been developed over the years and are currently in practice within the UK (Sawyer et al, 1997; While et al, 2004; Bennett et al, 2005; Tucker & Cabral, 2005). These may include a lifelong service provided by the paediatric team, a seamless clinic, which begins in childhood and continues into adulthood, and a committed follow-up service provided solely by the adult team. A breakdown of each of these models will be discussed, identifying their place within transitional care.

A lifelong follow-up service

In conditions with a limited life expectancy such as childhood cancers, some centres have favoured a lifelong follow-up service within the paediatric setting. Although this approach may be more appropriate in conditions with a limited life expectancy, it does not come without its own disadvantages. These could include making it more difficult for the young person to access information on adolescent issues such as fertility and contraception, or on vocational and benefits issues, or even making it impossible for the young person to develop more appropriate independent living (DH, 2006). These disadvantages and further aspects are discussed in more detail later.

Seamless clinics

A seamless clinic that begins in childhood and continues into adulthood has also been used successfully, with both the adult and the paediatric teams providing ongoing care and sharing knowledge and experience. Orr et al (1996) reported no negative impact on glycaemia control at the time of transfer from a paediatric to a young adult programme for young people with diabetes involving paediatric and adult providers. Evidence of the prevalence of adolescent-onset disease, the disproportionate disadvantage of the young adult age group and the significant morbidities associated with late adolescence provides further support for the development of young adult clinics (Dovey-Pearce et al, 2005).

Complete adult follow-up

A committed follow-up service may be provided within the adult setting with no direct input or continuity from the paediatric services. This may be simple, but in order to work well there needs to be a streamlined coordinated approach to transition with the inclusion of what constitutes a transition programme of care, for example specialist transition clinics held within the paediatric centre and a 'transition champion' to lead and coordinate the transition process for young people to ensure an effective handover to the adult services (Foster et al, 2001). As this process is relevant to most specialties within paediatric healthcare, it appears to follow the guidelines recommended by the DH (2006). However, such programmes need time, resources and commitment (RCPCH, 2003).

International initiatives

The 'On Trac' (Taking Responsibility for Adolescent/Adult Care) team at the British Columbia Children's Hospital in Vancouver, Canada, have developed a non-specific transition service for use within their hospital whereby the role of the dedicated and specifically trained healthcare professionals is to support and educate 14 subspecialty clinical teams who are providing care to adolescents aged 10–18 years. They do this by providing the tools and resources necessary to offer developmentally appropriate transition planning and coordinated care, and ensuring that all young people using the hospital go through the appropriate transition to the adult system (Paone et al, 1998). The On Trac model and clinical pathway offers a generic framework that can be modified to meet the needs of adolescents and families being cared for in primary and tertiary care centres. The Department of Health in Australia has taken a similar approach and has also, due to a larger geographical areas, developed 'transition coordinators'. Their role is to expand links for transition between children's hospitals and local general hospitals.

Ideal process for transition

A successful transition process provides health care that is uninterrupted, coordinated, and developmentally appropriate and psychologically sound, both before and throughout the transfer into the adult system (Rosen et al, 2003). Although many of these diverse models have been studied and described no single approach has been shown to be superior. However, a combination of all these models devised to meet the needs of a particular specialist service could provide the key to successful transition programmes within the UK. Box 6.1 gives an outline of the golden rules of transition, which should form the basis of any transition model.

Practical issues and problems

Although the philosophy of transition has been accepted both nationally and internationally for over a decade, the challenges of translating policy into practice remain in many areas. In a study carried out by McDonagh et al (2005), a transition policy was developed and implemented in a major UK paediatric hospital, but after 2 years of implementation across the trust it was found that only 5 of the 38 specialities had adapted this policy to meet their transitional needs. Current practice and initiatives indicate the evidence that policy and policy guidelines do not guarantee change or improvements. Unsurprisingly, under the current government and the National Health Service (NHS), the three main challenges to successful transition are time, training and money.

Box 6.1   Golden rules of transition

1. Transition preparation must be seen as an essential component of high-quality healthcare in adolescence.
2. Prepare early. In chronic conditions, transition timing should be outlined as soon as children enter the second decade of life, if not before.
3. Young people should not be transferred to adult services until they have the necessary skills to function in an adult service. Improving young people's self-management skills should be a central part of all transition programmes.
4. An education programme is needed for patients and parents that addresses medical, psychosocial and educational/vocational aspects of care and which is age and developmentally appropriate, culturally competent, responsive and comprehensive.
5. Timings of transfer to adult services should be after major educational and physical milestones. In best practice, young people should be managed in an adolescent clinic until they have finished school and finished growth and puberty.
6. A key worker should be identified for each individual.
7. A written transition policy should be agreed by all members of the multidisciplinary team and target adult services.
8. A written individualised healthcare transition plan should be in place by age 14 that is created with the young person and their family, and is subject to regular review and update.
9. There should be liaison personnel in both the paediatric and adult team.
10. A network of relevant local agencies and target adult services should be in place.
11. Administrative support should be available, including the provision of medical summary that is portable and accessible
12. There needs to be a training programme in adolescent health and transitional care for paediatric and adult team members.
13. Primary and preventive care involvement and provision should be in place.
14. Evaluation and audit must be undertaken.

Viner (1999), DH Vascular Programme Team (2006), McDonagh & Viner (2006).

Time and commitment

Lack of transition planning or late introduction to transition is widely identified in the literature as a major barrier to successful transition (Patterson & Lanier, 1999). The DH advocates that each specialist area should enlist a 'transition champion' whose primary role would involve coordinating and facilitating transition to the adult centres (DH Vascular Programme Team, 2006). The current financial pressures on NHS trusts make allocating 'transition champions' to each specialist area difficult and too costly to last. Therefore without the financial backing, time and commitment for this role, it is unlikely to be set up, and the transition process will be unsuccessful.

Unmet education and training needs

The current background of limited training opportunities in adolescent health training for both paediatric and adult healthcare providers will have a major impact on delivery of transitional care within the UK. McDonagh et al (2004) carried out a study looking at the training needs of health professionals in adolescent care and transition. A range of unmet education and training needs in adolescent health and transitional care was identified during the course of this study. This lack of time and training has been echoed as a major barrier to transition by many authors (Geenen et al, 2003; Shaw et al, 2004). Education of not only key staff but also young people and their families plays an important role in the success of the transition process and is largely discussed throughout this chapter.

Cost implications

There are no major studies that highlight the cost implications of transition services in the UK. However, Geenen et al (2003) reported lack of finance as a perceived barrier to transition in their study carried out in the USA. It appears that appropriate funding and financial incentives are key to supporting the implementation of promising practices and model policies on transition. Further research in this area is necessary in order to further identify the costs faced by the paediatric and adult services when developing a transition service and if these costs have implicated the establishment of such services. Personal experience would indicate this might well be widespread.

Lack of support

The DH Vascular Programme Team (2006) states that management and institutional support is essential at both ends of the transition process to ensure the concept is initiated, planned, implemented and adequately evaluated. Likewise, without the resources of administrative and secretarial support, the efficient organisation of appointments and transfer of medical records may be hindered, thus possibly jeopardising successful transition.

Key people involved

Milne and Chesson (2000) identify the importance of health professionals engaging the young people themselves when planning and coordinating their care. When transition plans developed with young people and their parents were implemented in a programme of transitional care, they were successfully completed by 95% and 92% of adolescents and their parents respectively, effectively identifying their needs (McDonagh et al, 2006).

Psychological aspects of transition

The developmental perspective

Adolescence is a time of challenge, conflict and negotiation as the young person strives to achieve the desired independence and autonomy whilst also maintaining close and supportive links with the nuclear family. It is a time when young people endeavour to create a sense of identity and self-understanding through social relationships with peers, self-reflection and thoughts on future expectations.

Those coping with illness face the same developmental challenges as their healthy peers but the challenge is exaggerated, and they may be particularly vulnerable to social isolation and the delayed development of peer support networks. For the young person with CHD, there may be concerns (real and/or perceived) about body image, low self-esteem, delayed physical development, being different or not 'normal', restrictions with regard to participation in social, sporting and academic activities, and anxieties regarding ongoing physical health needs, all of which compound the challenges already being faced. A further issue is the need to make the transition from paediatric to adult cardiac services, and in other disease groups the time of transition has been identified as one of increased vulnerability (Watson, 2000; Van Walleghem et al, 2006).

Engaging in risk-taking behaviours is a normal part of adolescent development, but the negative consequences of such behaviours in terms of non-adherence with medications or ignoring restrictions in activities can be serious for the young person with CHD. Within this population, an increase in hospitalisation surrounding the time of transition to adult programmes has been identified (Gurvitz et al, 2007), suggesting an increase in risk-taking behaviours and highlighting the importance of recognising the potential vulnerability of young people at this time and the need for them to achieve their goals of adolescence without adversely affecting their health.

Adolescents' understanding of their condition and its impact on their lifestyle

One key area for successful transition concerns young people's knowledge and under-standing of their condition. Young people with a chronic illness often have limited knowledge regarding their health condition and healthcare, which is often at least in part attributable to the fact that, when diagnosis occurs at a young age, the majority of diagnostic and prognostic medical information is directed at their parents (McDonagh & Kelly, 2003). Many young people with chronic conditions report numerous unmet information needs and difficulties, including receiving incomplete information, receiving conflicting advice, lacking confidence in doctors' knowledge, not understanding what was said and being refused information (Beresford & Sloper, 2000).

A number of adult studies of CHD have identified that a significant proportion of patients have limited knowledge about their condition and about issues such as symptoms of deterioration of the heart condition, risk factors for endocarditis and the appropriateness of different physical activities (Swan & Hillis, 2000; Moons et al, 2001; Chessa et al, 2005), and it is becoming increasingly evident that poor knowledge can lead to a lack of awareness of the importance of appropriate follow-up in adult clinics, sometimes with negative consequences. A crucial component of this is the young person's level of cognitive development. It is recognised that cognitive development may be delayed in some patients with CHD, those with cyanotic lesions being at greater risk of this (Wray, 2006; Karsdorp et al, 2007; McCusker et al, 2007), and this may have an impact on their ability to comprehend key aspects of their condition and treatment.

In contrast, some adolescents may have developed a high level of expertise about their condition and its management, and it is often these patients who are more willing to actively engage in the transition process. Despite their knowledge and understanding, adolescents/young adults may at times of deterioration in their phys-ical health need their parents to resume a more active caring role, and this should be seen as a normal response in the context of chronic illness.

Research indicates that chronically ill young people are as likely as their healthy peers to be sexually active and share similar patterns of contraceptive use and age at sexual debut (Suris et al, 1996). For the young woman with CHD, contraception is a particularly important area to address as there are a number of contraceptive methods that are contraindicated due to the risk of endocarditis or thrombosis. Qualitative studies have identified that fertility, contraception and pregnancy concerns are predominant among young women with CHD, further emphasising the need for adequate advice and guidance (Gantt, 1992). Pregnancy can pose a significant risk in women with high-risk lesions and poor functional class, and consequently preconception counselling and risk stratification are strongly recommended for all women with CHD of childbearing age (Earing & Webb, 2005). Such discussions clearly need to begin in the paediatric clinic and continue through the transition process into the adult clinic, although anecdotally this is not a topic that is dealt with particularly well in the paediatric setting. Within the context of increased independence and the likelihood of an increase in risk-taking behaviours, it is crucial that the topic of sexual activity forms part of the transition discussions.

A further concern raised by young people is that of employment. Research indicates that adults with CHD are more likely to be unemployed and are less likely to receive useful advice regarding potential careers. However, those who do receive careers advice are more likely to find employment (Kampius et al, 2002; Crossland et al, 2005), highlighting the importance of addressing the vocational needs and concerns of young people with CHD during transition.

The family perspective

For a successful transition to adult services to be achieved, it is vital that parents are also ready for their child to leave the paediatric environment. This can be particularly difficult for families because of the longstanding relationship that they have had with the paediatric cardiac team and the trust that they have built up with them. It is also a time of transition for parents, as they are expected to relinquish some of their parental authority and facilitate their child assuming more responsibility for his or her own care.

A study of parents of adolescents and young adults with CHD identified that their child's illness affected their ability to see them as a normal healthy teenager and made it difficult for them to have normal aspirations and set long-term goals for their child (Sparacino et al, 1997). 'Letting go' and leaving the security and familiarity of the paediatric environment can be as stressful, if not more so, for parents as for their children. It is well recognised that parental anxiety is not related to the severity of their child's heart condition (Davis et al, 1998; Lawoko & Soares, 2006), and particularly for those young people with less severe heart disease, high levels of parental anxiety can severely impede their progression through the necessary developmental and medical transitions.

The role of parental anxiety is an important factor to consider during the transition process, but it is also necessary to recognise that in some situations maintaining a degree of control of their child's care may, rather than being indicative of overprotectiveness, indeed be necessary in those situations where their child continues to be medically and psychologically vulnerable.

Moving into the adult environment and building relationships with the adult team

Moving from the security and nurturing environment of the paediatric clinic to the unfamiliar, more impersonal adult clinic can be a stressful and anxiety-provoking experience for both the young person and their parents. Patients have reported finding the change in the way in which care is delivered, as well as different treatment protocols, difficult to cope with, further heightening anxiety levels. One concern that young people often raise before making the transition is that they will be surrounded by 'old people' in the clinic or on the ward, and that the environment will not be geared to their needs. Learning to trust a new team and developing relationships with a different group of professionals can be very stressful for the less confident young person, and a reluctance to embrace change can result in an unwillingness to attend for follow-up. In a comprehensive evaluation of young adult patients with complex CHD initially treated at a specialist paediatric cardiac centre in Canada, fewer than half of the patients were found to have transferred successfully to adult care (Reid et al, 2004), the consequences for poor transition being potentially dire for some.

There is a wealth of evidence addressing non-adherence in the chronically ill adolescent population, and the time of transition can result in increased non-adherence (Watson, 2000; Annunziato et al, 2007), particularly if the young person has unmet informational, social, emotional or physical needs. A further issue for young people who have left full-time education and are not in receipt of welfare benefits is that of needing to pay for prescriptions. Evidence from studies in the UK (Jones & Britten, 1998; Schafheutle et al, 2002) and USA (Chisholm, 2004; Kennedy & Morgan, 2006) indicates that the financial burden of prescription charges is a contributory factor to non-adherence. If the need to pay coincides with transitioning to an adult centre and the loss of psychosocial support services in the paediatric centre, the young person can feel isolated and unaware of how to access help from the adult centre, further increasing the likelihood of an unsatisfactory transition.

The healthcare providers

It is also important to consider the impact of transition on the healthcare providers in both the paediatric and adult settings, and the resulting effect on the young person. It is the paediatric team who are the 'experts' in CHD and who have had the often lifelong relationship with the adolescent patient, so it is not surprising that many are reluctant to transition their patients to adult services. For those patients who do not want to make the transition, healthcare professionals' ambivalence surrounding transition may be exploited and can result in adult patients being treated in paediatric settings.

However, paediatric professionals do not have experience in dealing with adult-onset cardiac issues or in non-cardiac issues such as sexual health or employment counselling. In contrast, not all adult cardiologists are experienced in CHD and in particular may not have an understanding of the psychological factors associated with CHD or of the developmental issues associated with adolescence and the transition to adult care. One area that has been highlighted is the importance of adult cardiologists acknowledging adolescents' story of growing up with a chronic illness and hearing their concerns and fears, which is clearly fundamental to the development of a good relationship.

The process of transition can have a psychological impact on patients, families and healthcare providers. The planning and implementation of a successful transition programme and the provision of support to facilitate this are therefore crucial for the continued physical and psychological well-being of young people with CHD.

Support

Transition is a time of change affecting the relationships that young people and their families have with each other and with their healthcare teams. The key to a successful transition between paediatric and adult services is to enable young people and their families to manage this change.

The development of integrated, holistic care for young people with CHD in the UK has been slow and the need not widely recognised. Improvements in the management of CHD have led to the need for improved psychological and social care of young people with CHD (Kovacs et al, 2005). Young people and their parents need to be supported to develop confidence in managing their heart condition as well as to manage common minor illness (DH, 2004a, 2004b). As children enter adolescence, many begin to ask more questions and voice their own anxieties about the future. However, some are either too frightened to ask or simply do not want to know. Guidance and support are critical to enable adolescents to understand and articulate their feelings about the future. A sensitive and understanding approach is crucial, particularly when seeking to develop a new therapeutic and trusting relationship.

Published data suggest that transition is more successful in healthcare settings where a key worker or lead professional, usually a nurse specialist, has responsibility for transition arrangements between paediatric and adult care (Foster et al, 2001). The presence of a nurse specialist at the transition clinic is desirable to minimise anxiety for the young person and their family, to act as a point of contact and provide continuity of information, and to support and be responsible for coordinating transfer arrangements.

The views of young people

The author attended a transition workshop facilitated by the GUCH Patients Association during which young people with CHD from all over the UK discussed their experience of moving from paediatric to adult care. The majority had simply been transferred; few had any experience of transition. Understandably, these patients have high expectations about their care; the areas of concern they expressed related to the quality of communication and balance of power in the relationship between young people, their parents and health professionals. The knowledge and competence of the adult medical and nursing team is considered to be important, in addition to the need for someone such as a nurse specialist to relate to so their parents can stand back. This is important as many parents find it hard to let go and need support from the healthcare team.

Sparacino et al (1997) described the dilemmas of parents who have children with heart defects. The problems of normality, disclosure (whether to reveal the presence of a heart defect), uncertainty, coping strategies, social integration and impact on the family continue to be dilemmas for these young adults. Parents are rarely advised about when and how much information should be given to their child. They may be particularly vigilant about their maturing child's health, be overprotective and resist attempts for increased independence (Kovacs et al, 2005). Some parents need more counselling and support than others to help their offspring become more independent and take responsibility for the management of their own heart condition. Parents need support and guidance through the transition process to adapt to the change that is required in their role, from that of being actively involved in their child's healthcare to taking on a more supportive role. Parents require support in understanding the importance and outcome of the transition process, and it is important to include them. One way of easing the transition process with parents is to begin by initially having parents present during the entire visit to clinic and then gradually reducing the amount of time they are present during the consultation until the visits eventually take place without any parental presence (Tong & Kools, 2004).

Adolescents need support and encouragement to begin making decisions, maximising their strengths and abilities in order to begin taking more control of their lives. However, support is a nebulous concept, and although young people (Kendall et al, 2003a) and their parents report that they benefit from support (Kendall et al, 2003b), it is difficult to find any published evaluation of the effectiveness of the various methods in relation to the families of young people with CHD.

Support strategies

Nevertheless, young people undergoing health transition should have access to appropriate support such as education advice and health education (RCN, 2008). There are a variety of ways in which support may be offered. Education forms part of the process of helping young people and their families to cope with their heart condition and the way it affects their lives. Teaching young people how to cope with healthcare transition is part of the transition process. Learning through clear, honest, open communication of information, frequently repeated, is central to the process of change required in developing coping strategies and managing stress. Patients may require help to come to terms with changes in their condition and enable them to understand complex problems and treatments. The provision of timely information and support at critical times, such as the visit to the clinic when therapy may be adjusted, or when there is need for medical or surgical intervention, is essential to help the patient to adjust to the new situation in order to cope and understand.

Support should be tailored to individual patient need. The lead key worker/transition nurse needs to assess the quality of support networks available to the young person with CHD, recognise their social concerns and reinforce positive coping strategies when appropriate (Uzark, 1992). As young people develop, they move from using emotional coping strategies to problem-solving strategies (Children's Hospital Boston, 2009), which can be developed during the transition period.

Many young people, however, find it difficult to talk to adults, do not trust them or feel they do not understand and may prefer to seek support elsewhere. A number of internet support sites (see the end of the chapter) exist for young people, for example Youth2Youth, a national young person's helpline run by young people for young people. Other sites include the British Heart Foundation's yheart.net and YoungMinds. The GUCH Patients Association provides a national support network run by and for young people with CHD. The network allows similar experiences to be shared and, above all, encourages people to help and support each other.

During adolescence, the feeling of being different begins to emerge. Many young people with CHD perceive themselves to be different and struggle to be considered normal (Claessens et al, 2005). Visible signs such as cyanosis, finger clubbing, and thoracotomy and sternotomy scars, combined with a small stature and physical limitations, may distort the young person's perception of their body image and can hinder their ability to achieve full social independence (Tong et al, 1998). Youngsters may need support in ways to educate their peers about CHD and to maintain a peer network.

An awareness of psychosocial concerns and referral for appropriate mental health issues may be indicated for some patients who experience specific challenges that may affect emotional functioning, self-perception and peer relationships (Kovacs et al, 2005). Self-harming behaviour, panic attacks, anxiety and depression, eating problems, bullying and difficulty in coping with everyday life are issues that may affect some young people with CHD. The availability of psychological and psychiatric expertise for young people with CHD, particularly during the transition period, varies enormously across the UK and can be difficult to access. However, referral for appropriate assessment and therapy is important at the specialist CHD centre if it is available, or through the primary healthcare team.

Congenital heart defects are frequently associated with a number of learning disabilities. These patients may have complex support needs that need to be addressed, particularly if admission to hospital is necessary. Decisions about treatment should be made with the patient, the carer and the family. Close liaison with other relevant agencies, such as community disability teams, is important. There are specific medical concerns for youngsters with Down syndrome that occur at increased frequency during the transition period; these include weight gain, thyroid dysfunction, skin disorders, progression of pre-existing CHD, sleep apnoea and psychiatric disorders (Pueschel, 1996).

In the past, paediatric cardiologists may have acted as barriers to successful transitional care because they lacked confidence in their adult colleagues (Fox, 2002). ACHD is now a recognised speciality in the UK, with formal education programmes for doctors and nurses. However, transitional care needs to be included in education and training programmes for both adult services and children and young people's services. Adult healthcare teams need to understand young people's issues and needs as well as adolescent mental health issues (RCN, 2008). Workshops, study days and informal visits are ways of providing educational opportunities for people to learn about the transition process and services for young people and adults with CHD. Strengthening the links between paediatric and ACHD centres is critical.

The author has been involved in the development of a transition service where young people aged 12–18 years are referred by the paediatric cardiologists to the weekly transition clinic that takes place in the children's hospital. The paediatric cardiologists refer their patients to a dedicated paediatric cardiologist with a special interest in transitional care. A team from the ACH unit composed of adult congenital cardiologist, ACH nurse specialist and cardiac physiologist attend the clinic jointly. The team is able to develop a relationship with the young person and their family during the time they attend the clinic, which will continue once they have eventually moved to the adult unit. The nurse specialist is able to make an individual assessment of each young person and identify specific educational and/or psychosocial support needs and implement a plan of care. Protocols have been developed for the assessment of individual cardiac conditions; all necessary investigations are undertaken before the first clinic visit at the adult centre. During the transitional period, young people and their families will know how to contact the nurse specialist should the need arise. Following the last visit to the transition clinic, a full referral letter is written to the team at the adult unit with the most current and relevant results. The eventual transfer from paediatric to adult care should only take place during a period of medical stability. Every possible effort is made to maintain clinical continuity and help with the patient's journey, which can be difficult at times.

Summary

Despite the many challenges and barriers faced in transition, it is reasonable to assume that establishing an effective transition programme can be both time consuming and challenging. However, successful transition also brings with it many rewards and the end result will be extremely worthwhile for every young person, family and health professional involved.

References

Annunziato, R., Emre, S., Shneider, B., Barton, C., Dugan, C. & Shemesh, E. (2007). Adherence and medical outcomes in pediatric liver transplant recipients who transition to adult services. *Pediatric Transplantation*, *11*, 608–614.

Bart, W.M. (1983). Adolescent thinking and the quality of life. *Adolescence*, *18*, 875–878.

Beeri, M., Haramati, Z., Rein, J.J. & Nir, A. (2001). Parental knowledge and views of pediatric congenital heart disease. *Israeli Medical Association Journal*, *3*, 194–197.

Bennett, D., Towns, S. & Steinbeck, K. (2005). Smoothing the transition to adult care. *Medical Journal of Australia*, *182*, 373–374.

Beresford, B. & Sloper, P. (2000). *The information needs of chronically ill or physically disabled children and adolescents*. York: Social Policy Research Unit.

British Cardiac Society Working Party (2002). Grown-up congenital heart (GUCH) disease: current needs and provision of service for adolescents and adults with congenital heart disease in the UK. *Heart 8*(suppl1), i1–i14.

British Heart Foundation Statistics Database (2003). *Congenital heart disease statistics*. Oxford: BHF Health Promotion Research Group, University of Oxford, www.heartstats.org

British Medical Association (2003) *Adolescent health*. London: BMA.

British Paediatric Association (1985). *Report of the working party on the needs and care of adolescents*. London: BPA.

Bull, K. (1998). The Fontan procedure: lessons from the past. *Heart*, *79*, 213–214.

Chessa, M., De Rosa, G., Pardeo, M., Negura, G.D., Butera, G., Feslova, V. et al (2005). Illness understanding in adults with congenital heart disease. *Italian Heart Journal*, *6*, 895–899.

Children's Hospital Boston (2009). Information on the Transition Clinic, Adult Congenital Heart Service. Available at: http://www.childrenshospital.org

Chisholm, M. (2004). Increasing medication access to transplant recipients. *Clinical Transplant*, *18*, 39–48.

Christie, D. & Viner, R. (2005). ABC of adolescence. *British Medical Journal*, *330*, 301–304.

Claessens, P., Moons, P., Dierckx de Casterle, B., Cannaerts, N., Budts, W. & Gewillig, M. (2005). What does it mean to live with a congenital heart disease? A qualitative study on the lived experiences of adult patients. *European Journal of Cardiovascular Nursing*, *4*, 3–10.

Cross, K.P. & Santucci, K.A. (2006). Transitional medicine: will emergency medicine physicians be ready for the growing population of adults with congenital heart disease? *Pediatric Emergency Care*, *22*, 775–781.

Crossland, D.S., Jackson, S.P., Lyall, R., Burn, J. & O'Sullivan, J.J. (2005). Employment and advice regarding careers for adults with congenital heart disease. *Cardiology in the Young*, *15*, 391–395.

Davis, C.C., Brown, R.T., Bakeman, R. & Campbell, R. (1998). Psychological adaptation and adjustment of mothers of children with congenital heart disease: stress, coping, and family functioning. *Journal Pediatric Psychology*, *23*, 219–228.

Department of Health (1976). *Fit for the future: Report of the Committee on Child Health Services* (Court Report). London: HMSO.

Department of Health (2003). *Report of the Paediatric and Congenital Cardiac Services Review*. London: Department of Health.

Department of Health (2004a). *National Service Framework for children, young people and maternity services*. London: Department for Education and Skills/DH.

Department of Health (2004b). *Getting the right start: National Service Framework for children. Standard for hospital services*. London: DH.

Department of Health (2006). *Transition: Getting it right for young people, improving the transition of young people with long term conditions from children's to adult health services*. London: DH.

Department of Health Vascular Programme Team (2006). *Adult congenital heart disease. A commissioning guide for services for young people and grown ups with congenital heart disease (GUCH)*. London: DH.

Dore, A., de Guise, P. & Mercier, L.A. (2002). Transition of care to adult congenital heart centres: what do patients know about their heart condition? *Canadian Journal of Cardiology*, *18*, 141–146.

Dovey-Pearce, G., Hurrell, R. & May, C. (2005). Young adult's suggestions for providing developmentally appropriate diabetes services: a qualitative study. *Health and Social Care in the Community*, *13*, 409–419.

Earing, M. & Webb, G. (2005). Congenital heart disease and pregnancy: maternal and fetal risks. *Clinics in Perinatology*, *32*, 913–919.

European Society of Cardiology (2003). Management of grown up congenital heart disease: the task force on the management of grown up congenital heart disease of the European Society of Cardiology. *European Heart Journal*, *24*, 1035–1084.

Foster, E., Graham, T.P., Driscoll, D.J., Reid, G.J., Reiss, J.G., Russell, A. et al (2001). Task force 2: special health care needs of adults with congenital heart disease. *Journal of the American College of Cardiology*, *37*, 1176–1183.

Fox, A. (2002). Physicians as barriers to successful transitional care. *International Journal of Adolescent Medicine and Health*, *14*, 3–7.

Gantt, L. (1992). Growing up heartsick: the experiences of young women with congenital heart disease. *Health Care Women for Women International*, *13*, 241–248.

Gatzoulis, M.A. (2006). Adult congenital heart disease: education, education, education. *Nature Clinical Practice Cardiovascular Medicine*, *3*, 2–3.

Geenen, S., Powers, L. & Sells, W. (2003). Understanding the role of health care providers during transition of adolescents with disabilities and special health care needs. *Journal of Adolescent Health*, *32*, 225–233.

Greenaway, B. (2008). Looking out for the 'lost' congenital heart patients. *British Journal of Cardiac Nursing*, *3*, 158–160.

Gurvitz, M.Z., Inkelas, M., Lee, M., Stout, K., Escarce, J. & Chang, R.K. (2007). Changes in hospitalization patterns among patients with congenital heart disease during the transition from adolescence to adulthood. *Journal of American College of Cardiology*, *49*, 875–882.

House of Commons Health Committee (1997). *Hospital services for children and young people, fifth report*. London: HMSO.

Jones, I. & Britten, N. (1998). Why do some patients not cash their prescriptions? *British Journal of General Practice*, *48*, 903–905.

Jordan, A. & McDonagh, J.E. (2006). Recognition of emerging adulthood in UK rheumatology: the case for young adult rheumatology service developments. *Rheumatology, 46*, 188–191.

Kampius, M., Vogels, T., Ottenkamp, J., Van Der Wall, E., Verloove-Vanhorick, S., & Vliegen, H. (2002). Employment in adults with congenital heart disease. *Archives of Paediatric and Adolescent Medicine, 156*, 1143–1148.

Karsdorp, P.A., Everaerd, W., Kindt, M. & Mulder, B.J. (2007). Psychological and cognitive functioning in children and adolescents with congenital heart disease: a meta-analysis. *Journal of Paediatric Psychology, 32*, 527–541.

Kendall, L., Sloper, P., Lewin, R.J.P. & Parsons, J.M. (2003a). The views of young people with congenital cardiac disease on designing the services for their treatment. *Cardiology in the Young, 13*, 11–19.

Kendall, L., Sloper, P., Lewin, R.J.P. & Parsons, J.M. (2003b). The views of parents concerning the planning of services for rehabilitation of families of children with congenital cardiac disease. *Cardiology in the Young, 13*, 20–27.

Kennedy, F. (2007). Congenital heart defects in adults. In Hatchett, R. & Thompson, D.R., eds. *Cardiac nursing: A comprehensive guide.* 2nd edn. Edinburgh: Churchill Livingstone. pp. 335–356.

Kennedy, J. & Morgan, S. (2006). A cross-national study of prescription nonadherence due to cost: data from the joint Canada–United States survey of health. *Clinical Therapeutics, 28*, 1217–1224.

Kools, S., Tong, E.M., Hughes, R., Jayne, R., Scheibly, K., Laughlin, J. & Gilliss, C.L. (2002). Hospital experiences of young adults with congenital heart disease: divergence in expectations and dissonance in care. *American Journal of Critical Care, 11*, 115–125.

Kovacs, A.H., Sears, S.F. & Saidi, A.S. (2005). Biopsychosocial experiences of adults with congenital heart disease: review of the literature. *American Heart Journal, 150*, 193–201.

Lawoko, S. & Soares, J.J. (2006). Psychosocial morbidity among parents of children with congenital heart disease: a prospective longitudinal study. *Heart and Lung, 35*, 310–314.

McCusker, C.G., Doherty, N.N., Molloy, B., Casey, F., Rooney, N. & Mulholland, C. et al (2007). Determinants of neuropsychological and behavioural outcomes in early childhood survivors of congenital heart disease. *Archive of Diseases in Childhood, 92*, 137–141.

McDonagh, J. & Kelly, D. (2003). Transition care of the pediatric recipient to adult caregivers. *Pediatric Clinics of North America, 50*, 1561–1583.

McDonagh, J. & Viner, R. (2006). Lost in transition? Between paediatric and adult services. *British Medical Journal, 332*, 435–436.

McDonagh, J., Southwood, T. & Shaw, K. (2004). Unmet adolescent health training needs for rheumatology health professionals. *Rheumatology, 43*, 737–743.

McDonagh, J., Shaw, K. & Southwood, T. (2005). Translating policy into practice: development of a transitional care policy for adolescents with chronic illness. *Clinical Experience in Rheumatology, 23*, S88.

McDonagh, J., Southwood, T. & Shaw, K. (2006). Growing up and moving on in rheumatology: development and preliminary evaluation of a transitional care programme for a multi centre cohort of adolescents with juvenile idiopathic arthritis. *Journal of Child Health Care, 10*, 22–42.

Milne, A. & Chesson, R. (2000). Health services can be cool: partnerships with adolescents in primary care. *Family Practice, 17*, 305–308.

Moons, P., DeVolder, E., Budts, W., DeGeest, S., Elen, J., Waeytens, K. et al (2001). What do adult patients with congenital heart disease know about their disease, treatment, and prevention of complications? A call for structured patient education. *Heart, 86*, 74–80.

National Institute for Health and Clinical Excellence (2008) March. Prophylaxis against infective endocarditis. Clinical guideline 64.

Orr, D., Fineberg, N. & Gray, D. (1996). Glycaemic control and transfer of health care among adolescents with insulin dependent diabetes mellitus. *Journal of Adolescent Health, 18*, 44–47.

Paone, M., Whitehouse, S. & Standford, D. (1998). Challenges of transition: coping with a chronic condition. *British Columbia Medical Journal, 40,* 73–75.

Patterson, D. & Lanier, C. (1999). Adolescent health transitions: focus group study of teens and young adults with special health care needs. *Family and Community Health, 22,* 43–58.

Platt, H. (1959). *The welfare of children in hospitals.* London: HMSO.

Pueschel, S.M. (1996). Young people with Down syndrome: transition from childhood to adulthood. *Mental Retardation and Developmental Disabilities Research Reviews, 2,* 90–95.

Reid, G.J., Irvine, J., McCrindle, B.W., Sananes, R., Ritvo, P.G., Siu, S.C. & Webb, G.D. (2004). Prevalence and correlates of successful transfer from pediatric to adult health care among a cohort of young adults with complex congenital heart defects. *Pediatrics, 113,* 197–205.

Reid, G.J., Webb, G.D., Barzel, M., McCrindle, B.W., Irvine, M.J. & Siu, S.C. (2006). Estimates of life expectancy by adolescents and young adults with congenital heart disease. *Journal of the American College of Cardiology, 48,* 349–355.

Rosen, D., Blum, R., Britto, M., Sawyer, S. & Siegel, D. (2003). Transition to adult health care for adolescents and young adults with chronic conditions: position paper of the Society of Adolescent Medicine. *Journal of Adolescent Health, 33,* 309–311.

Royal College of Nursing (2004). *Adolescent transition care: guidance for nursing staff.* London: RCN.

Royal College of Nursing (2008). *Lost in transition. Moving young people between child and adult health services.* London: RCN.

Royal College of Paediatrics and Child Health (2003). *Bridging the gap: health care for adolescents.* London: RCPCH.

Sawyer, S., Blair, S. & Bowes, G. (1997). Chronic illness in adolescents: transfer or transition to adult services? *Journal of Paediatric and Child Health, 33,* 88–90.

Schafheutle, E., Hassell, K., Noyce, P. & Weiss, M. (2002). Access to medicines: cost as an influence on the views and behaviour of patients. *Health and Social Care Community, 10,* 187–195.

Shaw, K., Southwood, T. & McDonagh, J. (2004). Developing a programme of transitional care for adolescents with juvenile idiopathic arthritis: results of a postal survey. *Rheumatology, 43,* 211–219.

Somerville, J. (1997). Near misses and disasters in the treatment of grown-up congenital heart patients. *Journal of the Royal Society of Medicine, 90,* 124–127.

Sparacino, P., Tong, E., Messias, D., Foote, D., Chesla, C. & Gilliss, C. (1997). The dilemmas of parents of adolescents and young adults with congenital heart disease. *Heart and Lung, 26,* 187–195.

Suris, J., Resnick, M., Cassuto, N. & Blum, R. (1996). Sexual behaviour of adolescents with chronic disease and disability. *Journal of Adolescent Health, 19,* 124–131.

Swan, L. & Hillis, W. (2000). Exercise prescription in adults with congenital heart disease: a long way to go. *Heart, 83,* 685–687.

Therrien, J., Warnes, C., Daliento, L. et al (2001). Canadian Cardiovascular Society Consensus Conference 2001 update: recommendations for the management of adults with congenital heart disease—Part III. *Can J Cardiol, 17,* 1135–1158.

Tong, E.M. & Kools, S. (2004). Health care transitions for adolescents with congenital heart disease: patient and family perspectives. *Nursing Clinics of North America, 39,* 727–740.

Tong, E., Sparacino, P., Messias, D., Foote, D., Chesla, C. & Gilliss, C. (1998). Growing up with congenital heart disease: the dilemmas of adolescents and young adults. *Cardiology in the Young, 8,* 303–309.

Tucker, L. & Cabral, D. (2005). Transition of the adolescent patient with rheumatic disease: issues to consider. *Clinical Paediatrics, 52,* 641–652.

Uzark, K. (1992). Counselling adolescents with congenital heart disease. *Journal of Cardiovascular Nursing, 6,* 65–73.

Van Walleghem, N., MacDonald, C. & Dean, H. (2006) Building connections for young adults with type 1 diabetes mellitus in Manitoba: feasibility and acceptability of a transition initiative. *Chronic Diseases in Canada, 27,* 130–134.

Veldtman, G.R., Matley, S.L., Kendall, L., Quirk, J., Gibbs, J., Parsons, M. & Hewison, J. (2000). Illness understanding in children and adolescents with heart disease. *Heart, 84*, 395–397.

Viner, R.M. (1999). Transition from paediatric to adult care. Bridging the gaps or passing the buck? *Archives of Disease in Childhood, 81*, 271–275.

Warnes, C.A., Liberthson, R., Danielson, G.K. et al (2001). Task force 1: the changing profile of congenital heart disease in adult life. *J Am Coll Cardiol, 37*, 1170–1175.

Watson, A. (2000). Non-compliance and transfer from paediatric to adult transplant unit. *Pediatric Nephrology, 14*, 469–472.

While, A., Forbes, A. & Ullman, R. (2004). Good practices that address continuity during transition from child to adult health care: syntheses of the evidence, *Child: Care, Health and Development, 30*, 439–452.

Wray J. (2006). The effects of hypoxia on the cognitive development and behaviour of children and adolescents with congenital heart disease. *Developmental Science, 9*, 368–378.

Websites

British Heart Foundation: http://www.yheart.net/meet

Grown Up Congenital Heart Patients Association: http://www.GUCH.org.uk

YoungMinds: http:// www.youngminds.org.uk

Youth2Youth: http://www.youth2youth.co.uk

7 The information jigsaw

Suzie Hutchinson, Jo Wray, Paula Banda, Michael Cumper, Julie Wooton

Clinical teams plan a treatment pathway for their patients following a diagnosis of congenital heart disease (CHD), but whilst the children's medical care continues, it is important to remember that each child's experience includes living a life with their disorder, and that their life is not lived in isolation. They have a family, friends, peers, teachers and bosses, and ultimately may have families of their own. This chapter will explore how children, their families and all others involved in their life learn to cope with the lifestyle pathway that is affected by the disabilities that CHD can create.

The beginning of the journey

Expectant parents approach their mid-trimester scan as an opportunity to see their growing child and take home a picture that they can show to their family. Learning that your child has a problem with their heart proves devastating for many parents, especially as they have not prepared themselves for this eventuality. Even families whose children are able to undergo correctable heart surgery are left feeling isolated, first by a lack of knowledge about the disease, and second by the feeling that they are totally alone as they cope with this potentially life-changing condition. They are frightened of the risks for their baby and the effects that the diagnosis will have on their life.

> We were invited to a fetal cardiac scanning training day for our 20-week scan – we didn't even know what fetal cardiac scanning meant, and went along because it was on a Saturday so it was more convenient, and the letter said that we'd have a more detailed scan with extra pictures of our baby. We were totally unprepared for the devastating information that was to follow: our baby had a major heart condition, and the consultant couldn't be totally sure of the diagnosis at this stage – it could have been a condition which, although very serious, could be fully corrected through surgery. The other possibility was a non-correctable condition that the medics describe as 'not compatible with life'. We didn't want to be told this information, and we didn't want to have to make the decisions which came with it. (Isabel, the mother of a child with tricuspid atresia)

Antenatal diagnosis

Families learning that their unborn child has a heart defect have to ask themselves many questions before they choose to terminate or continue with the pregnancy.

Whichever treatment path the expectant parents take, they need a great deal of non-directive information and support (Rempel et al, 2004).

> When you are referred to the hospital, you know there is a potential issue, but absolutely nothing prepares you for hearing the diagnosis, in our case pulmonary atresia and a small right ventricle. We were given three options – termination, comfort care or a three-stage 'palliative' surgery; our baby's heart would never be fixed, and we were told there was a possibility that our baby's heart condition might be the result of a chromosome abnormality. We were totally devastated.
>
> We were given the option of having an amniocentesis there and then, so we did; we felt we needed to fully understand the extent of our baby's condition. We left the hospital numb. The disappointing thing was the lack of support we were given after the test. First, we did not realise the number of chromosome conditions: we assumed they were just testing for Down syndrome, Edwards, Patau and DiGeorge, and that they were going to contact us in 2 or 3 days with the results of these, but it actually took 3 weeks to get a full result. During this time, we felt in limbo, isolated and alone, and were jumping every time the phone rang. (The parents of a child with pulmonary atresia following an antenatal diagnosis)

Once expectant parents have made their treatment path decision, they need to be supported by the most appropriate team. This may be the children's hospital service, specialist information charities or organisations like ARC who specialise in offering support through antenatal diagnosis and termination.

> Our obstetrician advised us to contact Little Hearts Matter for further information about the condition. He gave us a booklet from the charity which explained the condition and its implications, and gave us something to show to other family members when we were trying to explain what was going on.
>
> We will never forget the first Little Hearts Matter Open Day we attended. Matthew was 3 weeks old and was in intensive care – we had no idea when, or even if, he would ever get off the ventilator. We were able to talk to parents who understood how we felt, and although they couldn't reassure us about Matthew, they could tell us of their own similar experiences, and how many children face additional hurdles even once they are through their first surgery. We also found a new hope for Matthew's future – seeing the children with heart conditions playing with their heart-healthy siblings and not being able to tell who had the conditions and who didn't was like a light at the end of the tunnel; assuming he made it through these difficult early weeks, there was a good possibility of a reasonable quality of life for him. (The mother of a child with complex non-correctable heart)

Throughout the rest of the pregnancy, it is important for parents to continue to build a relationship with their unborn child and gradually gain a greater understanding of the treatment path to come.

Postnatal diagnosis

Many parents will discover that their child has a heart condition after the birth. Although their pregnancy is unhindered by worry, following the birth of their child they have to come to terms with the diagnosis as well as trying to get to know their new baby. All the fears that are initially explored during the pregnancy with an antenatal diagnosis are experienced amidst all the plans to offer treatment. In the case of a life-threatening condition, this can lead to a disassociation with the child as parents fear developing a bond with a child whom they may lose.

> After the initial decision to go ahead, we wondered what we had done. What sort of quality of life would our son have? (The mother of a child with a right-sided single-ventricle disorder)

At whatever stage it happens, the time of diagnosis can create a crisis for parents as they struggle to cope with a host of emotional and practical demands. Parents have described a whole range of feelings, ranging from shock, devastation and anger to guilt, sorrow and depression. There may also be a period of mourning for the loss of the child that they thought they were going to have as they begin a period of adjustment and acceptance of the diagnosis and its implications. As parents look for answers that will help them understand why this has happened to them and how they will cope with the life ahead, they look to anyone to help them learn more.

It is important that clinical teams recognise families' need for information. Referring parents to recognised accurate sources of support and information helps them to gain the strength for the birth of the child and the initial treatment. An opportunity for families to speak to others who have been through the same experiences helps them to feel less isolated. Written information should follow every discussion about the diagnosis and treatment. Pictures of the heart with explanations written for a parent audience is essential. Clear facts about treatments and lifestyle expectations help families to paint a clearer picture of the effects of the diagnosis. They will need to spend time explaining this information to other family members and any other children.

It is important to remember that the information jigsaw is different for every family. Some parents only want a minimal explanation of the condition, whilst others seek more and more information; each family builds their own information jigsaw. It is important that all members of the care team have an up-to-date understanding of the heart conditions and possible treatments; many community clinicians are unaware of recent changes in treatment.

> I am the kind of person who wants to understand every detail of what is going on, and have spent a lot of time looking for information from all sorts of places including cardiac charity information sites, parents and medical resources. (The mother of a child with a complex tricuspid atresia)

The hospital experience

Hospitals, although seen as places of healing, are also places of mystery and fear. Very few parents are able to prepare themselves for the sight of their child in the intensive

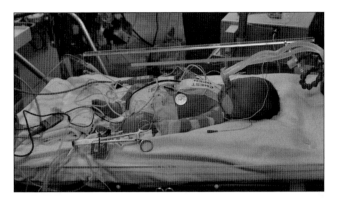

Figure 7.1 A child in the intensive care unit

care unit (Figure 7.1) even if they have had an opportunity to visit the department before their child is there for care.

In the case of a newborn baby, both parents are working to get to know their new baby at the same time as learning about the treatment and care that they are receiving. The mother is recovering from a delivery, and her hormone levels are in disarray. This is a very emotional time for families who may also have had to travel to a treatment centre many miles from their home and their normal support resources.

The care of the parents must also be considered at this time. The mother will need medical support post delivery; the father will be trying to offer support to his child and his partner, and may also be juggling the care of other siblings whilst informing grandparents and friends. He may also have to balance hospital visiting with work as the family income may depend on his continued employment. The role of the cardiac liaison nurse is extremely important at this time as he or she is the parents' advocate and works to link services and communication within the hospital.

Throughout the hospital stay, it is important that parents are continually included in the practical care of their child. Even in the intensive care unit, nurses will work to involve parents as much as possible. Even breast milk can be collected to be used as the baby's feeding develops. It is also important that parents are kept up to date with all changes in their child's condition and treatment.

The hospital becomes your entire world – it is hard to believe that life as normal is carrying on outside the four walls of the hospital 'institution'. As the weeks pass, you become quite used to the hospital routine and start to feel more comfortable in there, to the extent that the long-awaited discharge home can be quite a shock in many ways.

Despite the staff's best efforts, I didn't feel that Matthew was 'our' baby until quite a long time after we had brought him home. I remember having a conversation with an ITU nurse who asked me whether I worked or was a full-time mother – my reply was that I was a full-time hospital visitor! When Matthew was 2 months old, we took him home for a weekend on 'home leave' – it felt like we had been lent a baby for the weekend. (The parent of a child with single-ventricle disease)

Family relationships

Coming to terms and learning to live with the diagnosis, whether this is made ante-natally, postnatally or later in childhood, requires a period of adjustment that can put a strain on parents' own relationship.

> We just sat there, watching him, frightened to take our eyes off him for a second. But we had no time for each other and I found myself irritated by everything he [her partner] did – even though I knew it wasn't his fault. (The mother of a 3-month-old baby diagnosed at 2 days with CHD)

At the same time, some parents report that their relationship is strengthened as a result of their child being sick and that they are able to support each other very well.

> When she [his partner] is down I am up, and when I am down she is up. Although it is hard, we cope with it together, and there is no doubt it has brought us closer together. (The father of a 13-month-old at assessment for heart transplantation)

Encouraging parents to make time for themselves and each other is important. Parents often feel guilty about leaving their sick child, and in some cases it can help to give them 'permission' to take a break from caring for a few hours so that they can spend time with their partner away from the hospital environment.

A sick child in the family also has an impact on other family members, including siblings and grandparents. Other children in the family can be an additional source of stress – or comfort – for parents.

> I felt so guilty about my other little girl. She got sent from pillar to post; she didn't understand what was happening and then when she saw me she was so clingy, which made it hard to leave her again and go back to the hospital. (A mother talking about the impact on her healthy 3-year-old daughter)

> Even though he was only 2 years old he sensed my sadness and he just came up and put his head in my lap, trying to comfort me. (A father talking about his older child after he arrived home from leaving his wife and baby in hospital)

Other children may also need support to help them cope with the changes that having a sibling with heart disease can bring. They can often feel left out and resentful, and it is therefore important for them to feel involved as much as possible. This involve-ment can extend to the hospital environment, where encouraging parents to include their other children where appropriate can help to alleviate feelings of resentment in the siblings and also help parents to maintain some perspective on normality (Rempel et al, 2004).

The next steps

For most parents, gradually learning to understand their child's heart problem and treatments gives them back some of the control that the diagnosis took away. They begin to understand the process. Coupled with an involvement from the beginning in their child's general care, they are able to retain their position as parents, and they also gradually enter the treatment team circle. For many children, one treatment provides a cure and further involvement with the hospital team is on an outpatient basis, whilst others have to prepare themselves for a lifetime of care and further treatment with the ongoing uncertainty of whether they will survive into adulthood.

Stepping from the hospital environment into life at home can leave parents feeling vulnerable. The liaison nurse service helps to bridge care from the hospital into the community. Links with health visitors and general practitioners can help to ensure that the community medical team are able to continue care once the child is at home. This information exchange should be maintained throughout the child's life to provide continuity of care. Often the child's parents know far more about their child's condition than the community medical team do. It is even more important that these families have a referral process where they can seek and find support and information at all times. Most often, this support is found with medical team based at the cardiac centre.

Parents gradually learn to care for their child at home, furnished with information about lifestyle:

- the signs to look for when assessing their child's health: signs of heart failure;
- medications;
- advice and support related to feeding;
- immunisation requirements;
- plans for further treatment;
- advice about their child's crying.

> Feeding takes over your whole life. Taking our baby home being fed through a nasogastric tube was so different from my ideal of breastfeeding to the age of one! We needed to learn how to use the equipment for overnight pump feeds, and were doing 3-hourly feeds during the day. Each feed needed to be given over an hour, to try to reduce Matthew's vomiting, and he needed to be kept still and upright for an hour after each feed – so that didn't leave much time for anything else before getting ready for the next feed. (The mother of a child with tricuspid atresia)

Added information is often available through support and information organisations, which are also able to link parents who can share their problems and lifestyle solutions.

For many families, the stress and worry associated with having a child with complex heart problems is not the only added stress that such conditions create. The added expense of hospital visits and the need to take time away from work during treatment periods adds to families' worries. When inpatient treatment has been completed, the need to attend clinics regularly, even if their child has had corrective surgery, can be a stressful time for parents and bring back memories of fear and uncertainty.

It is important for staff to be aware of this and to recognise that, for some families, it can be an anxious time even when the child is well. It is widely acknowledged that the severity of the heart condition does not necessarily dictate how families will cope, and some parents whose children have a relatively minor heart condition can experience more difficulties and exhibit more stress than parents whose children have complex disease. Help to access allowances that will help with the added costs is often available from the hospital social work department or from social services in the community.

Parents will gradually take on the lead care role for their child.

> When the child is older, hospitalisation has a very different impact, both on the family and on the child. By this time, they will have built up relationships with different family members, and it seems even harder to let them go for surgery than when you let your precious newborn baby go. Matthew was in hospital for 10 weeks when he was 4 – I will never forget taking him out of hospital for a couple of hours for a church service (it was just before Christmas) and him saying 'the fresh air smells lovely' – this really brought home to me how much a long hospital stay was impacting on him in so many ways. (The mother of a child with tricuspid atresia)

Whilst successful surgery is what every parent hopes for, adjusting to having a well child can also be stressful. Parents have reported not knowing how to cope with their feelings of redundancy now that their child is well.

> Suddenly I felt redundant. He didn't need me any more. He just wanted to get on with his life, but what was I to do now? It was so hard to let him be 'normal' – he had never been normal before and I didn't know how to cope with him. (The mother of a 6-year-old child 12 months after surgery for CHD)

For some parents, particularly those of older children, the change in their child's behaviour after a period of time in hospital, and especially after surgery, can be difficult to manage, and they may need more support to cope with this. Parents also have to adjust to the changes in aspects such as their child's activity levels and desire for independence, which may be markedly different from before surgery. As one parent said:

> He was always such a quiet child before, staying inside and reading his books. Suddenly, now he has all this energy and he wants to be outside playing football with the other children. That has been a real shock for me – I never really realised what his heart condition was stopping him from doing. (The father of a child with hypoplastic left heart syndrome)

Health professionals have a key role to play in giving parents information about what they might expect when their child is in hospital and afterwards when they get home. Knowing that the changes they might see in their child's behaviour are normal and to be expected can make it much easier for parents to cope and will help them to feel more prepared and in control of the situation. For some older children, too, it can be difficult to adjust to being 'well' and the changes that come with that, in terms of the way in which others perceive them and the different expectations others have of them.

As the children grow, they continue with their treatments, but they also have to face many challenges in their everyday lives.

Exercise

One of the greatest challenges for children or young adults with complex heart disease is that they are unable to exercise at the same level as their peers. For many children, especially boys, this area of their lives may be extremely frustrating. It proves a challenge to ensure that they are able to take part in sport without pushing themselves beyond their safe health boundaries. Boys tend to compete with their peers in the sports arena, so care has to be taken to ensure that those with complex heart conditions have an opportunity to meet their competitive needs in other areas of their lives (Kendall et al, 2003).

Education

As children grow through childhood, they gradually gain more knowledge and independence through education. For many children born with a heart problem, their schooling is the same as others of their age, but children born with the more complex non-correctable disorders face many challenges at each stage of their school life (Shillingford & Wernovsky 2004; Shillingford et al, 2008). With care and team planning, it is possible for the children to take part in all areas of school life, but it is important for the parents to build a good relationship with the school and ensure that the targets that are set for the child are achievable.

In many cases, it is necessary to introduce formal assessment and educational support. This can take the form of an Individual Education Plan or an Educational Statement.

Every child is different, and as they grow their needs within the school environment will change, so regular formal assessment of their needs must be encouraged.

> My heart condition isn't as strong as a normal human being's. It isn't that I don't think that I'm normal, it's just that I've got something different than everyone else. You can't take that any other way I'm as independent as I can be. (Jack, aged 13, describing his heart)

Medication

Many children have to take medication every day of their life. For some, the medication affects what they can do. Anticoagulation therapy restricts a child's activity because of the risks of bleeding and bruising. No contact sports can be played, care must be taken in climbing the ropes in gym, and the child needs to be excluded from playground games.

Even the taking of medication whilst at school creates new hurdles with school bureaucracy. In extreme cases, children need oxygen therapy at home and school.

> What people don't realise is that every day reveals a new challenge. My son may not be having an operation or an investigation, but even going to school, attending a friend's party or planning a family holiday takes more thought, effort and worry than it would for other families. (Clare, the mother of Will, a 14-year-old boy with hypoplastic left heart syndrome)

More than just the heart

For some children, their cardiac condition is not their only problem: 10% of children born with complex heart disease are also born with another physical or developmental disorder. Common diagnoses are Down syndrome, 22q deletion (DiGeorge syndrome) and Edwards syndrome. Each of these diagnoses brings a plethora of lifestyle challenges, so the management and care of these children must be planned to ensure that each child is able to access as many services as possible in an efficient and organised fashion.

> The journey to Bristol is again a blur. Dan travelled in the ambulance and we were told to drive down separately. When we arrived, we went to the intensive care unit. We waited in the parents' waiting room for what seemed like ages, and then the cardiac consultant came to explain what he had found. He used a model of a heart to explain that Dan has tetralogy of Fallot. He also went on to explain that he also felt that Dan showed signs of DiGeorge syndrome. This was way too much information. I can remember thinking 'right, let's deal with the heart problem first'. Little did I know that the heart defect is as a result of the DiGeorge. He said that Dan would experience blue spells until he was about a year old and then he would need surgery. (The parent of a child with a number of diagnoses)

It is also important to plan who will lead the care as mixed messages often occur when there are many clinicians involved in the management of medical conditions.

It is often helpful to identify a more general paediatrician who can keep an overview of all care and take a lead in the organisation of community-based services such as developmental support and speech therapy.

Adolescence and independence

All children grow from childhood into adolescence and then independent adulthood. This is no different for children born with a heart condition, but for some the process is more complicated.

Adolescents think themselves invincible. Many of them test life to its limits by taking non-prescribed drugs, drinking excessive alcohol, trying sexual experimentation and driving at speed. Learning that you are vulnerable and dependent and that your life span is not the same as your friends' is a very hard lesson. Some adolescent girls will discover that having children is not advisable and that there are restrictions in their choice of contraception. Adolescent boys in particular will discover that many physical jobs, like the army or emergency services, are impossible (Crossland et al, 2005).

Young people need support and information that helps them reach a mature safe independent adulthood. It is important to help them understand their limitations as well as to encourage them to take a full part in as many areas of life as they can.

They need guidance on the choices that they need to make so that they can take part in life but also keep themselves safe.

> Matthew, a 17-year-old young man with tricuspid atresia, was in the emergency department again. When asked what had happened, he explained that his mates had decided to go skiing at the local snow dome, but as it was summer they were in jeans and tee-shirts, so Matthew had collapsed with the cold at the bottom of the slope and had had to be brought to the hospital by ambulance.
> 'The ambulance crew freaked out at the colour that I was,' Matthew explained. 'I was very purple at the time.' Only after he explained that he was always blue did the paramedics relax a little. As Matthews's liaison sister, it was my job to

talk to him about how he should take more care of himself. Matthew's answer was why should he bother if he was going to die anyway? It was extremely important to allow Matthew the opportunity to talk through his fears and frustrations. He did not like talking to his parents as they worried about him all the time and he did not want to add to their fears. (A member of the liaison staff at Birmingham Children's Hospital)

Seeking out services that have been developed for disabled young people can help teenagers to explore their restrictions and solutions to their problems. It also helps them to meet with other young people experiencing similar problems, forming their own support network. Information websites, chatlines and interactive games sites can help young people explore their heart disease from home.

Transition

There are now more adults than children who were born with a heart condition, which is a great testament to the care given by medical staff, parents and carers, as well as the determination and fortitude of the young people themselves. As well as having the aspirations, hopes and fears that all teenagers have, those with lifelong heart conditions have the added pressure of beginning to take responsibility for their own health and well-being. At what age this transfer of responsibility for their own health should begin is open to debate, but it is essential that parents and carers as well as health professionals plan *with the young person* their journey through this process.

Parents know their child, but they may not know their child as a young adult, an individual with their own reasoning, logic and expectations. Allowing the young adult to gain the knowledge to make informed decisions about the myriad of choices they may have to make is one of the first steps in letting go, preparing the young person for adulthood. To achieve this, knowing what the young person wants to know is essential.

A focus group with young people between the ages of 12 and 18 was held in Manchester to try to find out what information young people with grown-up congenital heart (GUCH) defects want. They were able to say what they would like to know at each age and what their concerns were about their health. Medication, tattoos, (medical) contact numbers, where to go in hospital and the effects of alcohol were just a few things mentioned (GUCH, 2008). However, many will not want to let their parents or others know what they want to know – let alone gain information from them. Some will push their own limits and purposely rebel against any advice relating to their restrictions.

I think we're all guilty of ignoring some things our docs say! I was told I shouldn't go above 6,000 feet, but I've skied loads of times at over 9,000! Still here and loved every minute! I'm not condoning ignoring doctor's advice, but isn't life a risk anyway? (A young adult with complex congenital heart disease)

Others will not want to know anything about their health and refuse to start accepting any responsibility.

I was born with heart disease and since then I have run from it, ignored it and fooled myself I was the same as others. Every visit and check up with the doctor

> I just went along to keep the family happy, took no note and brushed it all off each time. (A young adult with congenital heart disease)

Fears about being different from their peers is one of the biggest problems young adults feel they have.

> I always felt so lonely and different from others and I hated it. (A young woman with tricuspid atresia)

Lack of control or anger over their condition can lead some individuals with GUCH to self-harm. Worries about relationships, scars, palpitations during intercourse and a host of other problems assail young GUCH individuals.

> I have also 'self-harmed' when I was 13 for about a year, and I'm just 16 now. Like Lisa [who also posted on this website message board], I only felt guilty when my friends noticed it, but that never stopped me. However, looking at the scars now, I am ashamed. They remind me of a dark place I don't want to go back to, but it took me a year to realise that. I don't know if I regret doing it, because it has kind of made me stronger, but I hate the scars. (A teenager on a GUCH website message board)
>
> Here's the shizzle. I'm 17 and have a long-term boyfriend. I know he wants our relationship to go further and I think I do too. … I am very self-conscious about my (very obvious) scars and would like advice on how to broach this with him. (A young woman with complex congenital heart disease seeking support on the GUCH website)

An open, honest, non-judgemental attitude from all adults will help ease the anxiety of GUCH individuals going through the transition to adult care services and make them stronger adults at the end. Support is essential, from parents, peers, medical staff and other young people with GUCH, which will help to alleviate feelings of isolation and loneliness. Information is available from a variety of sources and should be used to help young people equip themselves with whatever knowledge they want or feel they need.

> Looking back on it, it just happened. I made it to adulthood. I guess my parents and I should have had a bit of a celebration really, given what we had all been through up to then, but it just happened. It was better that way.

Bereavement

Sadly, one of the consequences of CHD is that many children die along the treatment path. Although surgery and medical treatments have improved dramatically over the past 30 years, there are still some heart conditions that cannot be fully treated and some children who are unable to survive surgery.

The death of a child is the most difficult thing that families have to come to terms with. Again, it can leave parents feeling isolated. In an effort to comfort a family, it is important that carers do not say, 'I know how you feel' unless they too have lost a child.

Two things made me so mad. The first one was the blood on the sheet. He was lying on a dirty sheet and I just wanted them to take it away. The second thing was that the nurse kept putting her arm around me and saying, I know how you feel. How could she! Her child hadn't died. I got so cross. In fact I shouted, and it was only when the liaison nurse, who I knew really well, came to help me that I calmed down. (A mother just hours after her new baby died)

It is important that explanations about the death are, where possible, given to parents by the medical team. This information may need to be reiterated many times because parents may not be able to remember all that is said at such a stressful time. Offering families an opportunity to attend an appointment with the doctor 6 weeks after the death of their child will give them time to compile questions and an opportunity to clarify any areas of care where they feel that they lack information.

Parents should be allowed to spend time with their child both before and after he or she has died. At all times, the families should be consulted about the way forward: Would they like a minister present? Would they like to wash and dress their child? Would they like photographs and hand and foot prints taken? Some parents like all of the family to visit, whilst others like to spend the time with their child in private.

I knew when it was right to leave the hospital. We washed and dressed Connor and then took him to the rainbow room. The nurses said that we could visit again at any time, but in my heart I knew that I had said good bye. (The father of a 2-year-old boy)

It is important to remember that there is no wrong way for a family to grieve and no wrong way for them to approach coping with a death, but it is also helpful for carers to introduce possible sources of support such as the taking of photographs or the building of a memory box that may well help families in the future and may not have been thought about during times of stress. The families of babies often need help to build memories if their child was only alive whilst in hospital – stress-filled memories may be all that they have (Little Hearts Matter 2008; Morrow, 2008).

All these treasures help me to keep the memory of Jessica alive. I know that I will never forget, but they helped and reassured me in the early stages of grief. (Penny, a bereaved mother, following the loss of her baby with hypoplastic left heart syndrome)

The death of an older child or young adult is still the death of a child and no more or less devastating for a family. There may be many more memories, but equally there may have been many more hopes for the future.

It felt like I was in a very large pot of treacle. The more I tried to swim to the side, the more the treacle pulled me down. Without the help of my doctor, I would not have found my way out of the depression that was getting on top of me. (The mother of a child who died at the age of 10)

All families need an opportunity to mourn at their own rate. Many couples grieve separately and experience the different emotions of grief at different times. Often, it can help to seek the support of others who have had similar experiences, and sometimes parents need professional support as they experience one of the most challenging pathways. It is important for clinical teams to understand that parents will never 'feel better', but with support they can regain a good and happy life.

> Ten years on, I still think of Andrew every day. Having looked after him for 11 years, I learnt that I could be a very good carer. I trained to be a nurse, and now I work with sick adults. His life has affected and moulded mine, and he will be with me for ever. (The mother of Andrew, who died age 11 having a heart transplant.)

Conclusion

Looking back through this chapter, it becomes clear that the voices that matter are those of the children, young adults and their families. They want to know what is going on either with their own health or with that of their child. They want to understand the condition, the treatments and any of the lifestyle changes that the condition may create in their everyday life. Members of the clinical team need to look at the many ways in which they can include the patient and their family in the decision-making, treatment-sharing and lifestyle control that come with every diagnosis, whilst at the same time they need to offer their information in a caring and supportive manner. This will help each and every family build their own information jigsaw.

For some, the puzzle will only need four pieces; for others it will need many more. Every family is different.

References

Crossland, D., Jackson, S., Lyall, R., Burn, J. & O'Sullivan, J. (2005). Employment advice regarding careers for adults with congenital heart disease. *Cardiology in the Young, 15*, 391–395.

GUCH (2008). *What teenagers want – and when!* Available at: http://www.guch.org.uk

Kendall, L., Sloper, P. & Levin, R. (2003). The views of young people with congenital heart disease, on designing the service for their treatment. *Cardiology in the Young, 13*, 3–6.

Little Hearts Matter (2008). *From us to you*. Birmingham: Little Hearts Matter.

Morrow, A. (2008). *Despite intense grief following the death of a child – bereaved parents have a low divorce rate*. Available at: http://www.About.com

Rempel, G.R., Cender, L.M., Lynam, M.J., Sandor, G.G. & Farquharson, D. (2004). Parents' perspectives on decision making after antenatal diagnosis of congenital heart disease. *Journal of Obstetric, Gynaecologic and Neonatal Nursing, 33*, 64–70.

Shillingford, A.J. & Wernovsky, G. (2004). Academic performance and behavioral difficulties after neonatal and infant heart surgery. *Pediatric Clinics of North America, 51*, 1625–1639, ix.

Shillingford, A.J., Glanzman, M.M., Ittenbach, R.F., Clancy, R.R., Gaynor, J.W. & Wernovsky, G. (2008). Inattention, hyperactivity, and school performance in a population of school-age children with complex congenital heart disease. *Pediatrics, 121*, e759–e767.

Further reading

Contact a Family. *No time for us*. Available from: www.cafamily.org.uk/publications (see also the main website for additional information).

Index